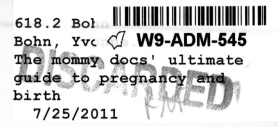
THE
MOMMY DOCS'
ULTIMATE
GUIDE TO
PREGNANCY
AND BIRTH

THE MOMMY DOCS' ULTIMATE GUIDE TO PREGNANCY AND BIRTH

Yvonne Bohn, MD · Allison Hill, MD · Alane Park, MD

with Melissa Jo Peltier

Da Capo
∞
LIFE
LONG

A Member of the Perseus Books Group

Copyright © 2011 by Yvonne Bohn, Allison Hill, Alane Park, and Melissa Jo Peltier

Editorial production by *Marra*thon Production Services. www.marrathon.net

Illustrations by Victoria Parr
Research by Ben Stagg

Design and production by Jane Raese
Text set in 10-point LinoLetter

Cataloging-in-Publication Data for this book is available from the Library of Congress.

ISBN 978-0-7382-1460-3 (paperback)
ISBN 978-0-7382-1478-8 (e-Book)

First Da Capo Press edition 2011

Published by Da Capo Press
A Member of the Perseus Books Group

www.dacapopress.com

Note: This book is intended only as an informative guide for those wishing to know more about health issues. In no way is this book intended to replace, countermand, or conflict with the advice given to you by your own physician. The ultimate decision concerning care should be made between you and your doctor. We strongly recommend you follow his or her advice. Information in this book is general and is offered with no guarantees on the part of the authors or Da Capo Press. The authors and publisher disclaim all liability in connection with the use of this book.

Da Capo Press books are available at special discounts for bulk purchases in the U.S. by corporations, institutions, and other organizations. For more information, please contact the Special Markets Department at the Perseus Books Group, 2300 Chestnut Street, Suite 200, Philadelphia, PA, 19103, or call (800) 810-4145, ext. 5000, or e-mail special.markets@perseusbooks.com.

We would like to thank all our patients for being a part of our lives and allowing us to be a part of theirs. Through taking care of you, we've learned so much more than how to practice medicine. By helping you through your hopes and fears, we've learned the importance of relationships and trust. Great doctors are made, not born—and we believe our patients are our best teachers.

contents

DELIVERING MIRACLES

NOTHING IN THIS WORLD—nothing at all—compares with delivering a new human life into the world.

Take it from us. We're a team of ob-gyns—Dr. Allison Hill, Dr. Alane Park, and Dr. Yvonne Bohn—who also happen to be moms. You may know us from our cable television reality show, *Deliver Me*, which aired for three seasons on the Discovery Health Network and is now airing on the Oprah Winfrey Network (OWN). You can also check out our blog at MommyDocs.com on all matters dealing with pregnancy and women's health.

We did the math, and between the three of us, we've delivered more than ten thousand babies. And yet each time we do it, the excitement surrounding the event simply can't be put into words. Just imagine this scenario: You are awakened from a sound sleep at 3:00 a.m. and your car keeps stalling and then you're practically in tears on the freeway, driving eighty miles an hour to get to the hospital. You may be worried about your own child at home with the sniffles or your husband, who's feeling a little neglected. But after you're in the delivery room and the action begins, you are right there in the thick of it with the mother, and it's the Big Show. The moment right before the baby comes out, you can feel your heart beating right along with the baby's, and the adrenaline rush could beat the thrill of any extreme sport on earth.

Being medical doctors, moms, and veterans of every imaginable childbirth scenario, we wish every expectant mom could feel the same thrill of adventure and discovery that we feel, from the moment we take on a new patient to the culmination of birth, when we're holding a new life in our arms.

But in our combined forty-five years of experience, we've noticed a trend that conspires to make pregnancy and childbirth stressful, frustrating experiences for women, when they should be exciting and joyful times. We've witnessed far too many women struggling through pregnancies that seem traumatic and nerve-wracking—not because of medical high-risk factors such as diabetes or lupus, which in our experience are challenges but surmountable ones—but from a simple lack of information or outright misinformation. For a variety of reasons, urban legends and old wives' tales seem to thrive in the world of pregnancy. Some of these myths and half-truths are perpetuated on the pages of the most popular and trusted pregnancy guides, blogs, and Web sites on the market. The result is plenty of confused and often terrified moms-to-be who can't find fact-based advice and answers they can trust.

> "Is it true that I can't touch a cat for nine months?"
> "Is my best friend right when she says that eating sushi will harm my baby?"
> "Why can't I wear high heels?"
> "My mom says I shouldn't raise my arms over my head after the seventh month. Is she crazy . . . or am I?"

These questions may sound ridiculous on the surface—but they are very serious to a frightened pregnant woman.

The fact is, we answer questions like these every day. We're truly grateful that our patients trust us enough to ask them. But sometimes, we're privately astonished by the misconceptions that make otherwise smart women lose sleep during the nine months of their pregnancy.

After checking out some of the other information out there that we believe may be as much a part of the problem as the solution, we decided it was time to pool our vast wealth of shared knowledge and experience and write our own book, based on the most up-to-date medical research available and filtered through the lens of our daily lives, both as busy ob-gyns and as dedicated moms.

Our Experiences

We've just celebrated the twelfth anniversary of our OB-GYN private practice. Before that, our partnership was forged at Los Angeles County Hospital, a veritable war zone of illness, accidents, and injuries in the gritty heart of downtown Los Angeles. The Residency Program of the University of Southern California Medical School required each of us to spend four years at County. As it turned out, our tour of duty at County was the best preparation on earth for the work we do now.

At County, we rarely saw any low-risk, regular moms. Instead, for four years, we took care of only medically complicated pregnancies. A group of midwives in the hospital managed the low-risk moms on an entire floor dedicated to natural, vaginal births. The chief of obstetrics at County instructed the midwives to guide us through our first deliveries. He said to us, "In the next four years, you're probably never going to get to do this. I want your first experience to be with a midwife, so you know what it's like to be a part of a regular, normal labor and birth."

After that, our real training began. In a typical day, each of us would help deliver as many as twenty-five babies. We were flying by the seat of our pants half the time, but we were doing it together. Every shift, we dealt with high-risk pregnancies, sick moms, and very sick babies, making split-second, life-or-death decisions several times a day.

Those four years gave us a solid foundation of knowledge and experience for dealing with every kind of complication that can happen in a pregnancy or during birth. It would be hard to think of a scenario that one of us hasn't dealt with in our careers. We want you to know that given the right team of people and specialists, we can take care of you even if you have high-risk complications.

Why We Became Doctors

Dr. Allison Hill

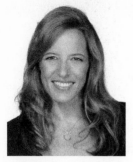

As a teenager, I was extremely uncomfortable during my first gynecological exam because the doctor was an older gentleman who had been in practice forever. He didn't do anything wrong, but I had lots of questions about very personal topics. And I thought, "There's no way I would ever tell this guy what's on my mind. It would be like talking to my grandfather." I remember walking out of there that day and thinking, "I could do this better. I think I could make women feel more comfortable than what I just went through." That idea stayed with me.

The field of OB-GYN and women's health issues inspires me. It deals with the most intimate concerns in a women's life, such as sex, hormones, sexually transmitted diseases, birth control . . . and having babies. The experience you have with your gynecologist or your obstetrician is an extremely personal one, and I value the relationships I get to have with my patients.

A Midwestern girl at heart, having been born and raised in central Illinois, I moved to LA for my residency and never looked back. Now I am a single mom to two great kids—Luke, eight, and Kate, six. Both were born prematurely and, as a result, taught me a lot more about nurturing than any textbook could. These days, they have me running all over town, as the soccer team mom, Cub Scout den mother, and all-around chauffeur. In my spare time, I am a runner and a yogi—two things I love to do alone to get away from the chaos of my everyday life.

Having traveled to places such as Ethiopia, Costa Rica, St. Lucia, Mexico, and Indonesia to work on projects that promote women's health, I am excited to bring home the simple ideas of preventive care for women with the Mommy Docs Foundation. Our goal is to provide free health care to women in underserved communities in Los Angeles and, ultimately, other parts of the United States.

Dr. Yvonne Bohn

My mom became mentally ill when I was about twelve. I became interested in medicine because I naively wanted to try to save her and people with her problems. During my studies, I found that I excelled at activities that involved my hands, such as procedures, neurosurgery, and general surgery. However, these were still male-dominated fields, which made me un-

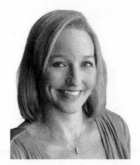

comfortable. Then I discovered that being an ob-gyn would allow me to do surgery in a field surrounded by women. With gynecology, I help women with their general health; with obstetrics, I have the exciting benefit of delivering babies.

My other jobs—as mother and wife—are just as rewarding as the thrill of being an ob-gyn. The daily love and joy from my eight-year-old son, Ryan, and nineteen-month-old daughter, Kylie, make me a better doctor, able to more deeply understand the importance of healthy babies and families. Bob, my husband of thirteen years, has been by my side since I met him in college, cheering me on when I was accepted into medical school and seeing me through the long hours of residency and private practice. Without his dedication as a husband and father, I would not be able to do what I do every day.

I believe exercise and staying fit are keys to a healthy and productive life, so in my limited spare time, I am a runner, hiker, spinner, and "boot camp" addict. I love to cook and garden; feeding family and friends fresh, delicious, and healthy home-cooked meals is another of my passions. I also find the time to volunteer at my son's elementary school teaching gardening and science.

Along with Allison and Alane, I am committed to sharing our talents by providing women's health care and education to the underserved and financially struggling women of Los Angeles through the Mommy Docs Foundation.

Dr. Alane Park

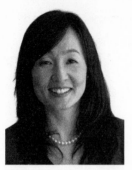

Doctors and the medical professions have been a part of my life for as long as I can remember.

I was born in Seoul, Korea and spent summers visiting my maternal grandfather, a pediatrician who was the kind of beloved, old-school neighborhood doctor you only read about these days. During cold season, he would sometimes see more than a hundred kids a day.

My grandfather lived in a two-story house, and he had converted the first floor into his medical office, small laboratory, and pharmacy. I loved sneaking downstairs to watch all the action and to witness my grandfather effortlessly working at the profession he so clearly loved. My uncle lived with us while he was studying for his entrance exams for medical school. When I would go to his basement room to announce that dinner was ready, I would often find him asleep over a pile of books.

Despite this early exposure to the medical field, I did not realize I wanted to be a doctor until much later in life, after college. Before I took the plunge into medical school, I tried my hand at research in the hopes of becoming a professor or a science teacher. When long hours in the laboratory lacked the human contact I craved, I realized that medicine would allow me to blend both my love of people and science. During medical school, I looked forward to my OB-GYN rotation because it was the perfect combination of everything that excited me: interaction with women, surgeries, and babies.

Becoming a mom and trying to be a good partner to my husband have been the best and hardest things I have ever accomplished. Every day, my two boys, Matthew, nine, and Max, five, teach me to become a kinder, more patient human being. My husband, who has been with me since I was a teen, has weathered both sunshine and storms with me over the past twenty-seven years. In addition to a busy OB-GYN practice and driving my boys to sports and school activities, I am involved with a charitable organization called Milk and Bookies that promotes literacy and inspires children to start early in giving back to their communities the way my partners and I want to give back through the Mommy Docs Foundation.

Being a doctor and a mom are vital parts of who I am; they are my calling.

Three Peas in a Pod

Our OB-GYN practice is successful for several reasons. First, we're friends who genuinely enjoy each other's company. Our families even get together in our off-hours (except that we rarely have off-hours at the same time).

Because we survived the cauldron of LA County Hospital together, perhaps it's no surprise that the three of us have emerged with similar work styles and work ethics. We trust each other's knowledge, surgical skills, and people skills. If one of us goes out of town and a patient calls with a problem, we don't worry if she's going to be treated well because she will be treated by one of us!

We are all at the same stage of our lives. We all have small kids, and we know that someone will cover for us if we have to, say, go to a soccer game. We all feel incredibly comfortable together, as if our childhood friends were our business partners.

Many pregnant women are shocked to discover that they could see one doctor throughout their pregnancy, but if that doctor is sick or out of town on delivery day, she might be having her baby with a doctor she's never met. (See the movie *Knocked Up* for a fictional version of this scenario.) In truth, few doctors are available 365 days a year. Our patients meet all three of us and know that they will be in good hands regardless of which doctor is there when the big moment comes.

One of our goals for this book was to create a handy guide that could act like a trusted ob-gyn for you, our readers, almost as if the three of us were beside you every step of the way to answer your most pressing questions.

Why Women Trust Us

Recently, Allison saw a woman named Lila who had developed high blood pressure in her pregnancy and became quite ill. Allison told her, "The same thing happened to me. Here's what I did, and these were the results." The look of relief on Lila's face said it all—she was doubly reassured to hear from both a doctor and a mom who had survived the same complication.

Our patients are comfortable with us because we're just like them. We're wives and working moms and have our own small kids, so chances are that at least one of us has experienced the issues a patient is curious about. None of our pregnancies were glitch-free: Allison had preeclampsia, Alane had vaginal tearing on one delivery, and Yvonne had placenta previa, a potentially serious complication. We all struggled with the first weeks of having a new infant at home, the challenge of breastfeeding, and maintaining our careers. But we all made it through. We're moms of beautiful, healthy kids, and we are confident that we can get our patients through whatever challenges may face them. We treasure being able to share our personal stories with the women who trust us to care for them and deliver their babies. And when we share details of our experiences, especially with first-time moms and dads, we bond with our patients.

Our approach to medicine is to be one part ob-gyn, one part fellow mom, and one part psychologist to our patients. Pregnancy brings with it so many emotions. Our patients trust us with the most personal areas of their body, so they're often willing to share the intimate details of their lives, even when those issues might not have anything to do with gynecology. We know if there's a death in the family, if a husband is cheating on them, or if their mother is making them crazy. They tell us their problems before they tell anyone else. On the other hand, some women are afraid to speak about certain issues, even when we can sense that something is going on. When we're concerned, the three of us get together and compare notes on certain patients. We wonder, "Does she seem different to you? Is she like this with you or is she like this just with me? Is something going on in her life? Does she seem unhappy?" We try to figure out what is wrong because these problems can have an effect on the physical part of her pregnancy.

LA County Hospital is a melting pot, and it was there that we first experienced some of the powerful cultural issues and pressures that influence a pregnant woman. Every culture has biases and myths that we have learned to treat with respect but to help dispel when necessary. For example, the Hispanic community has a traditional opposition to epidural anesthesia. We have to help moms understand that it is a safe form of pain relief that might be necessary to complete a vaginal delivery, which is also often a cultural imperative. Respecting a woman's culture, familial traditions, and personal vision for her birth experience is an important part of our jobs. We also make sure that each pregnant woman feels as if she is an individual during this crucial time in her life. At the same time, we step in and educate women when the realities of their pregnancies clashes with their ideal fantasies.

Countering Meddling and Fear Mongering

What is it about seeing a pregnant woman that makes everyone think they're an expert or that they need to share their own birth horror stories? Our patients tell us tales of random people who just stroll up to them and say things such as, "Oh you shouldn't do that." "Aren't you doing yoga?" "Have you watched this movie?" "Are you really going to drink that espresso?" "Haven't you read that article that's going around the Internet?" It seems like everyone's been deputized to dole out unsolicited obstetric advice.

Although well meaning, these so-called suggestions can have devastating effects. Moms break down in our office and tell us that their pregnancy seems to lurch from one set of fears to another. These women say, "I feel like I can't even enjoy being pregnant anymore, like I need to be wrapped in a bubble where nobody can touch me." They are overwhelmed by the amount of information out there and their inability to separate fact from fiction.

We can't measure the exact physical toll such worries take, but we know that stress is not beneficial to the body. We want this book to help reduce needless fears and concerns. The process of pregnancy has so many beautiful aspects; we don't want you to be robbed of a positive experience due to the misinformation of friends, relatives, coworkers, and even perfect strangers.

In our area of medicine, patients will choose to listen to their grandmothers or their Aunt Delores rather than their doctors. Can you imagine a patient with a heart condition saying to her cardiologist, "Well, I know you're recommending that I should have a bypass, but my old college roommate says I'd be better off eating 75 grams of protein a day instead?" Of course not. The unfortunate truth is that in the not so distant past, traditional medicine often let female patients down. Hospital policies were rigid, and pregnancy was looked at as a disease. Women—particularly pregnant women—often felt they weren't being listened to, and for good reason. We're happy to tell you that our profession really has changed with the times. Modern OB-GYN practices are more progressive, flexible, and patient-centered than ever before. And our own patients know that we have been through the same experiences they're going through and will listen to their concerns.

Pregnancy is not a disease. We'd like this book to be a safe place for any mother-to-be to step out of the fear-mongering world and get solid information. We want you, our readers, to feel reassured that you can take simple steps to an easier pregnancy and a healthier baby. Even if you have a health condition such as chronic hypertension or diabetes (both of which put you at higher risk for possible complications), it's highly likely that you'll have a healthy baby in your arms if you follow solid medical advice and take good care of yourself.

Some of our patients have had cancer and chemotherapy in their pasts but went on to have normal, healthy pregnancies. One mom-to-be with a severely irregular heartbeat and a pacemaker had been told that she shouldn't ever try to have children. She sought the advice of specialists and now has a beautiful baby girl. Every case is unique, but medicine has advanced to the point where even high-risk pregnancies aren't as risky anymore. We want you to know that you can have a good outcome. Take it from us—we've delivered thousands of healthy babies to moms who, on paper, might not have been the ideal candidates for pregnancy.

How to Use This Book

We've organized this book in a way that we hope is easy to read and even entertaining for all new mothers and parents-to-be. Chapters follow the order of pregnancy, with reference information inter-spersed with simple explanations and anecdotes from our practice, our patients, and ourselves. Because most pregnancies progress nor-mally, we saved the detailed information on high-risk pregnancies for last. The majority of women will never deal with these issues. For those who will, we hope to allay your fears and concerns with a clear, concise description of each complication, its causes and risk factors, and how medicine can improve the chances that a high-risk condi-tion will result in a healthy mom and baby. Remember, each one of us went through a complication in one of our pregnancies, and we're here to write about it, with our healthy kids waiting at home.

We've also provided a chapter on some of the emotional issues we've seen during the thousands of pregnancies we've handled; chapters on coping with miscarriage and fertility; and a chapter on the most frequently asked questions and common myths that we hear. We're grateful that our patients find us a safe haven to whom they can talk about their fears and concerns—as well as their hopes and dreams—for their babies.

chapter one

PREPARING FOR
PREGNANCY

▶ ▶ ▶ "WE'RE READY TO HAVE A BABY!"

How could one simple sentence be such a life-changer? A new patient named Ginger uttered those words with a cautious smile. Ginger had just moved to Los Angeles from Milwaukee after getting married the year before. Both she and her new husband were in the graphic arts business, so LA seemed the perfect place to start their careers. Now that their new jobs were finally gaining momentum, the time seemed right to tackle life's next milestone: parenthood.

As we talked more about her future plans, Ginger confessed that she harbored a few troubling fears. She had two sisters who were moms; the first had given birth by cesarean, and the second had a preterm delivery. Ginger was afraid that a problematic pregnancy would be her fate as well. I explained to her that she was not at an increased risk just because it happened in her family.

Ginger then shared more of her own medical history. She had problems with her Pap smears in the past and had surgery on her cervix five years ago. She feared that these past gynecological issues might make it difficult to conceive or carry the baby to term. When I told her that the chances were good that her fertility and pregnancy would not be affected, she breathed a sigh of relief.

"So what do I do next?" she asked. My recommendations were short and to the point—get started on her prenatal vitamins and enjoy her alone time with her husband. Being "ready" to have a baby often means letting go of unfounded fears and just jumping in. There is never a *perfect* time to start a family, but if you approach the experience with the right attitude, it can be a time of challenge, excitement, learning, and, most importantly, a time to affirm the beauty and miracles of life.

—Allison ◀ ◀ ◀

Before You Get Pregnant

During our years in practice, we've seen an increasing number of patients who visit their doctor for preconceptional counseling. During this visit, your doctor can recommend a prenatal vitamin, explain the timing of intercourse to maximize fertility, review your medical problems, take a family history, and perform a basic physical exam and tests. More importantly, a preconceptional visit gives both you and your doctor a chance to control the things you can control in a pregnancy and increase your chances for a healthy baby.

Take Prenatal Vitamins

Surprisingly, perhaps the most important time to take prenatal vitamins is before you even get pregnant. We recommend that our patients start a comprehensive prenatal vitamin formula—or at least take the proper amount of *folic acid*—two to three months before they try to conceive. Luckily, many cereals are fortified with folic acid and it is found in its natural form, metafolin, in orange juice, spinach, asparagus, and pinto beans. An average American diet provides 200 to 250 micrograms of folic acid daily. However, because the recommended amount of folic acid in pregnancy is 600 micrograms, women of child-bearing age should add a multivitamin or prenatal vitamin to their regimen.[1] Most multivitamins contain 400 micrograms of folic acid, and prenatal vitamins have 800 to 1,000 micrograms (1,000 micrograms is equivalent to 1 milligram).

Low levels of folic acid are linked to the development of birth defects such as neural tube defects (NTDs) and cleft lip and palate. *Spina bifida,* a NTD, results from the incomplete closure of the baby's spine, or neural tube, which occurs during the fourth week after conception. Quite often, women don't even know that they're pregnant at that time. Affecting one to two babies per thousand, spina bifida causes paralysis and deformities of the legs. Similarly, folic acid plays a role in facial development, and women with low levels have a higher risk of having a baby with cleft lip and palate, which occurs in one in seven hundred infants. Neural tube defects and cleft lip and palate are birth defects a mom-to-be can help prevent. Consuming the correct amount of folic acid prior to pregnancy and during the first trimester decreases the incidence of these birth defects by 75 percent. Following is the recommended folic acid intake:

Mothers at low risk: 0.6 milligrams per day
Mothers on seizure medication: 4 milligrams per day
Mothers with a previous fetus with a neural tube defect:
   4 milligrams per day[2]

Some new prenatal vitamins and supplements contain the natural, active form of folic acid, metafolin. Folic acid is synthetic and must be broken down by enzymes in the body to be active, but metafolin does not require these metabolic steps. About half the population has an enzyme deficiency that limits the ability to metabolize folate. A blood test can be performed to see whether a patient has an abnormality in the gene that metabolizes folic acid. For these women, metafolin is a better choice.

The other ingredients in prenatal vitamins are similar to a general multivitamin: B-complex vitamins, vitamins C, D, and E, and the minerals zinc, iron, calcium, and copper. Some also contain a stool softener and DHA, an omega-3 fatty acid. The brand that you use is a personal decision. The variety on the market now is impressive: You can find chewable vitamins, vanilla-flavored vitamins, two small pills versus one large pill, and some with ingredients to alleviate nausea. We recommend finding something that doesn't make you nauseous, is easy to swallow, and tastes good.

If you're already pregnant and didn't load up on prenatal vitamins, relax. Remember, at least 50 percent of pregnancies are unplanned and everything still turns out fine because most women get the vitamins they need through their diet. But if you have the opportunity to plan and start prenatal vitamins in advance, you can increase the chances of having a healthy baby.

Maintain a Healthy Weight

"Doctor, I'm thinking about having a baby but I'm concerned that I'm too heavy. Is this something I should worry about?" The answer to this question is an unfortunate, yet definite, yes. Losing weight is difficult, but returning your body to a healthy weight before pregnancy is one of the best things you can do for yourself and your baby.

● ● ●

The statistics on obesity are staggering. Only about one-third of American women are of a normal weight. One-third are overweight, with a body mass index, or BMI, of 25 to 30, and one-third are obese, with a BMI greater than 30. As a result, our perceptions of normal weight have been dramatically skewed. Many health providers don't even notice when a woman is overweight, but this carries many increased risks as well.

The consequences of obesity in nonpregnant women are well known—diabetes, high blood pressure, stroke, certain cancers, joint problems, and liver and gallbladder disease. And now, the health risks of obesity on pregnancy are clear as well, as described in the following sections.

Infertility: Women who are overweight have a higher chance of infertility. Specifically, many overweight women do not have monthly menstrual cycles because they are not ovulating. Medication can be given to help with ovulation, but just a 5 to 10 percent reduction in body weight can cause ovulation, and regular menstrual cycles, to resume.

Diabetes: An overweight mother is four times more likely to develop gestational diabetes. This form of diabetes can lead to extremely large infants, who are more likely to have birth injuries or who will require cesarean delivery.

Preeclampsia: Obese mothers are twice as likely to have high blood pressure related to pregnancy, which can increase their chance of blood clots, stroke, and premature birth.

Cesarean risk: When delivering a baby vaginally, we like to say that it's "all about the push." Women carrying extra weight, especially in the midsection, have less muscle tone and thus less strength with which to push out their babies. In addition, the extra fat deposits within the birth canal make it much more difficult for the baby to slip through.

Many patients ask us what they can do to avoid a cesarean delivery. Maintaining a healthy weight is high on the list. Just look at these statistics. The chance of a cesarean delivery is

- 11 percent for women of normal weight;
- 18 percent for overweight women; and
- a whopping 43 percent for obese women.

In addition, obese women who have a cesarean have a higher risk of blood clots, bleeding, and infections after surgery.

Birth defects: In obese women, the risk of spina bifida is twice that seen in normal-weight women. The risk for cleft lip is 20 percent higher, for heart defects, 30 percent higher, and for hydrocephalus, 60 percent higher.

Birth defect detection: Ultrasound is our best tool in obstetrics, yet this technology is limited by the distance the sound waves need to travel. For overweight women, three or more inches of fat on the abdominal wall can limit the detail of what we can see, so subtle birth defects may go undetected.

Pregnancy symptoms: Even the more mundane symptoms and discomforts of pregnancy, such as heartburn, carpal tunnel syndrome, back pain, pelvic pressure, and headaches, occur far more often in obese mothers.

● ● ●

Public health officials are concerned because the maternal mortality rate in the United States has been on the rise in recent years. A major contributing factor is the increase in obesity. *Of all maternal deaths, two-thirds are related to complications of obesity.*[3]

Clearly, one of the best things you can do before becoming pregnant is to get your body to its healthiest weight. First calculate your body mass index as follows:

$$BMI = \frac{weight\ (lbs.)}{[height\ (in.)]^2} \times 703$$

Then talk to your doctor about a weight loss plan *before* putting yourself and your baby at unintended risk. We'll talk more about diet and exercise during pregnancy in Chapter 2.

Get Immunized

Prior to conception

We advise our patients and their family members to be properly vaccinated prior to pregnancy. These vaccinations not only protect the pregnant women from contracting infectious diseases but also protect their newborns by passing the immunity from mom to baby.

Inactivated vaccines can be administered before and during pregnancy. Live attenuated vaccines should be given 4 weeks or more prior to conception.

During pregnancy

Many vaccines, including those for influenza, whooping cough (pertussis), pneumonia, and tetanus, are safe, even if you are already pregnant. However, because of the theoretical risks to the fetus, we avoid giving live attenuated vaccines—such as measles, mumps, rubella (often given in one vaccine as MMR)—to pregnant women.

The following is a list of the most common vaccines and their safety in pregnancy.

Vaccine	Safe in pregnancy	Type of vaccine
Influenza–injection	yes	Inactivated
Influenza–nasal spray	no	Live
MMR (Measles Mumps, rubella)	no	Live
Pneumococcus	yes	Inactivated
Meningococcus	yes	Inactivated
Tetanus/Diphtheria/ Pertussis	yes	Toxoid/inactivated
Varicella (Chickenpox)	no	Live
Hepatitis A	yes	Inactivated
Hepatitis B	yes	Inactivated
Rabies	yes	Inactivated
Human Papilloma Virus (HPV)	no, under investigation	Inactivated

The flu vaccine needs special mention, since pregnant women who contract the flu may be at risk for serious complications. Therefore, all pregnant women in any trimester should receive the injectable form of the flu vaccine during the months of the flu season between November through March.

After delivery

All vaccines listed above are considered safe after the delivery of your baby and while breastfeeding.

For details on vaccines, please refer to the Website for the Centers for Disease Control and Prevention at http://www.cdc.gov/vaccines.

Conceiving after Thirty-Five

More frequently than ever, women are waiting until they are older and more settled into their lives before trying to conceive a baby. *Being an older mom does not necessarily make the pregnancy high risk.* However, women who are over thirty-five have a higher incidence of chronic medical conditions, such as high blood pressure, diabetes, or thyroid problems. Although these can complicate any pregnancy, they are more frequent in older moms. On the other hand, a very healthy forty-year-old woman who keeps herself in top shape will probably not put herself at any additional risk.

The second issue for women over thirty-five is the increased risk of chromosomal abnormalities such as Down syndrome. This birth defect is directly related to a mother's age. The age of the father does not influence the risk.

There is no reason why an older mom shouldn't have a baby—in fact, each of us had at least one child after we turned thirty-five. Genetic testing is also available, as we discuss in Chapter 2.

However, after you reach your early forties, it becomes increasingly difficult to become pregnant with your own eggs. After age forty, the chance of conceiving goes down to less than 5 percent per month, and the risk of miscarriage increases to 35 percent. Although we all know women who have had spontaneous healthy pregnancies in their early to mid-forties, the odds decline rapidly during this decade. When you start making decisions about family planning, it's important to remember that the "biological clock" is very real, indeed.

Optimize Your Health

As mentioned, preconceptional counseling involves sharing your gynecologic history and undergoing a pelvic exam. Your doctor will inquire about your menstrual cycles. Are they heavy? Are they regular? Are they painful? Irregular cycles may indicate that you are not ovulating and that you may need medication to help you get pregnant. Heavy or painful periods are associated with fibroids or endometriosis, which may also influence fertility. If you have a history of a sexually transmitted infection, such as chlamydia or gonorrhea, or a severe pelvic infection, you may have scar tissue that prevents pregnancy. This problem can be further evaluated by using a special X-ray called a hysterosalpingogram (HSG) to see whether the fallopian tubes are open. During the pelvic exam, the doctor will check for the presence of uterine fibroids and ovarian cysts. If either is discovered, surgery may be required before you attempt to become pregnant.

Ideally, all existing medical conditions—diabetes, chronic hypertension, lupus, thyroid disease, seizure disorder, and any other chronic medical issues—should be well controlled *before* conception. Doing so will minimize the chance of pregnancy complications such as birth defects, miscarriage, and preterm delivery.

Diabetes

Diabetes is a metabolic disease characterized by elevated blood sugar levels. A woman with preexisting diabetes will have fewer complications during pregnancy and childbirth if her blood sugar levels are well controlled. Generally, blood sugar levels are controlled with insulin, but they can also be controlled with oral medications. A blood test called Hemoglobin A1C will tell us how a woman's glucose control has been for the last three months. The higher the Hemoglobin A1C, the greater the risk of miscarriage and birth defects (nervous system and heart defects). Ideally, the Hemoglobin A1C should be in the normal range before pregnancy.

Asthma

Asthma is a common lung disease where the air passages spasm, decreasing oxygen flow. In pregnancy, it is particularly important to keep oxygen flowing to the baby. Complicating the picture, as pregnancy progresses, many women feel increasingly short of breath because of the physical pressure of the uterus under the diaphragm. In addition, the rise in estrogen levels can increase nasal congestion and mucous production. Therefore, before and during pregnancy, women who have asthma need to use oral medications and inhalers to open their airways. Although many pregnant women are hesitant to use their medications because of fears of harming the baby, most drugs for asthma are Class B or C and are considered safe. (See the upcoming Figure 1-1 on page 28 on the safety of drugs in pregnancy.) Women with asthma should be encouraged to use their inhalers regularly, take antihistamines if needed, and treat upper respiratory infections early to prevent exacerbation of asthmatic episodes.

Seizure Disorder

Seizure disorder, or epilepsy, is a condition in which the brain's electrical activity is abnormal, resulting in convulsions. Before becoming pregnant, women with seizure disorder need to see their neurologists to evaluate their seizure-preventing medications. The goal is to find the lowest dose and least number of drugs to prevent the convulsions. Uncontrolled seizure activity can lead to lack of oxygen, which is dangerous to a baby's development. If a woman has not had a seizure for many years, her neurologist may decide to discontinue her medications. If she remains seizure-free after conception, she may be able to stay off them during the entire pregnancy.

Although some seizure medications are considered safer than others, all carry the risk of causing birth defects. The risk of birth defects for mothers on seizure disorder medication is two to three times higher[4] than for the general population. Still, in most cases, doctors agree that the risk of the medication is lower than the risk of uncontrolled seizures.

Thyroid Disease

The thyroid gland, which is located in the neck, produces a hormone that regulates the rate of your body's metabolism. *Thyroid disease* is categorized into two disorders—hyper and hypo—depending on whether too much or too little of the hormone is produced. Thyroid disease should also be treated before you become pregnant. Untreated *hypothyroidism* (underactive thyroid) can lead to *anovulation* (impaired egg release) and ultimately infertility. Women with hypothyroidism may present with symptoms of fatigue, constipation, muscle cramps, slow heart rate, dry skin, cold intolerance, and deepening of the voice. If pregnancy does occur and hypothyroidism is not under control, moms-to-be run the risk of pregnancy complications, including preeclampsia, placental abruption, anemia, postpartum hemorrhage, cardiac dysfunction, low birth weight, and stillbirth. During pregnancy, the amount of thyroid medication needed may change, so thyroid levels should be monitored routinely by blood tests. Because a woman's thyroid can change dramatically after birth, blood tests should be checked again at six weeks postpartum.

Hyperthyroidism (overactive thyroid) is most commonly caused by Grave's disease, an autoimmune disorder in which the body makes thyroid-stimulating antibodies, increasing the levels of thyroid hormone. Hyperthyroidism is diagnosed with the help of blood tests measuring TSH (thyroid stimulating hormone) and free thyroid hormone. If uncontrolled, symptoms include a rapid heart rate, bulging eyes (exopthalmus), increased body temperature, and weight loss. In pregnancy, a woman with uncontrolled hyperthyroidism is at increased risk of preeclampsia, heart failure, preterm delivery, miscarriage, and placental abruption. In addition, thyroid-stimulating antibodies can cross the placenta and overstimulate the thyroid gland of the fetus, leading to growth restriction, stillbirth, hypothyroidism, or goiter.

Hyperthyroidism can be successfully treated with drugs before and during pregnancy. With antihyperthyroidism drugs, as with all drugs in pregnancy, the goal is to use the lowest dose possible to control the disease. Babies born to mothers on such drugs may have low thyroid levels, so they will be screened for this.

Because thyroid disease affects one out of eight women and the effects on the fetus can be severe, women with symptoms should be screened with a TSH blood test before or during pregnancy.

▶ ▶ ▶ THYROID DISEASE IS FOREVER

Sonia, a quiet, unassuming woman, came to us for her first prenatal visit ten weeks' pregnant. During our discussion of her medical history, she casually mentioned that she had been previously diagnosed with hypothyroidism but that she was no longer on medication for her disease. Sonia was totally unaware that hypothyroidism is a chronic disease and requires lifelong medication. Sure enough, on that first visit, our tests revealed that she had uncontrolled hypothyroidism.

We immediately referred her to an endocrinologist who restarted her thyroid medications. Throughout her pregnancy, we monitored Sonia's thyroid levels regularly and adjusted her medications as needed to keep the disease under control. Her pregnancy was uneventful and she delivered a healthy seven-and-a-half-pound boy.

After her baby was born, however, Sonia stopped taking her medication again because she felt fine. When she came to see us for a follow-up gynecological appointment four months later, she looked completely different. Her face was swollen and she had gained a significant amount of weight. We remarked on how beautiful her son was, but she did not seem happy or smile. We thought this was strange because she had been so upbeat and cheerful during her prenatal care and the immediate postpartum period. She then said to me, "Doctor, ever since I had my baby, I can't swallow and I'm having a hard time talking." We checked her thyroid and the levels were dangerously low. She had developed a condition called macroglossia where her tongue had swelled, impairing her ability to speak. She had gained twenty-two pounds in four months. Her untreated thyroid disease was responsible for these changes.

The endocrinologist who again treated her said that Sonia's case was one of the most severe she had ever seen. Without immediate medication, the condition could be life threatening. Thankfully, Sonia was compliant with her treatment and has gone on to be a wonderful mother to her son.

—Yvonne ◀ ◀ ◀

Chronic hypertension

Chronic hypertension is a disease in which the resting blood pressure is consistently higher than 140/90. Affecting 30 percent of the adult population, high blood pressure is another condition that should be controlled before conception takes place. Women with hypertension have an increased risk of preeclampsia and growth restriction of the fetus. Again, the goal is to be on the lowest dose of the safest drug. Specific antihypertensive medications are safer than others and some should definitely be avoided when pregnant. At a preconception visit, your doctor can change your medication or adjust your dose. The antihypertensive medications used most commonly in pregnancy are methyldopa, labetolol, and nifedipine.

Cardiac conditions

Women who have had previous heart disease, heart surgery, an irregular heartbeat, or cardiomyopathy should have a complete exam including echocardiogram with a cardiologist before trying to conceive to ensure that their hearts are strong enough to withstand the changes of pregnancy. If the structure of the heart is normal and is not enlarged, most of these women can undertake pregnancy safely.

Cancer

Thankfully, cancer is relatively rare in women of childbearing age. The most common types are breast cancer, lymphoma, and thyroid cancer. In the past, it was thought that elevated hormones from pregnancy might increase the risk of cancer recurrence, but current data does not support that theory. In general, pregnancy after cancer is considered safe for mother and baby. However, a woman should wait some time after treatment to evaluate for any recurrence before attempting pregnancy. The amount of time depends on the type and severity of the disease, and should be discussed with an oncologist.

▶ ▶ ▶ NEVER SAY STERILE

"That's impossible!" Laurence was an assertive, take-charge thirty-two-year-old, and nearly every word she spoke rang of certainty. "There's no way I could be pregnant!"

Laurence, one of our regular gynecological patients, was a proud and courageous cancer survivor. In her early thirties, she'd been diagnosed with breast cancer and had undergone a lumpectomy, radiation, and chemotherapy. Although these treatments ultimately saved her life, the chemotherapy had suppressed her ovarian function, and she stopped menstruating. Her oncologist had told her that she was now sterile and would never become pregnant.

Yet here she was, sitting in Allison's office. A routine appointment to check out her abdominal pain had revealed that she was sixteen weeks pregnant. After she got over her shock, Laurence cried tears of joy. She was elated and couldn't wait to tell her husband.

Laurence went on to deliver a healthy baby girl. Following her pregnancy, she had follow-up mammograms and breast exams and still did not have a recurrence of her cancer. Since that time, she has gone on to deliver two other children—another daughter and a son. Both are healthy and thriving and she is still cancer free.

◀ ◀ ◀

One choice for women who receive the diagnosis of cancer before they have finished bearing children is egg preservation. Until recently, this technique had very low success rates, but those rates have improved significantly with advances in medical technology. Egg preservation, or egg freezing, involves completing the first portion of an IVF (in vitro fertilization) cycle. A woman takes hormones to stimulate the growth of multiple eggs, which are removed through a minor surgical procedure. Instead of being fertilized with a partner's sperm as in IVF, the eggs are frozen and stored for future use. Because cancer treatments can shut down egg production, women who may need to undergo chemotherapy or radiation should consider this process before starting treatment.

Because Laurence was young when she had her chemotherapy treatments, her ovarian function returned. This is not the case for all women, which is why egg freezing is sometimes an option. With the support of her oncologist, a cancer survivor may get pregnant and go on to have a healthy baby without any increased risk of recurrence.[5]

▶ ▶ ▶ A SECOND OPINION

Eileen was a thirty-nine-year-old social worker who was in remission from leukemia for three years. Her disease was controlled with an oral chemotherapeutic agent. Because of her age and the fact that she had been on chemotherapy, she didn't think she could get pregnant. When her home pregnancy test stick showed a positive result, she was thrilled.

Filled with joyful anticipation, she went to see an obstetrician in her area. He came out into the waiting room and, before even examining her or taking her full history, declared right then and there that she must terminate the pregnancy because she had been on chemotherapy. End of story.

Devastated by his pronouncement, Eileen nevertheless decided to seek a second opinion and came to see Yvonne, who did an ultrasound and discovered a healthy eight-week pregnancy. Eileen reported that she'd stopped her chemotherapy drug immediately after she found out she was pregnant. Yvonne told her that the pregnancy seemed normal at this stage and if Eileen decided to continue, all three of us would support her 100 percent. Her oncologist agreed, and felt it was safe for her to discontinue her oral medication because she had been in remission for some time. Follow-up ultrasounds later in the pregnancy did not reveal any abnormalities in the fetus from the medication.

Eileen went on to deliver a healthy baby boy. To this day, she is so grateful she sought out a second opinion, and thanks Yvonne for helping bring her son into the world.   ◀ ◀ ◀

These days, most serious medical conditions can be monitored and treated during pregnancy with great success. The mom-to-be must commit to understanding her disease and, ideally, optimizing her health before getting pregnant. She needs to find a supportive team of medical professionals who can address the high-risk nature of her pregnancy. Sure, maybe she'll need a few more visits to the doctor than a mom without any medical problems, but ultimately she too can have a happy pregnancy and deliver a healthy baby.

Avoid Risky Medications

Obviously, it's against every law of medical—or human—ethics to give a pregnant woman a risky medication to study whether or not it could possibly hurt her fetus. That's why determining the safety of medications in pregnancy is so difficult and such an inexact science. Most information on the safety of medications comes from either observations or animal studies. Based on this information, the FDA has set up a classification system for all medications. See Table 1-1 for informa-

Table 1-1: Drug Classifications[6]

Category	Interpretation
A	Adequate, well-controlled studies in pregnant women have not shown an increased risk of fetal abnormalities in any trimester of pregnancy.
B	Animal studies have revealed no evidence of harm to the fetus, but there are no adequate and well-controlled studies in pregnant women. Or animal studies have shown an adverse effect, but adequate and well-controlled studies in pregnant women have failed to demonstrate a risk to the fetus in any trimester.
C	Animal studies have shown an adverse effect, and there are no adequate and well-controlled studies in pregnant women. Or no animal studies have been conducted, and there are no adequate and well-controlled studies in pregnant women.
D	Adequate, well-controlled, or observational studies in pregnant women have demonstrated a risk to the fetus. However, the benefits of therapy may outweigh the potential risk. For example, the drug may be acceptable if needed in a life-threatening situation or for a serious disease for which safer drugs cannot be used or are ineffective.
X	Adequate, well-controlled, or observational studies in animals or pregnant women have demonstrated positive evidence of fetal abnormalities or risks. The use of the product is contraindicated in women who are or may become pregnant.

tion on drug classes in pregnancy. Most medications fall into the B or C class, and these classes are used in pregnancy if the benefit or the need for the mom is greater than the potential risk to the fetus. Drugs in class D are usually not used. Class X drugs are known *teratogens,* which means exposure to these while pregnant has been directly related to birth defects. An example of a class X drug is isotretinoin (previously known as Accutane), a medication used to treat severe acne. Women who are prescribed isotretinoin must use some form of contraception to ensure they don't get pregnant while taking it.

Certain conditions may require that a woman continue medications while pregnant. Again, the golden rule for medication use in pregnancy is to use the lowest dose, the safest drug, and the least number of medications to control symptoms. If you don't have to take a medication, don't. Figure 1-1 on page 28 shows some of the medications that can be safely used in pregnancy.

Antidepressants are the most commonly prescribed class of drugs in the United States, with more than 10 percent of Americans using one daily. A few small studies had previously suggested slightly higher risks of miscarriage, preterm delivery, and birth defects in women who used antidepressants during pregnancy. However, more recent and larger studies do not confirm these findings. In cases when the antidepressant is taken just before delivery, withdrawal symptoms—such as irritability and difficulty feeding—have been observed in the newborn. However, in serious cases of depression, if the mother discontinues her medication, the risk for return of the disease is high and, in some cases, can be life threatening. Therefore, the current recommendation is to continue antidepressant therapy with the safest drug at the lowest possible dose required to relieve symptoms. A pregnant woman with depression needs to work with her therapist, psychiatrist, and obstetrician to determine her best course of treatment.

Preconception Testing for Genetic Diseases

Another feature of the preconceptional counseling visit is surveying the patient's family history, looking for patterns of disease that may have a genetic link. If a specific gene has been identified, we can screen for it in the patient, and sometimes in her partner as well.

Figure 1-1: Safety of Drugs and Medications During Pregnancy

CATEGORY	SAFE FOR USE DURING PREGNANCY
Pain relievers	Regular Tylenol, Extra-strength Tylenol
Decongestants	Benadryl, Sudafed, Afrin nasal spray, TheraFlu, Tylenol Cold, Claritin
Cough medicines	Robitussin DM, Vicks Formula 44, Halls cough drops
Antacids	Tums, Maalox, Mylanta, Pepcid
Laxatives	Metamucil, Colace, Citracel, Milk of Magnesia, Dulcolax
Hemorrhoids	Tucks, Anusol HC, witch hazel, Preparation H
Antibiotics	penicillin, ampicillin, Keflex, Macrobid, Flagyl
Herbs	cranberry, echinacea
Yeast infections	Monistat, Gynelotrimin

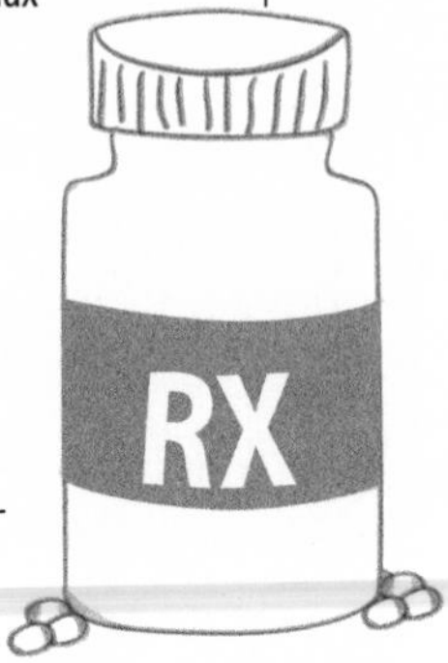

CATEGORY	NOT RECOMMENDED FOR USE DURING PREGNANCY
Pain relievers	Motrin, Advil, Aleve
Antibiotics	Ciprofloxacin, tetracycline, doxycycline
Herbal supplements	Black cohosh, feverfew, garlic, ginseng, St. John's Wort, goldenseal
Migraine medication	Imitrex, Amerge
Antihypertensives	Captopril, Benazepril, and Lisinopril
Acne medication	Isotretinoin
Blood thinners	Coumadin
Anti-anxiety medications	Xanax, Ativan, and Valium

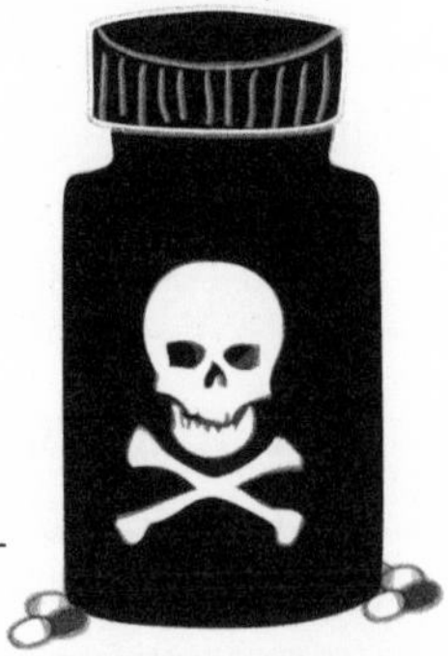

Genetic diseases can be divided into two groups: autosomal recessive disorders and autosomal dominant disorders.

Autosomal Recessive Disorders

In *autosomal recessive disorders,* a single gene defect has been identified that causes the disease. To be affected with the disease, a person must carry two copies of the abnormal gene, one inherited from the mother and one from the father. When someone has only one copy of the gene, they are not affected and are called a carrier. If both parents are carriers, there is a 25 percent chance that their child will have the disease.

When testing for these diseases, we first screen the mother with a blood test. If she is found to be a carrier, then we screen the father. If he is also a carrier, we can test the fetus using amniocentesis to see whether he or she inherited the disease. The most common autosomal recessive disorders are cystic fibrosis, sickle-cell anemia, and Tay-Sachs disease. Certain ethnic populations are at higher risk for these disorders, as shown in Table 1-2 for diseases related to ethnicity. In the following sections, we provide examples of the most common autosomal recessive disorders for which we currently screen.

Cystic fibrosis

Cystic fibrosis is an inherited disease that affects a baby's lungs and digestive system. A defective gene causes the body to produce unusually thick, sticky mucous that clogs the lungs, causing life-threatening

Table 1-2: Genetic Disorders Based on Ethnicity

Ethnic Group	Genetic Disorder
All ethnic groups	Cystic fibrosis
African American	Sickle-cell anemia
Ashkenazi Jew	Cystic fibrosis, Canavan disease, Gaucher disease, Fanconi anemia, Bloom syndrome, Tay-Sachs, Familial dysautonomia, Niemann Pick, Mucolipidosis IV
Cajun, French-Canadian	Tay-Sachs
Mediterranean	Beta-thalassemia
Southeast Asian	Alpha-thalassemia

infections and difficulty breathing. The gene also prevents the body from breaking down and properly absorbing food and nutrients. Those afflicted with cystic fibrosis also suffer from poor growth and infertility. According to data compiled by the Cystic Fibrosis Foundation, infants born in the United States in 2008 have a life expectancy of 37.4 years. The American College of Obstetrics and Gynecology recommends that all pregnant women should be screened for cystic fibrosis because it is the most common genetically transmitted disease. The carrier rates for cystic fibrosis in different ethnicities follow:

Caucasian	1:25
Hispanic	1:46
African American	1:65
Asian	1:95

Sickle-cell anemia

Sickle-cell anemia often affects African Americans as well as people whose families originate from Africa, South or Central America (especially Panama), the Caribbean islands, Mediterranean countries (such as Turkey, Greece, and Italy), India, and Saudi Arabia. People with sickle-cell anemia have red blood cells that contain abnormal hemoglobin, the protein that carries oxygen. The abnormal hemoglobin makes the cells have a crescent, sickle shape, hence the name sickle-cell. These cells don't move easily through the blood vessels. Instead, they form clumps, blocking blood flow and causing lack of oxygen to the tissues, serious infections, and organ damage. Symptoms include bone pain, abdominal pain, breathlessness, fatigue, poor eyesight, and even blindness. People who are afflicted with sickle-cell anemia typically survive but live with chronic pain, illness, and hospitalizations.

Thalassemia

Thalassemia is another form of anemia that is often seen in Asians, African Americans, and Middle Easterners. As with sickle-cell anemia, thalassemia sufferers are born with an abnormal form of hemoglobin. The disorder results in excessive destruction of red blood cells. Shortly after birth, babies suffer from severe anemia and failure to grow. Blood transfusions are the main therapy. Most women who survive are infertile and their life expectancy is usually shortened.

Tay-Sachs

Tay-Sachs is caused by a genetic mutation that creates an enzyme deficiency of hexosaminidase A. Infants with Tay-Sachs disease have developmental delays, seizures, coarse features, swelling, an enlarged liver and spleen, an enlarged tongue, and cherry-red spots in the eyes. Death usually occurs in the first or second year of life. Tay-Sachs usually affects the Ashkenazi Jewish, French-Canadian, and Cajun populations. It is estimated that one in twenty-seven Jews in America are carriers of the Tay-Sachs gene. Tay Sachs disease currently has no treatment, so the emphasis is on preconception testing and determination of carrier status. Like other autosomal recessive disorders, the disease can be detected in the developing fetus through either chorionic villus sampling or amniocentesis.

Autosomal Dominant Disorders

Autosomal dominant disorders need just one defective gene to cause the disease, not two. This means if a parent has the disease, there's a 50 percent chance that the baby will inherit it as well. There are no carriers. Neurofibromatosis is an example of an autosomal dominant disease. It affects the development and growth of nerve cell tissue, causing multiple disfiguring tumors. You may know neurofibromatosis by it's more common name, Elephant man's disease.

▶ ▶ ▶ WORTH THE RISK?

One of the most difficult decisions for a parent-to-be with a genetic disorder is whether it's worth the risk to reproduce, potentially passing on his or her condition to the next generation. A few years ago, a picture-perfect couple—a pretty, red-headed wife and a tall, fair-haired husband who worked in the music business—came to us for preconceptional counseling. The husband had neurofibromatosis, but he had a very mild form of the condition. The only obvious irregularities in his otherwise impressive appearance were his two different colored eyes (one green and one brown) and a prominent white streak in his hair. He did not have any tumors or disfiguration, yet he told us firmly that there was no way he was going to father any children. He didn't want to take the chance of his child inheriting the disease. He knew that even though he wasn't affected severely, any child of his could be.

The couple wanted to be parents, so they made the decision to rely on sperm donation and had four beautiful children that way. The first two were singleton (single baby) pregnancies; the third insemination resulted in twins. This man is a dedicated and loving father to his large family in every way that matters—just not biologically. He chose this path to spare his children from a potentially devastating disease and never regretted his decision.

The benefit of these preconception screening tests is obvious—they can prevent serious genetic disorders from being passed on to future generations and empower a woman with important medical knowledge. The downside, however, is that these diseases are rare overall and the exams are costly. Just the cystic fibrosis screening alone is $600. Most insurance companies cover the basic tests, but for someone who is not insured, these costs can be prohibitive and might scare away some of the very people who could benefit the most from them.

Talking about genetic diseases and disorders is scary and disquieting for all prospective parents. But it's important to remember that even if you carry the gene for one of these disorders, there remains a 50 to 75 percent chance (depending on whether the gene is recessive or dominant) that you will bear a normal baby. In cases where parents want to avoid the risk altogether, a sperm or egg donor is an option. And even in cases where a child is born with an abnormality, the joy that the child can bring to his or her family can end up to be the greatest and most surprising gift of all.

Getting Pregnant Takes Time

▶ ▶ ▶ TAKE YOUR TIME

Chelsea and her husband decided it was time to have a baby. She came in for preconceptional counseling and eagerly started her vitamins and discontinued her birth control pills. Barely a month later, she called Allison in a panic, because she had her period. Desperate to know what she was doing wrong, she chronicled what had happened in the last cycle, what she had eaten, when she had sex, and a litany of other life details.

Allison gently reassured her that even though she was young—in her late twenties—the process of getting pregnant usually takes time, even up to a year. After two more months of unsuccessfully trying, however, Chelsea was so frantic that she scheduled an appointment to come back to the office. At this visit, she was tearful as she insisted that she undergo a full workup to find out what was wrong with her. Again, Allison tried to impress on her the complicated processes that go on in the body to make a baby: The success rate is only 20 percent per month!

Allison reviewed Chelsea's ovulation charts and encouraged her to keep trying. Sure enough, in month five, Chelsea got the good news she was longing for.

◀ ◀ ◀

Getting pregnant can take time. After a month or two of trying to conceive, patients will tearfully beg us to tell them what they are doing wrong. Our usual answer? "You're not doing anything wrong." Under normal circumstances with everything working perfectly, the odds of a couple getting pregnant during a given month is only 20 percent. That's a one-in-five chance. Within three months of trying, 50 percent of women will become pregnant, within six months, 75 percent, and within one year, about 85 percent. That leaves only 15 percent considered subfertile, a topic we describe in Chapter 8.

Birth Control and Pregnancy

myth: Taking birth control pills can cause birth defects and infertility.

FACT: No, it doesn't. The hormones in the birth control pill have not been shown to cause birth defects even if taken when a woman is unaware that she is pregnant. In addition, fertility rates are not affected by previous pill use.

There's a misconception that the hormones in birth control pills are toxic to developing fetuses, so a woman should stay off the pill for several months before she tries to conceive. Birth control pills are metabolized very quickly. They're out of your system just a few days after you take your last pill, and you might start to ovulate the first month that you no longer take them. There's no danger if you get pregnant during the first cycle off pills. Some patients have missed pills, unknowingly become pregnant, and continued to take their pills for months before realizing what was going on. There was no increased incidence of birth defects in these babies.

If a woman is faithfully taking her pill every day, the failure rate of the birth control pill is less than 1 percent. When women do get pregnant on birth control, some degree of human error is usually involved, with the typical failure rate closer to 7 percent. For example, if you don't pick up your pills from the pharmacy on time and miss a dose within the first five days of the new pack, you're at the greatest risk for conception. That's often how women on the pill end up pregnant.

We recommend that you discontinue your pill only when you are truly ready to go the distance, because many women do get pregnant right away. For some women who have been taking oral contraception for many years, it may take one to three months to resume ovulation, but there's no way to predict exactly how long it will take.

Future fertility is not influenced by birth control use. With more than fifty years of data about the pill, we can now definitively say that it has no long-term effect on your ability to get pregnant. When a woman has been on the pill for many years and then decides to conceive, she may find that her fertility rate is lower simply because she is older.

Note that although birth control pills are very effective, on some rare occasions they may fail and you could get pregnant. Don't worry, though, because this *will not* cause you to have a miscarriage or create birth defects in your baby.

If you get pregnant while using the intrauterine device (IUD), go to your doctor immediately and he or she will remove it for you as long as the string is visible. If left in place, an IUD can increase your chances of either miscarrying or getting an infection that can lead to a miscarriage. Often, if the IUD is removed early, you will go on to have a normal pregnancy. An IUD does not cause birth defects.

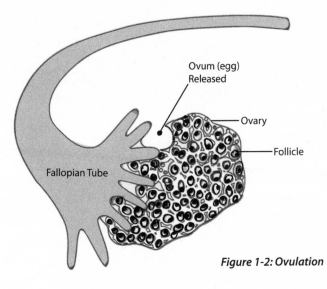

Ovum (egg)
Released

Ovary

Follicle

Fallopian Tube

Figure 1-2: Ovulation

Get an A in Ovulation 101

Let's go over a few things about your ovaries and ovulation. A woman has two ovaries that lie between the uterus and the pelvic wall. Inside the ovaries are tiny cysts called *follicles* where your eggs live. On average, you are born with two million follicles with eggs in them. Throughout your life, starting from birth, these follicles will steadily disappear and die. By the time you reach puberty, you will have about three hundred thousand eggs left. From this gigantic pool of eggs, a follicle (or sometimes follicles) will be selected each menstrual cycle to be "the chosen one" to ovulate. We do not know how this selection process happens, nor can we influence which egg is chosen.

Ovulation means the egg is released from its follicle in the ovary in response to a surge in lutenizing hormone (LH) from the brain (see Figure 1-2). After you ovulate, the egg moves into the fallopian tube where it can be fertilized by a sperm. Usually, only one egg is released, and if fertilized, you have a singleton pregnancy. If the fertilized egg splits into two within seven to ten days, you end up with identical twins. If two or more eggs are released simultaneously and multiple eggs are fertilized, you end up with fraternal multiples. For example, if three eggs ovulate and three different sperms fertilize the eggs, you will have fraternal triplets.

Check Your Timing

myth: When counting your menstrual cycle or figuring out when ovulation occurs, start counting from the day your menstrual bleeding ends.

FACT: Wrong! The first day of the menstrual cycle is the day you begin bleeding. This is considered cycle day one.

Many women think that the start of their menstrual cycle is the day that their period ends. Because we actually count day one as the *first* day of bleeding in a typical twenty-eight day cycle, most women will ovulate on day fourteen, or usually a week after menstrual bleeding ends. If a woman counts fourteen days from the *end* of her menstrual bleeding, she will always miss ovulation and will have difficulty becoming pregnant. Using a calendar, a computer program, or even a smartphone app to track your menstrual cycle are simple ways to ensure that you are sexually active at your most fertile time.

Know Your Cycle

When women come in for preconception advice, many of them don't know how to predict their ovulation. One simple way to do this is to utilize the calendar method. First, we advise them to determine the length of their cycles. A cycle is measured from the first day of menstrual bleeding to the next first day of menstrual bleeding. This is a process you can check over the course of several months. Remember to always count the first day of menstrual bleeding as the first day of your cycle.

Women's cycles can be different lengths. The first half of the cycle—from the first day of your period to ovulation—varies from woman to woman. The second half of the cycle—after ovulation—is fixed at fourteen days. Is your cycle twenty-four days? Is it thirty-two days? When you are certain of the total number of days, subtract fourteen from that number and that is your day of ovulation. So, for a typical twenty-eight-day cycle, women ovulate on day fourteen, and for a thirty-two-day cycle, on day eighteen. Remember to count day one as the first day of bleeding.

Before women ovulate, their estrogen levels go up, which thins the cervical mucous. The mucous looks like the clear white gel of fresh egg whites. That's a sign that ovulation is about to happen within the next few days, and that's when you should start trying to conceive.

myth: If you have intercourse in the missionary position, you will increase your chances of having a girl.

FACT: Millions of sperm are released in each ejaculate; half will produce boys and half will produce girls. While "girl" sperm are more dense and heavier than "boy" sperm, they have an equal chance of getting to the egg, no matter what position you happen to be in at the moment.

During ejaculation, approximately two hundred million to three hundred million sperm are deposited into the vagina. Fewer than two hundred live sperm actually make it to the egg because the majority of them die during the swim (see Figure 1-3). Sperm can be found in the fallopian tubes approximately five minutes after intercourse or artificial insemination. On the other end of the spectrum, living sperm have been found in the fallopian tubes as long as four to five days after intercourse.

Within two to three minutes of ovulation, the finger-like projections of the fallopian tube, called fimbria, direct the egg into the tube, where fertilization occurs. The egg lives for only one to two days after ovulation. Therefore, the most fertile time of the menstrual cycle is five days before ovulation and two days after—a total of seven days. Science shows us that, like a groom waiting at the altar for his bride, it's best to have the sperm there first, ready to fertilize the next egg that comes down the aisle.

myth: Lying still for thirty minutes and tilting your pelvis will increase the chances of you conceiving.

FACT: Although getting in this position is not harmful, it will not increase your chances of conceiving. The sperm swim under their own power, using the whip-like motions of their tails. Gravity does not play a role.

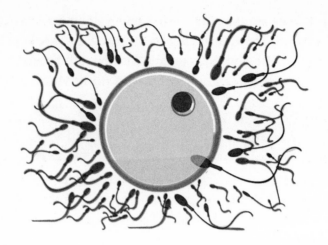

Figure 1-3: Fertilization

Time Ovulation with Temperature and Ovulation Kits

Aside from using the calendar method, another way to determine the time of ovulation is to monitor your *basal body temperature,* the lowest temperature attained by the body during rest. To do this, you need to check your body temperature when you are completely at rest, generally first thing in the morning at the same time each day. Your body temperature goes up at least 0.4 degrees within twenty-four hours after ovulation. You must use a special basal body thermometer that reads only from 96 to 100 degrees with clearer calibrations so you can more specifically determine your temperature.

Every day during your cycle, take your basal body temperature and plot it on a chart. If you are ovulating, you will see a rise in temperature *after* ovulation that persists for at least ten days. After you have charted two to three cycles, you should be able to calculate when you are ovulating. You can use this information in the *next* cycle to make sure you are sexually active during the fertile time.

Basal body temperature charts help women understand their menstrual cycle and fertility. However, the process of predicting ovulation in future cycles can be challenging. You must take your temperature at the same time every day, before you get out of bed or even speak. If you are sick or have slept less than five hours, the chart may not be accurate. While we applaud women who want to get a better sense of how their bodies operate, we've seen this process lead to extra stress and frustration for some of our patients and their partners.

Ovulation predictor kits may be easier to use, although they are more expensive than a basal body thermometer. You can buy the kit at your local pharmacy. Beginning on a day that's specific to your cycle, you urinate on a test stick every day for up to ten days. Roughly twelve to forty-eight hours *before* you ovulate, the luteinizing hormone (LH) will surge, and the test stick will reflect this change. When you have a positive result, you're about to ovulate and should have sex that same day and the next day.

Reduce Stress

myth: Stress itself causes infertility.

FACT: While extreme stress can cause periods of anovulation (missing your period), it rarely causes long-term fertility problems. Instead, stress can lead to lower sex drive and unhealthy habits such as overeating and difficulty sleeping, which can contribute to difficulties getting pregnant.

When a couple makes the decision to get pregnant, the previously pleasurable act of intimacy can suddenly become a stressful obligation. We tell our patients to relax when they are attempting to make a baby. If you are prone to anxiety and find that the process of trying to get pregnant pushes your nerves to the limit, take a deep breath and consider this: The pressures you are putting on yourself might be what's keeping you from getting pregnant.

Your body is a complex machine designed to adjust and protect itself in times of great stress, such as famine, disaster, or war. Often, that survival mechanism signals your body to shut down unnecessary systems to conserve energy and preserve life. During times of extreme stress, many women will stop ovulating. We've even seen women stop ovulating when they cram for college exams or experience a sudden illness. People who are grieving the death of a close family member have been known to go a few months without having a menstrual cycle. The body instinctively understands that extremely traumatic periods in life are not the optimum times to reproduce. However, this anovulation is usually temporary and normal fertility will resume as soon as the stressful event has passed.

We counsel our patients that getting pregnant should not feel like a science project; this is the time for you and your partner to be close and to connect with one another. Our advice is to slow down, relax, and remember that you have a one in five chance in any given month. Your best shot at getting pregnant may be to just enjoy the process.

▶ ▶ ▶ WHEN SEX STOPS BEING FUN

Allison had a patient named Shannon, a thirty-six-year-old literary agent, whom she had known for many years. Shannon and her husband had been married for nine years before they finally decided it was time to start a family. At her annual exam, Shannon excitedly told Allison that they were ready to go and that she would stop her birth control the next cycle. A month went by, another, and then another. Shannon called in a panic. How could it be that something she was trying to avoid for so many years now wasn't happening when she wanted it? Allison explained to her that perfectly healthy women have only a one in five chance per month of conceiving. They discussed timing, ovulation, and when to have sex.

Allison heard from Shannon again three months later. With frustration, Shannon said that this was becoming tedious and it wasn't fun for her or her husband because the whole timing thing had become really crazy. She was doing everything humanly possible to conceive, including charting her basal body temperature, tracking her cervical mucous changes, *and* using ovulation kits! Month after month, she would wait for her period, then wait for ovulation, then wait again. When her period came, she felt an enormous letdown. Shannon's stress levels were getting out of control. She started wondering, "Whose fault is it? What's wrong with me? What's wrong with him?"

Allison responded that most likely nothing was wrong with either of them. She suggested that Shannon just look at the calendar to get a general idea of when she was fertile, and plan a nice getaway during that time—and relax. Although she didn't get pregnant the first time she took Allison's suggestion, she and her husband did let up on their overly intense conception rituals. They finally had some good news ten months after she stopped taking the pill.

Trying to conceive can be one of the most frustrating times of a woman's life, but ideally it can become a time that brings a couple closer and prepares them for the challenges that will lie ahead with a new baby.   ◀ ◀ ◀

Over-the-Counter Pregnancy Tests

The transport of the fertilized egg through the fallopian tube takes about three days. It takes another two to four days for the embryo to attach to the wall of the uterus. At the time of implantation—about seven days after conception—the pregnancy tissue starts producing the *hCG* (human chorionic gonadotropin) hormone in minute amounts. By the time you miss your menstrual cycle, hCG is detectable in your blood and urine.

Before the advent of prepackaged pregnancy tests, people could rely only on pregnancy symptoms—missed periods, sudden nausea, growing bellies—to alert them to the possibility that they might be expecting. In 1927, it was discovered that if the urine of a pregnant woman was injected into a rabbit, the ovaries of the rabbit would swell with cysts.[7] Unfortunately, the rabbit had to be killed and examined to know whether the cysts formed. Thus the famous phrase "the rabbit died" came to indicate that a woman was pregnant. In reality, the rabbit died whether the woman was pregnant or not. We're all grateful that ob-gyns no longer have to sacrifice bunnies. In the 1950s, researchers identified hCG as the hormone produced by pregnancy, and by the late 1960s, hCG could be detected in a simple (and nonlethal) test.[8]

Over the years, we've observed that many of our patients don't trust over-the-counter home pregnancy tests. However, those tests are the same as the tests performed in the doctor's office. The chemical reaction in the stick can happen only if hCG is present. Even a few days before the missed period, the over-the-counter pregnancy test is going to be positive. On average, women buy at least two kits and then still want to come to our office to verify. We tell our patients, "If you have a positive pregnancy test once, you are pregnant." We are happy to confirm it and we'll start your prenatal care on that first visit.

We find that many patients test too early. Some tests claim accuracy as early as day twenty-four or -five of your cycle. However, the amount of hCG in the blood at that point may not be measurable by current methods. Women can be heartsick with disappointment but turn out to be pregnant when they test again a week later. Remember, you will not have a measurable amount of hCG in your body until at least twelve days after conception. For this reason, it may be best to wait until the day of the missed period to do the test. As the sensitivity of hCG detection improves, an accurate test may be possible sooner.

Getting Pregnant the Second Time

If you conceived effortlessly the first time, the second should be a breeze, right? Most of the time, yes. However, if many years have passed since the first pregnancy, a woman's age may now be a factor in her ability to conceive. Also, after a couple has children, they may not find as much time or energy to have sex as they did before.

▶ ▶ ▶ MY SECOND TIME AROUND

My husband wanted children right off the bat, even back when I was in medical school in my midtwenties. I, on the other hand, felt unprepared. In my first year in private practice, after four years of medical school and four years of OB-GYN training, my husband was beginning to doubt that we were ever going to have a family. Then one day, I finally felt ready—or as ready as you can ever be.

When I decided it was time to have kids, I was thirty-four years old. I had a lot of advantages: I understood how my body worked, I had regular twenty-eight-day cycles, I had the textbook egg-white consistency cervical discharge around the time of ovulation, and I understood that it might take me a while to conceive. I had no expectations about getting pregnant my first try, but as luck would have it, I did! My first son, Matthew, was born thirty-eight weeks later. From the first time I held him, I was so grateful that we'd taken the plunge into parenthood.

When I turned thirty-seven, I saw forty approaching and knew what this meant: not that I couldn't have a baby, but that it might take me longer to conceive. I also knew the chance for miscarriage was higher. Still, because I became pregnant so easily the first time, I felt confident—maybe too confident. Almost a year of trying and many negative pregnancy tests later, my husband was asking me, "What's going on?" I thought, "Huh, this is strange." I literally had to look in the mirror and give myself the same pep talk I share with my patients: "It takes six months to a year for the majority of women to get pregnant. The chance is only 20 percent each time you try. Don't make it like a homework project. Enjoy your time with your partner."

Through our experiences, my colleagues and I often walk a mile in our patients' shoes. This was definitely one of those times, and one of those life lessons. A little over a year later, I finally had the positive pregnancy test I was anxiously waiting for, and thirty-seven weeks later, little Max was in my arms. Now, when my moms-to-be get flustered the second time around, I can confidently reassure them, "You know, I got pregnant the first time I tried with my first one, but it took me a little over a year with the second one. I know what you're going through. Just be patient."

—Alane ◀ ◀ ◀

Previous pregnancies can also give us insight into potential problems with a future pregnancy, so we obtain a thorough history of how the prior pregnancy progressed. Did they deliver at term? Did they have preeclampsia? Did they have an ectopic pregnancy or miscarriage? If we uncover any unusual patterns, we can speculate about how that problem may affect subsequent pregnancies.

▶ ▶ ▶ **SECOND TIME PREPAREDNESS**

A patient of mine named Hannah delivered her first baby with a different doctor. She had a normal forty-week course, and the delivery went smoothly as well. She went home from the hospital the day after her baby was born. That night, she had a seizure and was rushed by ambulance back to the hospital. On the ride there, she had a second seizure. Immediately, she underwent brain scans, tests of her heart, and blood tests. She was started on antiseizure medications.

Finally the diagnosis was made—she had *eclampsia,* which is the severe form of preeclampsia. (See Chapter 9 for more on high-risk pregnancies.) It usually occurs during pregnancy but can occur in the immediate postpartum period as well.

Understandably, her husband was terrified. He had witnessed his wife having a seizure and did not know the cause or whether she would survive. Hannah stayed in the hospital for a week and was stabilized with no further seizures. For the first few months at home, her husband feared every day that they would end up back in the hospital. Fortunately, the rest of her postpartum course was uneventful.

After a few years, Hannah and her husband decided they wanted to add to their family. They were predictably nervous when I first met them and relayed their story to me. I suggested that we try to find any underlying cause for her rare condition. We did a battery of blood tests, and it turned out that she has a blood clotting disorder called antiphospholipid antibody syndrome, which can predispose women to preeclampsia and eclampsia. She didn't know she had this condition during her first pregnancy. This time, as soon as she became pregnant, we were able to start her on blood thinners, which may reduce the risk of recurrent eclampsia.

This story illustrates why the history of previous pregnancies is so important. If you have been pregnant before, you need to tell you doctor any important details that might affect you the next time around.

—Allison ◀ ◀ ◀

After conception has occurred, the risk of miscarriage is about 20 percent, or one out of five. The majority of these are the result of a genetic abnormality in which the cells in the embryo do not divide correctly. It's important to know that after one such miscarriage, the risk of another miscarriage is *not* increased. A woman can try again after she has resumed her regular menstrual cycles. A recent study in the *British Medical Journal* revealed that women who had a prior miscarriage were more fertile if they conceived within six months of a previous miscarriage.[9]

If a woman has had three consecutive first-trimester miscarriages or a second-trimester loss, additional testing may be performed to determine if there is an underlying cause such as diabetes, thyroid disease, autoimmune disorders, and genetic abnormalities in the parents. In addition, any abnormalities in the uterus will be evaluated. Fortunately, many of these conditions are treatable. For women with recurrent pregnancy loss, the chance of eventually delivering a baby is 60 percent.

Choosing Your Doctor

One of the first and most crucial decisions of your pregnancy is to find the right health care provider to guide you through this remarkable journey. Ideally, this person will be the same one who delivers your baby, although that is not always possible (as described shortly). In our experience with thousands of moms-to-be—not to mention our own pregnancies—we've found that the relationship between a woman and her obstetrician can be perhaps the most intimate of any doctor-patient connection. Trust and openness are essential.

We recommend meeting with your potential doctor well ahead of conception to make sure you are comfortable with that person. Does the doctor answer all your questions? Is he or she easy to talk to? Is he or she willing to let you prepare or participate in your birth plan? These questions are the beginning of the process of choosing a doctor who will be the right fit for you. In Table 1-3, we have listed the top ten questions that we feel you should ask a potential doctor.

Table 1-3: Ten Questions When Choosing Your Ob-Gyn

1. Is the doctor board-certified?

2. Does the doctor listen to me and answer my questions?

3. Do I feel comfortable with this doctor and the office staff?

4. Is the doctor flexible? Is he or she willing to try different methods of care I am interested in, such as acupuncture, physical therapy, doulas, or midwives?

5. Is the doctor reliable in returning phone calls?

6. Is the doctor affiliated with my preferred hospital?

7. Does he or she take my insurance?

8. Does the doctor work at a hospital with a high-level NICU (neonatal intensive care unit)?

9. Is the doctor open to more natural childbirth philosophies? Does his or her philosophy match mine?

10. Does the doctor perform VBACs (vaginal birth after cesarean)?

Great rapport with your provider isn't everything, however. In addition, you need to select where you want to have your baby: in a local hospital, in a birth center, or at home. Women with special-needs pregnancies should also seek a provider who is aware of and supportive of those needs.

For example, a mom who wants a *VBAC* (vaginal birth after cesarean, an attempt at a vaginal delivery after cesarean delivery, see page 277) will need to find a doctor who is willing to perform one. (Some doctors and hospitals don't allow VBACs.) If you have high-risk medical problems, you may need to be cared for by a person who specializes in that type of pregnancies. If you are at risk for delivering preterm, your doctor must work at a hospital that has a *NICU* (*neonatal intensive care unit*) that can care for your baby. You may hope to have a purely natural delivery and find yourself interviewing a doctor who says, "If you're going to deliver with me, you must have an IV and be on the fetal monitor during the entire labor process." If you're not okay with that answer, you need to look for other options. Know what you want out of your pregnancy and what is important to you, and address those issues with your prospective doctor up front.

You may also want to find out about your doctor's call schedule. Does the doctor deliver all of his or her own babies? Does the doctor work in a group with several others whom you may not meet until delivery day? Although doctors and midwives would like to always be available for their patients, sometimes it's not possible. As a result, some women are caught by surprise when someone they've never seen before walks in and announces that they're there to deliver the baby.

Then there's the challenging issue of commercial insurance carriers. You may be limited to certain doctors based on your insurance plan and what it covers. We urge you to investigate these caveats well ahead of time because some doctors accept only certain insurance programs or plans. In addition, some hospitals will take only certain types of insurance. You may need to switch your insurance to get the doctor and hospital you desire. We know some moms who have resorted to paying out of pocket because they insisted on being treated by someone who was not covered by their insurance policy.

◗ ◗ ◗ BEING THERE

Each one of us has become attached to individual patients, and we tend to go out of our way to deliver them, even when we are not on call. For us, the delivery is the end of a forty-week relationship and the highlight of our attention and care.

When Gayle's first baby was born, she was delivered not by her doctor but by a doctor on call whom she had never met. "We were barely introduced, and then the doctor gowned up and put on his mask and gloves," Gayle remembers. "He seemed to want to maintain a distinct doctor-patient distance from me at all times, which left me feeling a bit abandoned and afraid." For her second pregnancy, a close friend of mine who knew Gayle referred her to our practice.

I saw Gayle from the start all the way through to the end. She was a delight. The day she went into labor, I wasn't on call and it was my morning off to take my daughter to her swimming lesson, but I canceled everything and rushed to the hospital to deliver Gayle. I sat next to her at her bedside and spoke quietly to her as she gently delivered her son. The experience was peaceful and intimate. Gayle and her husband were so grateful. I left the delivery room that day with a powerful reaffirmation of why I chose this job. The next day, I dropped in on Gayle while I was making my rounds. She was still marveling at how different her two birth experiences had been. She appreciated how personal the process had been the second time around.

—Yvonne ◖ ◖ ◖

As part of your research, make certain your physician is board-certified by the American Board of Obstetrics and Gynecology. To become board-certified, doctors must complete a four-year residency training program and pass a series of written and oral exams. Thereafter, they have to participate in an annual recertification process in which they are tested on the most current news in the field. This can help to reassure you that your doctor is up to date on the latest trends and ongoing scientific research.

A busy OB-GYN practice has no ordinary days. Anything can happen at any time, and sometimes things may seem a bit chaotic. If we meet a patient who has expectations that cannot be met, we try to explain why her wishes cannot be accommodated. If we cannot find a compromise, we refer her to another practice where we hope she will be happier. We do not take it personally. We want the patient to have a pleasant experience too. Sometimes, people's personalities don't always click and it is better for everyone involved to find the relationship that works best for them.

As a patient, there are some basic things you should expect from your doctor and staff, but keep in mind that doctors are humans, too. We work hard to be on time to see our patients, but it can be difficult because sometimes we are called to deliver a baby or suddenly deal with an unexpected emergency. Because we don't use a "take a number" or cookie-cutter approach to office visits, we never know exactly how long each visit will take. It could be a routine examination that's over in fifteen minutes, or we could find that one of our moms-to-be has a newly diagnosed medical condition. Perhaps she has just lost a parent or a close family member has been diagnosed with cancer. It's not unusual for a fifteen-minute office visit to turn into an hour-long encounter because a woman is having emotional difficulties. For this reason, managing time becomes a specialized skill in our profession.

However, all patients deserve to be alerted by a doctor's office staff if their appointment might be delayed. We believe that it's important to tell our moms why their doctor is running late and give them the option to reschedule or to see another doctor. Women should feel that their needs are being addressed.

▶ ▶ ▶ PLEASE LISTEN TO ME

"Please doctor. Just read the letters," Olivia begged Yvonne. The letters, one from her mother, another from her maternal aunt, were many pages long and detailed, describing their own long and difficult birth experiences. Both had very long labors that led to serious postpartum hemorrhages. Olivia had wanted her previous doctor to understand what they had gone through because she thought there might be something genetically wrong in her family that caused these traumatic experiences to happen. Now that she was pregnant herself, she was terrified that the same thing would happen to her.

Olivia was worried that her previous doctor hadn't read the letters carefully, so later in her pregnancy, she came to us.

After Yvonne read the letters from Olivia's mom and aunt, she immediately realized that both had excessively long labors and dangerous hemorrhages that potentially could have been prevented by either an earlier intervention or a cesarean delivery. We assured Olivia that if the labor process was abnormally long, she would be offered a cesarean.

All Olivia really wanted was for us—her doctors—to validate her concerns. A patient wants to know that her doctor is listening. Even if you might secretly think your idea or fear is the most ridiculous thing in the world, we believe it's important that your doctor listen to you and take your concerns seriously.

Olivia went on to have a healthy baby boy by cesarean delivery with no abnormal postpartum bleeding, and was very happy with the outcome. ◀ ◀ ◀

Choosing a Midwife

Some women may choose to use a midwife instead of a doctor. This is another important decision to make as early as possible in your pregnancy.

A *midwife* is a person who's been trained to assist a woman throughout her pregnancy and during childbirth. Midwives can deliver babies in the home, in a birth center, or at a hospital. In many countries around the world, most babies are delivered by midwives, and only complicated births and cesareans are delivered by an obstetrician.

During the years that the three of us were residents at LA County–USC Hospital, the volume of deliveries there was so high that only the most complicated or high-risk deliveries were performed by the ob-gyn residents. Midwives attended all the normal births, so we were trained in our first deliveries by midwives! We will always be indebted to these midwives, but particularly to a wonderful midwife named Rosemary, a strong Italian woman who was like the earth mother of the entire hospital. Unfailingly kind and supportive to both patients and medical students, Rosemary even brought delectable home-baked treats to help us through our long nights on call. It was Rosemary who taught all three of us how to deliver babies without cutting episiotomies. Today, when patients ask us "Do you do episiotomies?" we can honestly answer, "Almost never," thanks to her patience and care in training us on how to stretch the perineum and avoid tearing.

Thanks to our experiences with professionals like Rosemary, we are extremely respectful of the amazing women who choose to become midwives. If your pregnancy is low risk, working with a midwife can be a fulfilling experience. The best midwives know as well as many doctors the ins and outs of pregnancies, and they also know when to ask for help. When a complication arises and it's time to transfer a patient's care to a doctor or a hospital, they never hesitate. In general, midwives can perform only normal vaginal births for moms with low-risk pregnancies.

If you choose a midwife rather than an ob-gyn, we strongly recommend that you use one who has a good working relationship with a doctor. The midwife will be the only provider who will see you during your prenatal care and she will be the one attending your birth unless a complication occurs. However, she needs access to a doctor to whom she can transfer care in case the labor is going too long or you need a cesarean delivery.

If you are using a midwife at home, we also believe it's critical that you can get to a hospital immediately—in no more than ten to fifteen minutes—in case of emergency. If a crisis happens and the baby is in trouble, you have only a few minutes to get the baby out quickly before he or she suffers from low oxygen, brain damage, or even death. These complications are quite rare, however, because most women who choose a midwife have low-risk, normal pregnancies to begin with.

Depending on the midwife's training, the scope of her practice may be limited. For example, some midwives have been trained in the process of augmenting labor but others have not. She won't be able to perform an emergency cesarean delivery or even an operative vaginal delivery. If you have a complex vaginal laceration, she may not be able to repair it.

If you have a high-risk pregnancy or a significant medical issue, such as chronic high blood pressure or diabetes, we urge you to choose a doctor rather than a midwife. Most midwives will also transfer care if a woman is going to deliver preterm. When choosing your midwife, make sure you discuss her backup plans if any of these situations should occur.

▶ ▶ ▶ A MIDWIFE'S PERSPECTIVE

What would birth look like if no one was there to witness it but the woman in labor? Birth is undoubtedly one of the most profoundly mammalian experiences a female will experience in her life, and one that under most normal circumstances will unfold as the biological design dictates: without the need for medical intervention.

I began my path to midwifery after working for Gaia Herbs as an educator and working as a nutritional consultant. I had just finished reading a book called *The Red Tent* by Anita Diamant and was enchanted by the visuals of women holding space for the females of their tribe as they birthed their children. I knew then that if midwifery was still a profession, it was the path for me. As soon as I made the decision, I took a doula training with Carmen Bornn and then began an apprenticeship at the Hollywood Birth Center in Los Angeles. Since 2001, I have attended more than 550 births and worked with more than two thousand families.

Some studies show that when under the supervision and care of licensed midwives, women will receive exceptional prenatal and postpartum care, resulting in fewer premature babies, fewer interventions during labor and thus fewer cesareans, a higher incidence of breastfeeding, and less postpartum depression.

And why is this? Midwives are able to cherry-pick their clientele, dealing with a low-risk population, and then are able to focus on developing a relationship of what I like to refer to as *partnership care,* meaning that the clients become responsible for being involved in the type of care they are receiving. Because midwives typically have fewer clients, the care is more one-on-one, and a deep sense of intimacy and trust is created. Plenty of time is available to discuss questions and fears that arise during the pregnancy, and a lot of attention is focused on nutrition, hydration, and exercise, allowing high-risk conditions to be caught early, typically with enough time to do prevention. Also, midwives keep close tabs on their clients through the postpartum period, catching issues with breastfeeding or hormonal dips when they first appear, so that they can be remedied in their early phases.

Midwives typically practice in a hospital setting, at birth centers, or in the home. If you want emergency medical treatment available or pain medications nearby to fully relax into the process of giving birth, your preferred choice might be a midwife who works in a hospital setting. You could still receive the compassion and understanding that is typical with midwifery care, but in the setting that most supports your desires.

Midwives who work in birth centers not associated with hospitals (typically freestanding birth centers) are no different than those who work in a home-based birth practice. Some do both and will give their clients a choice as to where they feel most comfortable.

Licensed midwives undergo a lengthy training process and are licensed by the Medical board, the same licensing body that regulates and licenses doctors. Licensed Midwives and Certified Nurse Midwives are medical professionals certified in Neonatal Resuscitation and carry with them medical equipment that enables them to manage most of the emergencies that could happen in a hospital setting, such as bleeding, dehydration, infections, and babies that need help breathing. Clients of home birth or birth center midwives typically dictate what tests they will receive prenatally (such as ultrasounds or diagnostic testing for gestational diabetes), how instinctually they want to labor and give birth, and who is going to catch the baby. Parents decide many of the details; the midwife is there to support the choices the parents have made and make sure everything is happening safely.

So what determines if you are low risk and a good candidate for a home or birth center birth?

Risk is determined by many factors and varies from midwife to midwife and doctor to midwife. In my own practice, we look at several factors and assess someone by looking at the whole person. Health conditions such as heart disease, kidney disease, some autoimmune disorders, diabetes, and birth defects could rule someone out because of high risk. But we consider other factors, such as certain types of anemia and how the client cares for themselves. We take into consideration a woman's stress level, exercise, and nutrition, and we insist that our clients meet the obligations of their contracts in terms of educating themselves about birth, meeting their financial obligations, and coming to all their scheduled appointments.

I believe that birth is an issue of woman's rights and a baby's rights. Something so profound and simple is here before us, a miracle with boundless healing potential and profound beauty, waiting to be experienced and shared.

—Midwife Aleksandra Evanguelidi ◀ ◀ ◀

A Life-Changing Moment

We haven't read any science on this, but we see it in our patients' faces every day: Emotionally, something powerful happens when a woman finds out she is pregnant. The moment you see that positive pregnancy result on the urine dipstick or your doctor informs you, "Yes, the fertility treatment worked this time," your mindset instantly changes. Some women fret about that glass of wine they drank the previous night—will it harm the baby? Or they may suddenly want to stop all their medications, even if they have a splitting headache. Other patients immediately start to time travel with their unborn baby. They visualize a boy or a girl, dressed in freshly pressed, new clothes on his or her first day of school. They visualize dance recitals and soccer games, and the pressure of getting their child into the right college. In a matter of moments, they're already twenty years down the road.

We've been there ourselves, so we know that this kind of thinking is normal, but it can also be overwhelming. You'll have to traverse so many bumps in the road simply to get the baby into the world, let alone raise your child over the next eighteen years. As doctors and as moms, we advise our patients to try to take their pregnancy one stage—and if possible, one day—at a time.

We're here to help you do that in the following chapters.

chapter two

DIET, EXERCISE, AND YOUR PREGNANCY

IN OUR EXPERIENCE, when a woman discovers she is pregnant, she immediately feels a heightened sense of responsibility. Now that she is the incubator for a potential new life, every move she makes, every place she goes, and everything she eats or drinks is now under a new kind of scrutiny. Our patients come into our offices brimming with questions: "What do I have to know about nutrition?" "How should I take care of my body?" "What activities can be dangerous to my baby?" Many of these questions involve issues related to diet, exercise, and safety. Unfortunately, so many myths and fear-provoking stories on these topics abound that our patients often find themselves hopelessly confused about what is fact and what is fiction.

We try to reassure our patients about their anxieties surrounding these issues. The truth is, the secret to a healthy pregnancy doesn't have to be complicated. So take a deep breath, relax, and start by following the simple guidelines outlined in this chapter, and you'll be well on your way to a safe and more enjoyable pregnancy.

▶ ▶ ▶ SHE ATE WHAT?

"This is your exchange calling. You have an emergency!"

As obstetricians, we take our emergency calls very seriously. At any given time, we have patients who are on the verge of delivery. In addition, you never know whether a mom might deliver prematurely or whether someone has developed a potentially serious condition like preeclampsia. It's our job to be there, to reassure a mom who is scared and confused about what might be happening to her body.

That's why I took the urgent call from my patient Theresa one Saturday at two in the morning.

"I ate something terrible," sobbed Theresa, a thirty-four-year-old travel agent who had thus far been a model patient. "I think I should go to the emergency room to get my stomach pumped."

I asked Theresa to take a deep breath, slow down, and explain the situation. It turns out she had eaten a small piece of carpaccio (a thin slice of raw beef) during a dinner several hours earlier. Since then, she had been surfing the Internet and reading about the dangers of uncooked meat. Now Theresa couldn't sleep and was terrified that she may have damaged her fourteen-week-old fetus. She was considering trying to throw up the food or going to her local ER.

I reassured Theresa that such drastic measures weren't necessary. The likelihood that the meat she'd eaten was contaminated with toxoplasmosis or any other kind of bacteria was low. She'd ingested only a tiny amount, and the restaurant where she had the meal was reputable with an excellent hygiene record. "You can't take back what you've already eaten," I said, while giving her a list of the warning signs for food poisoning and instructing her to report to a hospital immediately if she experienced any of them. She hadn't experienced any symptoms; she'd just read about the dangers of eating raw meat in pregnancy—which are real—and let her fears take over. My advice to her was to watch her diet a bit more carefully in the future to avoid another such scare.

Theresa went on to deliver a healthy baby girl, with no complications.

—Yvonne ◀ ◀ ◀

Weight Gain

myth: When you're pregnant, you're eating for two!

FACT: No, you're not! Here's another myth we're happy to strike down: You don't need to eat twice as much when you are pregnant. Yes, you have a baby growing and developing inside you, but most women are stunned when we tell them that they need to *add only about 300 extra healthy calories per day* to their diet. Your pregnancy diet is really not that different from what you are already doing on a day-to-day basis—assuming you eat a reasonably balanced diet.

The ideal amount of weight gain during pregnancy depends on your starting point. If you start at a normal weight, you should gain about twenty-five to thirty-five pounds during the forty weeks. If you start underweight, you should gain about twenty-eight to forty pounds. If you're starting your pregnancy overweight, you should add only about fifteen to twenty-five pounds.

Many women struggle with the concept of gaining so many pounds in such a short period of time. Even with minor adjustments to their diets, some women find that they gain as much as ten pounds in a month due to the dramatic changes that pregnancy wreaks on their metabolisms. This rapid weight gain leaves them panicked that the pounds will continue to pile on at the same pace throughout their pregnancies. At the other end of the spectrum, some women who have been restricting their diets for years will use pregnancy as an excuse to eat whatever they want, sometimes gaining fifty to sixty pounds during the forty weeks. For still others, especially women who begin their pregnancy overweight, carrying a baby can be just the incentive they need to get their diet back on track and to take better care of their bodies. Ironically, these women may gain very little weight during the journey.

The pattern of weight gain varies from woman to woman. The most common scenario is a gain of *three to six pounds* in the first trimester, and about a *half a pound to one pound every week* in the second and third trimesters. However, not every pregnancy follows this schedule.

Some women gain nothing or even lose weight at the beginning. Others put on ten pounds in one month and then plateau for a number of weeks.

Know that your fetus is an efficient freeloader. In your body, your baby is absorbing everything it needs from you, even if you are not gaining weight. And when the weight gain starts, some women are afraid they will continue at the new accelerated pace for the rest of the pregnancy. Fortunately, this rarely happens. Women will go through plateaus of slower weight gain later as well. The end of pregnancy can bring larger interval gains due to water retention, sometimes adding three to five pounds in one week. This excessive swelling will disappear after the baby is born.

The best way to know how much you should gain is to calculate your body mass index (BMI). You can use an online BMI calculator or use the following formula:

$$BMI = \frac{weight\ (lbs.)}{[height\ (in.)]^2} \times 703$$

Underweight	BMI <18.5	Gain 28–40 pounds
Normal weight	BMI 19–25	Gain 25–35 pounds
Overweight	BMI 25–30	Gain 15–25 pounds
Obese	BMI >30	Gain 11–20 pounds

▶ ▶ ▶ **THE DREADED SCALE**

The most dreaded place in our office is the scale. Women can handle the pelvic exams, the blood draws, the Pap smears. But that scale puts people over the edge.

A talented hairdresser and first-time mom, Sylvia would flinch every time she came for an appointment when it was time for the weigh-in. She had been overweight before her pregnancy and had worked extremely hard to lose twenty pounds before she conceived. After she became pregnant, it seemed like the weight was flying back on at an unbelievable rate. Soon she had gained back all the weight she had lost. At one visit, to her horror, her weight surpassed that of her husband. Sylvia became more and more depressed and disappointed with herself.

We explained to Sylvia that, as long as she is making healthy food choices and not overeating, the pattern of any given woman's pregnancy weight gain is usually determined by nature and pretty much out of her hands. Some women's metabolisms shift in such a way that no matter what they do, the pounds stay on. All they can do is exercise moderately and make the best possible food choices. Sylvia struggled for most of the forty weeks with this concept. She had a healthy seven-pound baby girl, and then breastfed and exercised when she could. She was pleasantly surprised to find the weight came off again with relative ease. She learned that you can control some things when it comes to pregnancy weight gain but others are out of your hands. You just have to let go and let your body do what it needs to do to help your baby grow.

◀ ◀ ◀

Ultimately, if you follow a healthy diet, your body will gain exactly what it needs. The week-to-week numbers are not as important as the overall total and the growth of the baby. Your metabolism will shift to allow weight gains and plateaus as your baby's needs change. If we see that the baby isn't growing well, we may tell you to increase your calorie intake, maybe by adding a protein bar or shake. If the baby seems to be getting too big, we will recommend cutting out the extra snacks and watching the amount of carbohydrates you are eating. Carbohydrates include the obvious, such as cakes and cookies, but too much bread, rice, pasta, potatoes, and even fruit and fruit juice can also contribute to excess weight gain.

Figure 2-1 shows you how your pregnancy weight gain is distributed. Consider this—you are putting on only about *four to six pounds of your own fat* during your entire pregnancy. Everything else is weight that's related to the baby.

Undereating

Most moms have no trouble gaining the recommended amount of weight or more. However, we've also had patients who weigh themselves all the time, with the goal of trying to stay as thin as possible. One patient who was terrified of gaining weight distressed us so much that we firmly had to order her to eat more. We sometimes see

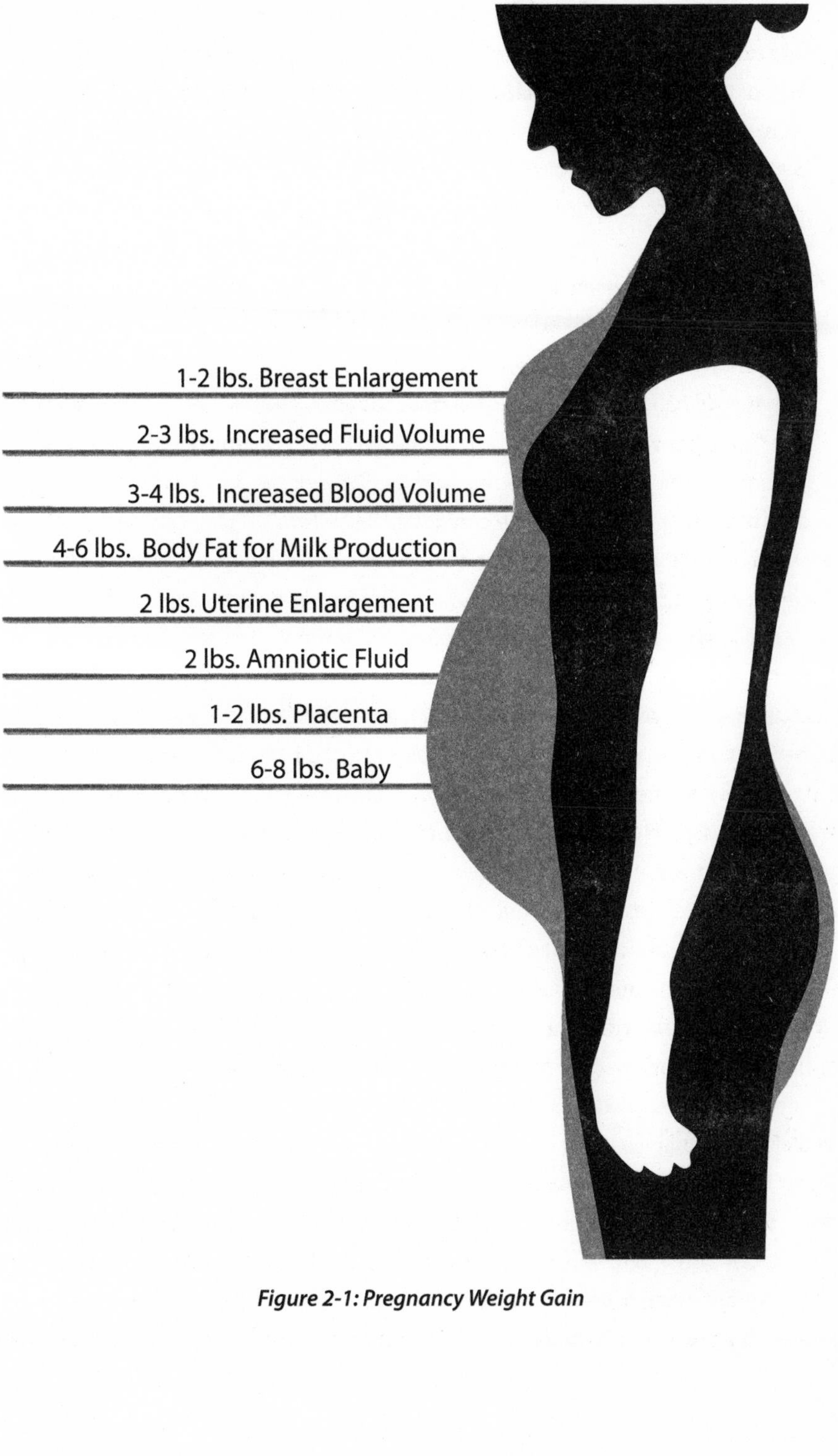

1-2 lbs. Breast Enlargement

2-3 lbs. Increased Fluid Volume

3-4 lbs. Increased Blood Volume

4-6 lbs. Body Fat for Milk Production

2 lbs. Uterine Enlargement

2 lbs. Amniotic Fluid

1-2 lbs. Placenta

6-8 lbs. Baby

Figure 2-1: Pregnancy Weight Gain

this behavior in women who have had a history of eating disorders or body image issues. In these cases, we try to reinforce that they need to eat a healthy, balanced diet for their own body as well as their baby's.

▶ ▶ ▶ THE GHOST OF AN EATING DISORDER

"Dr. Hill," said my nurse Patty, shaking her head and handing me a chart. "Your patient is ready for you, but she absolutely refuses to get on the scale to be weighed."

We've all had days like that, I thought to myself, heading into the examination room. But when I walked through the door, I caught my breath. Sitting on the edge of the table was a trembling, waif-like young woman who seemed to drown in the folds of her blue exam gown. Rachel was thirty-one years old, an assistant fashion magazine editor newly married to a nightclub promoter. This was her very first pregnancy and our first meeting as doctor and patient.

I decided that the best thing to do was to confront the issue of the scale directly. After she became more comfortable with me, Rachel came clean. She confessed that she had always dreaded this part of being pregnant. Rachel had been struggling with the devastating disease of anorexia for a long time but had finally reached a healthier weight in the last few years and was feeling that her life was starting to come into balance. While she understood that she would gain weight during pregnancy, she could not allow herself to step on the scale. She was terrified that she would again become obsessed with the numbers, as many anorexics do, and that it would send her back to her old patterns of self-starvation.

I made a deal with Rachel. I would get one baseline weight that first day—but I wouldn't tell her the number. From then on, I would measure the baby at each visit. If there was ever a problem with the baby's growth, she agreed to be weighed—again without me telling her the exact number. I would then advise her if she needed to eat more.

Throughout her pregnancy, her baby did grow, but at the lower end of the curve. She gave birth to a healthy son named Declan, who weighed just under six pounds. Rachel went through her entire pregnancy without ever knowing how much weight she gained.

—Allison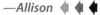

Your Diet

No matter how educated or sophisticated they may be, some of our patients are operating on the assumption that their babies are eating exactly what they eat. However, this is not quite the case. The growing fetus receives nutrition in basic forms—protein, carbohydrate, and fat—from the mother's blood. These nutritional building blocks are the products of the fully digested food from the mother. So if you eat an ice cream cone, your fetus does not devour a tiny fetus-sized amount of ice cream. Rather, it receives the protein, fat, and sugar from the food that has already gone through your digestive system.

Most healthy, normal-weight women need only about 300 more calories a day to support their developing fetus. On average, a typical woman consumes 2,000 calories per day when not pregnant. When you look at it that way, consuming 2,300 calories versus 2,000 calories isn't that much of a difference—*only 15 percent more calories per day*. To give you a sense of how little extra food you need to add to your pregnancy diet, here are some different food combinations that add up to approximately 300 calories.

Eggs and cheese
2 scrambled eggs
1 slice of Swiss cheese
Total: 305 calories

Yogurt and cereal with berries
1 container light vanilla yogurt
1 cup raspberries
1 cup cereal
Total: 300 calories

Dried fruit
1 cup of dried apricots
Total: 312 calories

Bagel
1 plain bagel
Total: 320 calories

Cereal with fruit
1 cup of cereal
8 ounces 2% milk
1 banana
Total: 290 calories

Cottage cheese with fruit and nuts
1 container cottage cheese
1 cup diced pineapple
20 whole raw almonds
Total: 290 calories

Stuffed potato
1 medium baked potato
2 tablespoons sour cream
2 tablespoons salsa
1 cup of melon
Total: 305 calories

Snack bar
1 protein bar (2 ounces)
Total: 250–300 calories

The goal for nutrition and physical fitness during pregnancy is to be *healthy*. This is not the time for dieting or exercising to the extreme. We recommend making as many good, healthy food choices as possible. Not gaining enough weight may cause growth problems for the baby, and gaining too much can make the last months of pregnancy very difficult because of the extra pressure on the hips, lower back, and knees, limiting mobility. In addition, the babies of moms who gain excessive weight tend to grow large, making delivery more difficult and dangerous. More than twenty studies have confirmed that newborns weighing more than eight-and-a-half pounds have a higher risk for diabetes and obesity in the future.

Regarding pregnancy diets, we simply recommend that you use your common sense. You do not need to be overly strict or chart your eating habits on a daily basis. People know when they're eating badly. We'll have a mom who spills out a confession: "Um, I ate a whole box of chocolate chip cookies the other night, is that okay?" Obviously, that's not healthy in the big picture, but one such incident isn't going to hurt the fetus either.

On the other hand, we also have some patients who need more specific rules when it comes to diet. You should think about what works best for you and be sure to communicate that to your doctor.

So, what is the best pregnancy diet? A basic one. Try to eat a variety of foods, as shown in Table 2-1. Consume more proteins, whole grains, and complex carbohydrates, along with fruits and vegetables. If you don't want to gain an enormous amount of weight, don't use your pregnancy as an excuse to load up on simple carbs such as processed foods, products containing white flour, and sugary snacks.

Table 2-1: Daily Diet Guidelines

Food	Amount	Examples
Fruits	1½ to 2 cups per day	1 cup = 1 cup fruit juice, 1 cup fresh fruit, or ½ cup dried fruit
Vegetables	2½ cups per day	1 cup = 1 cup vegetables, 1 cup vegetable juice, or 2 cups leafy greens
Protein	5 ounces per day	1 oz = 1 egg, ½ cup nuts, or 1 oz meat or fish
Dairy	3 cups per day	1 cup = 1 cup milk or yogurt, or 2 oz processed cheese
Grains	6 ounces per day	1 oz = 1 slice bread, 1 cup cereal, 1 tortilla or pancake, or ½ cup rice or pasta

Listen to your body's cravings. Some women require more weight gain toward the beginning of their pregnancies and others gain the weight at the end. If you are feeling famished all the time, you should listen to what your body is telling you and eat three full healthy meals. The Web site MyPyramid for Pregnancy & Breastfeeding at MyPyramid.gov is an excellent resource for diet guidelines geared to women who are pregnant or breastfeeding. Check out Table 2-2 for a summary of the changes we recommend you make in your diet when you become pregnant.

Table 2-2: Recommended Dietary Changes in Pregnancy

Nutrient	Nonpregnant	Pregnant	Increase
Calories	2,000	2,300	15%
Protein	40 g	50 g	20%
Calcium	800 mg	1,200 mg	50%
Iron	15 mg	27 mg	100%
Vitamin D	200 IU	400 IU	100%
Folic acid	400 mcg	600 mcg	50%

Note: g=grams; mg=milligrams; IU=international units; mcg=micrograms

▶ ▶ ▶ LISTENING TO MY BODY

"I always know when you're pregnant," my obstetrician told me in the hospital dining room as I reached for my banana. "You go from eating hamburgers and French fries to eating apples and bananas." It's true. It's like my body starts telling me, "Okay, enough of the junk food now." With both my pregnancies, in the first trimester I simply could not eat anything that wasn't good for me. It made me feel sicker. I craved raw vegetables and fruits. (But remember to wash those veggies and fruits thoroughly!) I wanted food crunchy, not cooked. It seemed to make my nausea feel better. Sometimes, our bodies are smarter than our heads.

—Alane ◀ ◀ ◀

Protein

Your growing baby needs protein to build its muscles and organs. This is why we recommend monitoring your protein intake.

Here's what you need to know. Prior to pregnancy, the amount of protein a woman needs depends on her ideal body weight, which is determined by her height. A rough estimate of ideal body weight is one hundred pounds plus five pounds for every inch over five feet. To calculate the recommended amount of protein for the nonpregnant state, multiply your ideal body weight in pounds by 0.43.[1] This tells you the grams of protein that you need daily. Pregnancy increases this requirement by 6 to 10 grams per day. An average woman is five feet, four inches tall with an ideal weight of 120 pounds. Her prepregnancy protein requirement will be about 50 grams per day. In pregnancy, add 6 to 10 grams of protein to her prepregnancy diet for a total of 56–60 grams per day. A pregnant five-foot-tall woman needs about 50 grams per day, and a woman measuring five-foot seven-inches needs 65 grams per day. For most women, 50 to 65 grams of protein every day should be fine.

Here are the formulas again:

Ideal body weight: 100 pounds + 5 pounds for every inch over 5 feet

Prepregnancy protein needs (in grams): Ideal body weight x 0.43

Pregnant protein needs (in grams):
(Ideal body weight x 0.43) + 6 to 10 extra grams

But there's a good amount of protein . . . and then there's *way more protein than you need*. Remember, with extra protein comes extra calories. We've heard all sorts of recommendations for pregnancy protein intakes, both low and high, including some that insist every pregnant woman must eat 75 grams or more of protein every day. Although some women may need larger amounts of protein based on the preceding formula, saying that every woman must consume that much may ultimately lead to an excessive calorie intake, a very large baby, and difficulty losing weight after the pregnancy.

Table 2-3 lists different protein sources. Choose a variety of items that work for you and enjoy yourself.

Iron

When you are pregnant, your body utilizes iron to make blood for the baby as well as to increase your own blood volume by 50 percent. You can easily become anemic if you aren't getting enough iron in your diet or through supplements. In addition, because we anticipate blood loss at the time of delivery, we will check for anemia while you are pregnant and recommend increasing your intake if you are found to be low.

Table 2-3: Sources of Protein[2]

Source	Serving Size	Calories	Protein (grams)
MEAT, FISH, AND EGGS			
Steak, lean	3 oz	184	28
Chicken breast, boneless, skinless	3 oz	142	27
Turkey breast, boneless, skinless	3 oz	132	25
Haddock	3 oz	95	21
Pork loin	3 oz	178	21
Trout	3 oz	144	21
Salmon	3 oz	120	17
Eggs, scrambled	2 eggs(122 grams)	204	14
Ham steak	3 oz	90	14
Veggie burgers, Boca	1 patty (71 grams)	90	13
Breakfast sausage, turkey	2 links (2 oz)	129	8.6
Egg, hard-boiled	1 egg (50 grams)	78	6
DAIRY			
Cottage cheese	1 cup (226 grams)	203	27
Feta cheese, crumbled	1 cup (150 grams)	396	21
Yogurt, nonfat plain	8 oz	127	13
Yogurt, lowfat fruit	8 oz	232	10
Milk, skim	1 cup (240 grams)	83	8
Cheese, swiss	1 slice (1 oz)	108	8
Cheese, cheddar	1 slice (1 oz)	114	7
Cheese, provolone	1 slice (1 oz)	100	7
Cheese, american	1 slice (1 oz)	94	5
FRUITS AND VEGETABLES			
Spinach, frozen	1 cup (190 grams)	65	8
Asparagus, frozen	1 cup (180 grams)	32	5
Potato, baked	1 large (312 grams)	188	5
Apricots, dried	1 cup (130 grams)	312	4
Avocado, mashed	1 cup (230 grams)	376	4
Dates, chopped	1 cup (178 grams)	502	4
Plums, dried (prunes)	1 cup (170 grams)	414	4
Banana, mashed	1 cup (225 grams)	134	2

Table 2-3 (*continued*)

Source	Serving Size	Calories	Protein (grams)
BEANS AND NUTS			
Soybeans	1 cup (180 grams)	254	22
Peas, split	1 cup (196 grams)	231	16
Baked beans	1 cup (254 grams)	239	12
Milk, soy	1 cup (245 grams)	132	8
Peanut butter	2 tablespoons (32 grams)	188	8
Tofu, cooked	120 grams	73	8
Peanuts, unsalted	1/4 cup (28 grams)	166	7
Almonds, whole unsalted	1/4 cup (28 grams)	163	6
Cashews, unsalted	1/4 cup (28 grams)	163	4
GRAINS			
Flour, enriched wheat	1 cup (137 grams)	495	16
Flour, whole-grain wheat	1 cup (120 grams)	407	16
Oat bran, raw	1 cup (94 grams)	231	16
Spaghetti, enriched	1 cup (140 grams)	221	8
Bagel, plain	1 bagel (89 grams)	320	7
Cereal (Grape-Nuts)	1/2 cup (58 grams)	220	7
Cereal (Raisin Bran)	1 cup (59 grams)	190	5
Muffin, English, multigrain	1 muffin (57 grams)	129	5
Oatmeal, steel-cut	1 serving (40 grams)	150	5
Rice, brown	1 cup (195 grams)	216	5
Rice, enriched white	1 cup (175 grams)	215	5
Bread, whole-wheat	1 slice (28 grams)	69	4
Tortillas, whole-grain	1 tortilla (32 grams)	100	3
Bread, white	1 slice (25 grams)	67	2
PROTEIN SHAKES AND POWDERS			
Protein powder, whey	1 scoop	120	24
Muscle Milk light	14 fl oz	160	20

In pregnancy, you need 27 milligrams of elemental iron a day. This amount is contained in most prenatal vitamins. Getting enough iron can be hard for some people. It is better absorbed when taken on an empty stomach or with vitamin C. Unfortunately, iron supplements can also cause constipation and stomach pain. Dietary iron is often better tolerated. Table 2-4 lists some of the best, most iron-rich foods.

Table 2-4: Iron-Rich Foods

Source	Serving Size	Calories	Iron (milligrams)
MEAT, FISH, AND EGGS			
Beef, lean, ground	3 oz	230	2
Beef tenderloin	3 oz	151	2
Steak, t-bone	3 oz	177	2
Chicken breast	3 oz	142	1
Egg, hard-boiled	1 egg (50 grams)	78	1
Turkey breast, boneless, skinless	½ breast	132	1
FRUITS AND VEGETABLES			
Spinach, fresh, cooked	1 cup	41	6
Apricot, dried	1 cup (130 grams)	312	3
Greens, beet	1 cup	39	3
Prune juice	1 cup	182	3
Figs, dried	6	285	2
Peas, cooked	1 cup	125	2
Potato, baked, with skin	1 medium	188	2
Greens, turnip, cooked	1 cup	29	1
Potato, sweet	1 (146 grams)	131	1
Pumpkin, cooked, mashed	1 cup	49	1
BEANS, NUTS, AND SEEDS			
Lentils, cooked	1 cup	230	7
Soybeans, cooked	1 cup	254	5
Beans, lima, cooked	1 cup	216	4
Beans, navy, cooked	1 cup	255	4
Beans, pinto, cooked	1 cup	245	4
Chickpeas	1 cup	286	3
Soy milk	1 cup	132	2
Tofu, cooked	120 grams	73	1

Table 2-4 (*continued*)

Source	Serving Size	Calories	Iron (milligrams)
BEANS, NUTS, AND SEEDS (*continued*)			
Cashews	1 oz	163	2
Seeds, pumpkin	1 ounce	148	2
Almonds, whole, unsalted	¼ cup (28 grams)	163	1
Seeds, sesame	1 Tbs.	50	1
Seeds, sunflower	1/4 cup	186	1
GRAINS			
Bran flakes	¾ cup	92	18
Wheat germ, toasted	1 cup	432	10
Cream of Wheat, cooked	1 cup	131	9
Oatmeal	1 packet (28 grams)	100	3
Spaghetti, enriched, cooked	1 cup	221	2

Calcium

All women—whether they're pregnant or not—need calcium to help maintain strong bones. During pregnancy, you need 1,000 to 1,300 milligrams of calcium a day. Calcium is also critical for bone development in the fetus. In Table 2-5, we provide a list of calcium-rich foods that can help you meet your daily requirement.

Table 2-5: Top Calcium-Rich Foods

Source	Serving Size	Calories	Calcium (milligrams)
Cereal, whole-grain Total	1⅓ cups	112	1,000
Cheese, ricotta	1 cup	339	669
Juice, fortified orange	1 cup	120	350
Yogurt, fruit	8 oz	232	345
Sardines	3 oz	177	325
Milk, nonfat	1 cup	83	299
Spinach (and similar dark leafy greens)	1 cup	65	291
Soybeans	1 cup	254	261
Cheese, swiss	1 oz	108	224
Tofu, cooked	120 grams	73	133

Vitamin D

Vitamin D regulates calcium and promotes bone growth and remodeling. It is also essential in building your baby's bones and teeth. More than 50 percent of women are deficient in this vitamin. Currently the recommended amount of vitamin D in pregnancy is 400 IU per day.

However, some recent studies have suggested that higher levels of vitamin D are greatly beneficial to pregnancy. For women who take 4,000 IU per day, there is a decreased risk of gestational diabetes, preeclampsia, and preterm delivery. We may see a change in the current recommendations in the near future.

Vitamin D is found in certain foods as well as produced in the skin in response to sunlight. Most prenatal vitamins contain 200–400 IU.

3 oz trout	645 IU
3 oz salmon	447 IU
3 oz canned tuna	229 IU
1 cup milk	117 IU
1 tablespoon margarine	60 IU

DHA

Docosahexaenoic acid (DHA) is an omega-3 fatty acid that is important for fetal brain and eye development. Extensive research has been conducted on DHA, showing increased IQ scores for children whose mothers took it during pregnancy. It is recommended that women take 300 milligrams of DHA per day during pregnancy, through dietary sources or supplements. The best source of DHA is oily fish. DHA supplements are made from fish oils or from micro-algae, and are now available in prenatal vitamins.

2 tsp cod liver oil	1,000 mg
3 oz salmon	650 mg
3 oz flounder	250 mg

Folic Acid

Folic acid, which is crucial for the development of the fetal spine, has already been discussed in Chapter 1 (see page 13). Every pregnant woman should be sure that her vitamin regimen contains the proper amounts of this nutrient.

Vegetarian and Vegan Diets

Women following a vegetarian or vegan diet can easily fulfill the pregnancy diet requirements by following a few simple guidelines. For vegetarians, it is easy to get protein through eggs, cheese, tofu, and whole grains. In addition, many iron-rich foods, such as spinach and soy beans, can replace meats in the diet. For vegans, the choices are more limited but can easily conform to healthy pregnancy diets. Vegans need to focus on beans, whole grains, and nuts to meet their protein requirements. In addition, they can receive the calcium they need through these grains, spinach and soy beans, or supplements.

Pregnancy after Gastric Bypass Surgery

Gastric bypass surgery, previously known as stomach stapling, is becoming more common. In 2009, 220,000 people underwent this procedure and more than 75 percent of them were women.[3] Although many morbidly obese women are infertile, after weight-loss surgery they may resume ovulation and become pregnant. The good news is that, after surgery, these women can have healthy pregnancies and babies. Morbid obesity can lead to multiple pregnancy complications, including diabetes, preeclampsia, and large babies requiring cesarean delivery. For this reason, weight loss before pregnancy is the ideal. (See Chapter 1, page 15.)

For women who have undergone gastric bypass or the lap band procedure, we recommend they wait until the period of rapid weight loss has passed—usually after the first twelve months—to ensure adequate nutrition for the baby. These moms will need to be monitored closely for signs of anemia, since iron absorption is limited after bypass. If adequate iron levels cannot be attained, some of these women may require blood transfusions. A nutritionist can assist in forming a diet plan that works best for these moms.

Foods to Avoid

Many women feel bombarded by scary stories in pregnancy. Don't eat this! Don't touch that! It's easy to feel like you need to wrap yourself in a bubble to avoid all the things that could harm the baby. Fortunately, the list of foods to avoid or limit is relatively short. Most people can continue to follow whatever healthy diet they did before pregnancy. However, there are some guidelines, as we outline next.

myth: Eating spicy food can cause a miscarriage or induce labor.

FACT: Although spicy food may increase heartburn, it is perfectly safe to eat during pregnancy. Eating spicy food has no relationship to pregnancy loss or labor.

▶ ▶ ▶ THE DODGER DOG DILEMMA

"He wouldn't let me eat my Dodger Dog!" Caroline complained. Caroline's husband, Danny, looked down sheepishly at his feet. The two of them had always appeared to be a close, happy, and communicative couple. Both teachers, they had arrived together for every prenatal visit and were planning to do natural childbirth. They functioned well as a team.

Now, with Caroline twenty-eight weeks pregnant, she reported this small blip in their previously smooth and joyful pregnancy. Danny had stopped her from eating her favorite baseball game treat the week before, and she really wanted to enjoy the hot dog she'd been craving when they returned to Dodger Stadium the following weekend for the playoffs.

Danny was concerned that hot dogs would be detrimental to Caroline's pregnancy. I told him we do not know of any harmful effects to a fetus from a mom eating hot dogs. I wasn't worried about Listeria (more on this shortly) because hot dogs are cooked. Danny informed me that he'd read something about the nitrites in hot dogs leading to cancer. I explained that there are no conclusive studies linking hot dog consumption to cancer. Are hot dogs an ideal pregnancy food? Certainly not! But from someone who enjoys an occasional hot dog herself, I reported to my patients that as long as Dodger Stadium was still cooking its hot dogs, Caroline had my permission to enjoy that occasional special treat.

—Yvonne ◀ ◀ ◀

Unpasteurized cheese: Do not eat soft cheeses such as brie, feta, blue cheese, and Mexican cheese *unless* they are made with pasteurized milk. Cheese made with unpasteurized milk can be contaminated with bacteria called *Listeria*. Listeria can cause flu-like symptoms, muscle pain, vomiting, and seizures. If a pregnant woman contracts Listeria, it can cause miscarriage, preterm labor, or stillbirth. Thankfully, Listeria is a very rare infection, affecting only about 2,500 people in the United States per year. If diagnosed, it can be treated with antibiotics. Hard cheeses and cheeses that are pasteurized or cooked are both safe to consume during pregnancy.

Raw meats: Uncooked meats carry the same risk factors for the bacteria Listeria as unpasteurized cheeses do. This can be avoided by cooking all meat to 160 degrees or higher. Raw meats also can carry *Toxoplasmosis gondii,* a protozoan infection most often hosted by cats (more on cats later, pages 85–86). The cysts from this organism can contaminate uncooked meat. After you ingest the contaminated meat, the infection may remain asymptomatic or cause a flu-like illness with fatigue, muscle aches, sore throat, and swollen lymph nodes. About 60 percent of moms with this illness will transmit the infection to their fetus, which can then suffer from intrauterine growth restriction (IUGR) (problems with fetal growth), nonimmune hydrops (swelling of the fetus), and hydrocephalus or microcephaly (poor brain development). If a mother is infected, she can be treated with the antibiotic spiramycin to prevent transmission to the baby. If the fetus becomes infected with toxoplasmosis, a combination of antibiotics can be used to try to prevent the associated birth defects. Obviously, the goal for this disease is avoid exposure in the first place, so avoiding uncooked meats is our most powerful tool for prevention.

Deli meats and hot dogs: Deli meats and hot dogs are cooked and then packaged. The risk with these foods involves potential contamination with Listeria before the packaging stage. If

HANDLING FOOD SAFELY

We feel that advice given by the USDA to prevent people from getting sick from infected food is sound and sensible. Here are their guidelines for safe food preparation:

1. Clean: Wash hands and surfaces often.
2. Separate: Avoid cross-contamination by keeping raw and cooked foods in separate areas.
3. Cook: Cook to proper temperature.
4. Chill: Refrigerate promptly.

these foods are reheated to 160 degrees or more, they are perfectly safe. Some people are concerned about the presence of nitrites in deli meats and hot dogs. The metabolites of nitrites have been implicated in some types of cancer,[4] but this association has not been proven. In addition, nitrites have not been linked to the formation of birth defects.

Fish: The concern with seafood is the mercury content, which can cause nerve damage in the developing fetus. We recommend that you avoid the types of fish that tend to be higher in mercury levels. These are big fish that eat smaller fish and concentrate mercury in their tissues.

Fish to avoid:

Shark
Mackerel
Tilefish
Swordfish

According to the FDA, pregnant women can eat two portions (12 ounces total) per week of

Shrimp
Salmon
Pollock
Cod
Tuna (light canned tuna). Limit tuna steak and albacore tuna
    to 6 ounces per week

Sushi: Although women in the United States have been told that sushi is taboo during pregnancy, those in other cultures continue to consume it regularly without a problem. No birth defects are related to sushi ingestion. As we've mentioned, any raw fish, like raw meat, could potentially contain bacteria or parasites. However, the risk of parasitic infections from sushi is quite rare (about forty cases in the United States per year).[5] Any cooked or vegetarian sushi is safe. And we recommend that our patients avoid sushi made with fish high in mercury.

Caffeine: How many women dread pregnancy because they think they must give up their daily cup of coffee? The truth is that caffeine in moderation—that's less than 200 milligrams per day—is fine. Caffeine in these amounts has not been associated with any birth defects or pregnancy complications. One 12-ounce cup of coffee contains 200 milligrams of caffeine. A can of cola has 35 to 55 milligrams; green tea, 25 milligrams; and a chocolate bar, about 35 milligrams.

Other Pregnancy Don'ts

Modern medicine has made today's pregnant women aware of some of the other dietary and environmental risks to their developing babies. However, there's still a lot of confusion and conflicting information.

Smoking Cigarettes

We recommend that you do not smoke cigarettes during pregnancy. Studies have shown that smoking increases your risks of having a miscarriage, preterm labor, premature rupture of your bag of water, lower birth weight infants, SIDS (sudden infant death syndrome), birth defects, and complications related to your placenta (placenta previa, placental abruption; see Chapter 9 for details).[6] Nicotine has a direct toxic effect on the fetus. In addition, it can compromise blood flow, thereby limiting the oxygen and nutrition that reaches your baby. So please, it's never too late to stop smoking.

Nicotine patches release small amounts of nicotine into the skin to help overcome nicotine addiction. Although the patches do contain the same nicotine that is toxic to a developing fetus, the overall amount of the drug is less than what you would consume from smoking cigarettes. In addition, other toxins in cigarette smoke are avoided with the patch. Although using a nicotine patch isn't ideal, it is definitely better than smoking and may help women on their path to quitting completely.

Drinking Alcohol

Will your baby have a birth defect because you drank one glass of wine at a dinner party and you had no idea you were pregnant? No, it won't. However, despite more than twenty-one thousand articles written on the subject, scientifically we have not been able to define a threshold below which alcohol use is safe for pregnant women. For this reason, most medical policymakers recommend total abstinence. At the same time, no studies show that light drinking—one to three drinks per week—is harmful.

Heavy drinking—defined as more than nine drinks per week—has been associated with fetal alcohol syndrome (FAS). *FAS* is a pattern of physical changes including low birth weight, characteristic facial features, and small brain size. In addition, there are mental changes, such as learning disabilities and retardation.

Using Illegal Drugs

Drug use of any kind (other than as prescribed by your doctor for a legitimate medical condition) is not recommended preconceptionally or during pregnancy. Drugs of all types have been associated with poor fetal growth, low infant birth weight, premature delivery, and drug withdrawal after birth.

Exercise

Women with uncomplicated pregnancies can exercise throughout pregnancy, right up until delivery. Ideally, women should participate in moderate exercise for at least thirty minutes a day, five to six days a week. (However, we may set special limits for some women with high-risk conditions, including preterm labor, premature rupture of membranes, vaginal bleeding, placenta previa, and preeclampsia. Every woman should discuss her exercise regimen and health history with her doctor during the first trimester.)

In the first trimester, most prepregnancy exercise regimens can be continued without modification. Many times, at the very beginning, people don't even know they're pregnant and go on their merry way, exercising as they normally do. Exercise can even help with nausea by releasing natural endorphins that can help moms feel better. However, some women feel too sick and fatigued to exercise. If you feel miserable, don't force yourself. Eventually, you'll feel better and you can pick up the pace again.

Women who never work out should not suddenly become gym rats. Instead, low-impact activities such as walking, prenatal yoga, and swimming are the most beneficial. For these women, the cardiovascular changes of pregnancy alone are stressful on their bodies. On the other hand, women who exercise regularly can continue on their current regimen because they're already starting at an adequate fitness level.

Whatever your exercise program, the key to safe activity while pregnant is to monitor your heart rate. You can check your pulse or pick up a reasonably priced heart rate monitor at a sporting goods store. In general, we recommend maintaining your heart rate at less than 140 beats per minute. If you cannot hold a normal conversation while you're exercising, you're probably overdoing it. Because the resting heart rate is already elevated in pregnancy, many women are surprised how a little exertion will raise the rate over 140.

Monitoring your heart rate is so important because when you exercise intensely, blood is shunted away from your uterus and the growing baby and sent to your working muscles. When your heart rate goes above 140, your muscles are receiving the majority of the oxygen. Although it is not harmful to exceed this limit occasionally, prolonged periods of intense exercise will decrease the oxygen supply to the baby.

▶ ▶ ▶ THE PERILS OF OVERDOING IT

Betsy was a pharmaceutical representative who had a long-standing passion for fitness. She did triathlons, practiced yoga, and played beach volleyball, all with a vengeance. After she became pregnant with her second child, however, she decided to cut back on some of these activities and try new exercise programs that would be more pregnancy-friendly.

The day Betsy went to her first spinning class, she was hooked. She went to the class three times a week and felt great. However, when she came in for a routine visit at thirty-two weeks, we noticed that the baby's growth was not as good as expected. Betsy confessed that she had been working out very hard and not monitoring her heart rate. We sent her for an ultrasound and found that the baby's belly was quite thin and the amniotic fluid level was low. We immediately broke the news to her: no more spinning. It seemed that her intense workouts had taken much-needed blood away from the placenta. While she knew it was the right thing for her baby, it was hard for Betsy to change her routine, but she did it. Within three weeks, the fluid level had improved and the baby started to grow again. She had to stay on bed rest until delivery, but thankfully, her daughter was born perfectly healthy.

Looking for a safe but effective exercise regimen for your pregnancy? Following are some of our favorites.

Prenatal Yoga and Pilates

All three of us are major fans of prenatal yoga (see Figures 2-2 through 2-5) and Pilates. Yoga has so many health benefits. Number one, it increases flexibility. For pregnant women who are carrying an extra load, keeping the body flexible will help prevent strains and injuries, and can also help prepare you for delivery. Yoga is also good for circulation and helps build strength in a way that is minimally stressful on the joints. Pilates is also a great strength builder that uses the body's own weight as resistance.

A good yoga class also gives a mom-to-be a quiet, focused time to become aware of her body, breathing, and general state of mind. Taking this quiet time can have a calming effect, which is especially important in the first trimester.

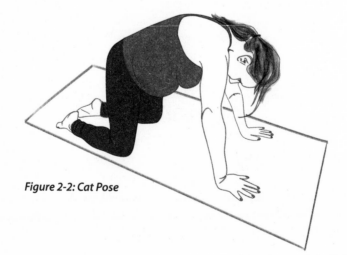

Figure 2-2: Cat Pose

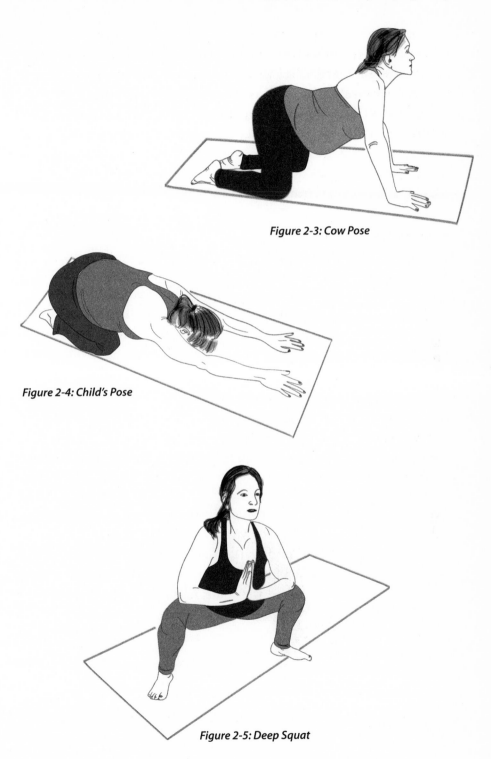

Figure 2-3: Cow Pose

Figure 2-4: Child's Pose

Figure 2-5: Deep Squat

Walking and Jogging

Walking and jogging may be the simplest activities to do while pregnant. In the first trimester, women can continue to run or jog at their prepregnancy pace. However, as the second trimester progresses, the intensity will need to come down to ensure the heart rate stays around 140. At this time as well, it becomes very difficult to jog because of the pressure of the growing uterus on the bladder. You may feel like you need to take a bathroom break every few blocks. For this reason, most women transition to walking at this time, either outdoors or on a treadmill.

Swimming

Swimming has proven to be an excellent exercise in pregnancy. There is no impact, so no extra stress on the joints. Swimming increases strength in the core muscles of the abdomen and back and also improves flexibility. Many women who swim say that it helps decrease the edema, or swelling, in their arms and legs, and that while in the pool, they often don't feel pregnant. And yes, it's okay to swim in a pool and in the ocean.

Circuit Training and Weight Lifting

If a woman has been doing circuit training or weight lifting before becoming pregnant, there's no reason why she can't continue. Circuit, or resistance, training is one of the best ways to maintain muscle strength. Doing circuit training at a slightly faster pace can also raise the heart rate so you get a cardiovascular workout as well.

Because the presence of progesterone causes the joints to loosen during pregnancy, we recommend that our patients use lighter weights with more repetitions during workouts. A simple guideline is to decrease the weight from your prepregnancy baseline by 25 percent.

Elliptical and Stair Climbing Machines

Elliptical and stair climbing machines have the advantage of a variable resistance that can be decreased to accommodate the needs of a pregnant woman. They are low impact and help to maintain muscle strength as well as cardiovascular endurance.

Spinning and Stationary Bike

Spinning is one form of exercise that can really send the heart rate soaring, so you have to be careful not to overdo it. However, one advantage to spinning or riding a stationary bike is that the resistance on the bike can easily be decreased and therefore the intensity can come down quickly. Again, you should maintain a heart rate of less than 140 beats per minute. Light to moderate exercise on stationary bikes is also good for moms who are having trouble with balance because of their growing bellies.

▶ ▶ ▶ MY EXERCISE UPS AND DOWNS

All three of us are advocates of a healthy, physically active lifestyle, and we each wanted to model this for our patients during our own pregnancies. During my first pregnancy with Ryan, I did it all—weight lifting, running, yoga, and spinning. I kept in shape right up until my delivery, and then I had an easy delivery and recovered quite quickly. In retrospect, however, I don't recommend running much after the first trimester because of the pressure you feel on the bladder. You constantly feel like you have to pee, which can be uncomfortable. I did love spinning and felt it was a pregnancy-friendly way of getting a good workout, right up until delivery.

For my second pregnancy, however, I had a different experience. After my IVF (in vitro fertilization) treatments, I was not allowed to do any strenuous exercise, so I only walked about three miles a day until I was twelve weeks pregnant. After I was out of the first trimester, I returned right away to my prior exercise routine of weight lifting and spinning. But at fourteen weeks, on a morning after I had lifted weights, I had an episode of heavy bleeding. I was so worried. I saw Alane the next morning and she found that I had *placenta previa*, where my placenta was very low, covering my cervix. This prompted me to go back to a walking routine and lighter exercise. My placenta previa was confirmed again at twenty-four weeks, and after that point, I wasn't allowed to exercise at all for the remainder of my pregnancy, for fear that it might trigger more bleeding.

I'm one of those people who get very upset when I can't exercise, but the time passed amazingly quickly and I didn't have any further bleeding episodes. I delivered my daughter safely at thirty-seven weeks.

We usually encourage our pregnant moms to exercise, but there are some cases where exercise must remain off-limits. You need to check with your doctor if you have one of the following conditions: preterm labor, cervical insufficiency, premature rupture of membranes, preeclampsia, or placenta previa.

—Yvonne ◀ ◀ ◀

Activities to Avoid

The most important physical activities to avoid are those that can be dangerous to your baby. Avoid contact sports such as basketball, soccer, and ice hockey because they may put you at risk for direct abdominal injury. In addition, watch out for any sport that requires balance, such as downhill skiing, waterskiing, surfing, snowboarding, or gymnastics. We also do not recommend any exercises where you could fall and hit your belly. These include mountain or road biking, rollerblading, and horseback riding. You can continue your routine abdominal exercises—sit-ups and crunches—into the first trimester. But as the uterus grows in the second trimester, it will soon become impossible for you to bend over your enlarged belly.

If you have a personal trainer or fitness instructor, always let him or her know that you are pregnant. Some gyms or studios have restrictions for pregnancy.

More Ways to Take Care of Your Body (and Baby)

Most women don't want to give up their beauty and personal routines just because they're pregnant. However, so many old wives tales and horror stories are circulating that some of our patients admit they are afraid to put on their makeup in the morning. Let's look at the real story.

Acne and wrinkle creams: Creams with Retin-A, a form of vitamin A used to treat acne and wrinkles, are Class C drugs. (For more on drug safety classes, see Table 1-1 in Chapter 1, page 26.) Only about 10 percent of the medication in these creams is absorbed into the maternal bloodstream. However, because no well-controlled studies confirming their safety exist, some obstetricians advise their patients to avoid these creams. The oral form of these vitamin A-based drugs, isotretinoin, cannot be used in pregnancy because it has been directly linked to birth defects.

For acne, topical treatments such as benzoyl-peroxide or certain antibiotic creams or solutions are considered safe.

Makeup, cleansers, moisturizers, and sunscreens: All of these products can be safely used throughout pregnancy. Creams and cleansers containing salicylic acid can be used only if the concentration is less than 2 percent.

▶ ▶ ▶ A SPOT OF TROUBLE

Every woman has her own individual area of vanity, and for Rebecca, it was her fair, smooth, and perfectly flawless skin. Pregnant with her second baby, Rebecca came to me in distress because she had developed a small, dark area of skin under her left eye. In the second trimester, some women can experience hyperpigmentation in their face, which we call "the mask of pregnancy" (see Chapter 4). Rebecca wanted to correct this problem right away and asked me about the safety of bleaching creams to fade her discoloration.

Although most of these creams are Category C, very few studies exist on their safety in humans. Therefore, I suggested to Rebecca that it would be better to use sunscreen and wear a hat to prevent the sun from highlighting and intensifying these already hyperpigmented areas. After the pregnancy is over, she would then be free to get more aggressive about treating those small brown spots.

—Yvonne ◀ ◀ ◀

Self-tanners: Self-tanning creams contain a dye that stays on the skin surface. They are considered harmless to pregnancy.

Tanning beds: Pregnancy increases skin sensitivity to the sun and can make burning more likely, even with the UVA rays of tanning beds. These rays can increase the risk of skin cancer but do not affect a fetus.

Hot tubs and saunas: During your pregnancy, you should not go into a hot tub or use a sauna. The increased core temperature can cause an elevation in the fetal heart rate and possibly cause harmful stress. In addition, a maternal temperature above 102 degrees Fahrenheit has been associated with spinal malformations in a fetus. A tub that is below 100 degrees should be fine for short periods of time.

Hot baths: If the bathwater is only slightly higher than your body temperature, soaking in a tub is okay. Hot showers are fine because you are not submerged in the water and are able to dissipate the heat easily.

Dentist visits: It is perfectly safe to have your teeth cleaned during pregnancy. Necessary dental X-rays are also safe if an abdominal shield is used. Having cavities filled and oral surgery (root canals) can be performed under local anesthesia such as novocaine. Certain antibiotics are safe too if the dentist recommends them.

Teeth whitening: Although there is no documented harm caused by whitening gels, the manufacturers recommend not to use them during pregnancy.

Hair dyes and perms: The truth is, only a very small percentage of hair dyes, perms, or straighteners are absorbed into the skin, so they are considered safe in pregnancy. Permanent dyes contain ammonia, which can have a very strong odor, causing nausea. For this reason, semipermanent dyes and highlights may be better during pregnancy.

Hair removal: Women may notice an increase in hair growth during their pregnancy due to rising pregnancy hormones. It is safe to shave, wax, and use laser hair removal.

Manicures, pedicures, and acrylic nails: No known birth defects are linked to the use of the products associated with these beauty treatments. Because these treatments often emit a strong odor, it is recommended to have them performed in a well-ventilated salon. In addition, be sure the salon sterilizes their instruments to avoid any potential infections. You can also bring your own instruments, if you want to be extra cautious.

Other Safety Issues

As modern women, we go through our busy daily lives exposed to many strange materials, chemicals, and substances that we may never even bother to think about—that is, until we become pregnant. Our patients have a myriad of questions about these day-to-day exposures, and we've heard a lot of myths and misconceptions about these topics, which we hope to dispel next.

Paint and paint thinners: There is no evidence that exposure to paint or paint thinners causes birth defects. However, many pregnant women find that their sense of smell is heightened, so the fumes from these agents may cause nausea. If you need to be in an area with fresh paint, we recommend keeping the area well ventilated.

Loud noises: Often we are asked if it is okay to go to a rock concert during pregnancy. Women are concerned that the persistent loud noise may damage the ears of the developing fetus. There's no need for concern in this case. Imagine being underwater in a swimming pool, and you'll get the idea of what it's like for your baby, floating in its protective sac of amniotic fluid. Although the baby can hear outside noises and may even react to a sound or vibration by moving around in the womb, the sound does not carry through the water at the same frequency as it would through air, and is not as loud. Therefore, you do not need to worry that your baby will need mini–ear plugs while you are at your concert.

Artificial sweeteners: These additives are calorie-free and add sweetness to foods. The most common—aspartame (found in Equal and Nutrasweet), Stevia, and Splenda—are considered safe in pregnancy by the FDA. Saccharin, found in Sweet 'N Low, is safe for general consumption but its safety in pregnancy has not been confirmed.

Cats and Other Furry Things

Cats or dogs will not hurt a developing fetus. However, cats can pick up an organism called *Toxoplasma gondii* by eating infected rodents or meat. These organisms are then excreted in the cats' feces. If a pregnant women handles the feces and contracts toxoplasmosis,

myth: You have to get rid of your cat when you become pregnant.

FACT: Cats themselves do not harm a developing fetus. However, cat feces can carry toxoplasmosis, which causes birth defects, so pregnant women should not be cleaning up after their cats or emptying the litter box.

serious birth defects or stillbirth may result. Therefore, pregnant women should avoid changing or cleaning their cats' litter boxes. (This warning goes for both outdoor and indoor cats equally. Although outdoor cats are more likely to encounter infected rodents, indoor cats can be exposed to mice or small rats as well.) You may still touch or hold any cat.

Toxoplasmosis is specific to cats. Dogs do not carry the same organisms in their feces so it is fine to pick up your dog's feces if you are pregnant. You can also get toxoplasmosis from eating meat infected with the organism, which is why you should not eat raw beef.

Mosquito repellents: Mosquito repellents contain the active ingredient DEET in various concentrations. These products can be safely used in pregnancy if the recommended safe dosage listed on the instructions is followed. There have been cases where mosquito-borne illnesses such as West Nile virus have been transmitted to a developing fetus, so prevention of these insect bites is extremely important.

Lice medications: Head lice are commonly seen in school children and are highly contagious. Infestation crosses all socioeconomic lines and often occurs at the beginning of a new school year. Pregnant moms may contract the lice from their school-aged children. Medications currently available from the pharmacy can be used safely to treat this annoying condition. These include Nix, Elimite, and Ovide, which are Category B drugs. In addition, Rid is Category C. There is no link between lice treatments and birth defects.

What's Okay—and Not Okay—for Your Baby

Our patients, especially our first-time moms, come to us brimming with questions and concerns about the do's and don'ts of early pregnancy. With the news bombarding us with environmental warnings and red flags practically every day, it's understandable that a newly pregnant woman would feel like she has to zip herself into a protective bubble to keep away anything that could be potentially harmful to her developing baby. The reality is, you and your baby are both pretty hardy. The world is not a dangerous place suddenly out to get you. Just remember to use your common sense—and enjoy your pregnancy, too.

Traveling in the First Trimester

myth: Never fly on an airplane during your first or last trimesters.

FACT: If you're traveling in a pressured cabin, flying itself will not harm your baby at any stage of your pregnancy.

We think this myth must have started when someone, somewhere got on a flight, went home, and had a miscarriage. The story spread like wildfire that the flight was the cause of her miscarriage. If you're someone who has to travel by air, we're happy to tell you that this activity is safe. Most airlines won't let you travel in the last month of pregnancy, but that's just because they don't want people going into labor on the airplane.

Being at altitude in a pressurized cabin is not dangerous in itself. The main concern—on an airplane or in any travel situation for that matter—is that sitting for a long time immobilizes the legs and increases the risk of blood clots. In pregnancy, that risk is increased even higher. We recommend that you walk up and down the aisles at regular intervals, at least every two hours. TED (thrombo embolic deterrent) hose or surgical support stockings can help decrease that risk as well.

Sex

Here's a question that we get asked every week, if not every day. In general, yes, it is definitely safe to have sex during pregnancy. For most normal, healthy pregnancies, you can have sex throughout the entire forty weeks—that is, if you're up for it!

myth: Having sex during pregnancy will hurt my baby.

FACT: Happily, it won't!

This myth has caused some amusing situations with our patients. Alane had a mom with increased libido whose husband was refusing to have sex with her because he was afraid it would hurt their baby. She said, "He won't believe me unless it comes out of my doctor's mouth!" and actually made Alane call her husband to reassure him. Some men—and women—don't fully understand exactly where the baby is positioned in the body. Some men think that the penis will poke the baby in the head or eye during intercourse and are petrified to have relations when their partner is pregnant. The cervix, which is the opening to the uterus, is at the end of the vagina and is at least two inches long. This is the barrier that keeps anything in the vagina safely away from the baby.

However, this free-sex rule has exceptions. When you have unexplained vaginal bleeding, placenta previa, preterm labor, cervical insufficiency, or any other extreme complication, usually your doctor will advise you to stop having sex.

Surgery

myth: You cannot have surgery when you are pregnant.

FACT: About 75,000 surgeries are performed safely on pregnant women every year. Most of these surgeries are directly related to the pregnancy, such as cervical cerclage placement; other types include surgery for ovarian cysts, appendicitis, and gallstones.

Most surgeries, especially those that are elective, should be avoided until after you've had the baby. While general anesthesia drugs are relatively safe, they directly pass to the baby. That means when you are put to sleep, your baby is also put to sleep. We want to minimize the exposure of the fetus to these medications unless absolutely necessary.

That said, if you have any cancer warning signs, such as a breast mass, you should definitely proceed with any necessary evaluations during the pregnancy. You should never delay a diagnostic procedure such as a biopsy, which usually requires just a local injection, not general anesthesia.

X-Rays

In general, pregnant women should avoid X-rays unless the benefit to the mother outweighs the risk to the fetus. But if an X-ray is required to check for a serious condition in the mom, it should be performed regardless of the fear of exposure to the baby.

The amount of radiation that can cause damage to a developing fetus is approximately 5 rads. (A rad is a unit of absorbed radiation.) It takes more than 100 rads to cause a miscarriage or stillbirth. Generally, if the radiologic study produces less than 5 rads, it is considered safe. A chest X-ray gives only 0.00007 rads, so you would need seventy thousand of them to cause an injury. Similarly, a dental X-ray is 0.0001 rads, requiring fifty thousand separate X-rays to reach the 5 rad limit. X-rays with the highest dose of radiation are CT scans of the abdomen or spine, which have 2.6 to 3.5 rads each. Don't worry if you received an X-ray at the dentist before you knew you were pregnant. Your baby will not be affected by these low-dose exams.

When it comes to ultrasounds and MRIs, neither of these radiologic exams use radiation, so both are safe at all stages of your pregnancy.

And for those of you who travel frequently by airplane and have to go through body scanners, try not to worry. The amount of radiation exposure during one scan is equivalent to 0.01 chest X-rays.

Accidents

Women's bodies are well designed to protect the fetus, especially in the first trimester. During these months, the uterus remains well within the shelter of the pelvic bones, so unless you actually break your pelvis, your baby is protected from any ordinary fall or impact. For example, if you are in a car accident, most pregnancies less than twelve weeks will not be affected because the uterus is shielded by the pelvic bones. Having said this, be safe, drive carefully, and always wear your seatbelt!

The truth is, pregnancy shouldn't be a restrictive time, but it is a time when most women realize that taking care of their bodies and modifying their lifestyles in a healthier way really matters. "I got away with terrible health habits most of my adult life," Catherine, one of our patients, told us. "I smoked, I gorged on junk food, and I drank way too much on the weekends. Getting pregnant gave me a new perspective on what I was doing to my body because all of a sudden I realized I was sharing that body with a very important new life. Pregnancy actually inspired me to change—and even after my son was born, I managed to make those changes permanent ones."

Catherine's story reminds us that, even after the forty weeks of pregnancy have passed, you're going to be a mother for a very long time, with a little one who will depend on you to be at your best.

Common Infections

> **myth:** If I get a cold or infection, it will go directly to my baby.
>
> **FACT:** Most infections do not cross the placenta. Even though the mom may be miserable, the baby is usually safe.

The most common infections in the first trimester are urinary tract infections, respiratory infections, and the stomach flu. In pregnancy, bladder infections (UTIs) often can be symptom-free. But because they can lead to more serious kidney infections, UTIs are treated with oral antibiotics.

Respiratory infections are also common. Most viral infections resolve on their own and are treated with supportive measures—fluids, acetaminophen, decongestants, and cough suppressants. However, if a mother has a persistent fever, she should contact her obstetrician because sometimes she may need IV fluids or antibiotics.

Gastroenteritis (stomach flu) may also affect pregnant women. It is an infection of the small intestine usually caused by a virus, such as norovirus or rotavirus. It spreads through contaminated food, water, or another infected person and causes nausea, diarrhea, fevers, and abdominal pain. Although this infection does not affect the baby, it can cause dehydration and make a mom-to-be feel miserable. Viral gastroenteritis has no cure, but most episodes resolve within a few days. Treatment is rest and drinking plenty of fluids. In severe cases, IV fluids may be necessary.

Viral Infection Exposure

Picture this: You are three months pregnant, and one day, your five-year-old brings home a notice announcing a chickenpox outbreak in her school. Many moms-to-be face this situation and are rightly concerned about exposure to viruses while they are pregnant. So which viruses can affect your fetus? What should you be worried about?

Chickenpox is caused by the varicella virus. It is highly contagious and manifests in small red spots all over the body. Most adults (95 percent) are immune to chickenpox because they were exposed earlier in life and have developed antibodies to the virus. Children are now regularly vaccinated against varicella.

If a woman is infected with varicella during pregnancy, she can develop severe pneumonia. For her unborn fetus, approximately 2 percent can develop skin scars, growth problems, and mental retardation if the infection occurs before the twentieth week. Before pregnancy, if you are unsure whether or not you've had chickenpox, your doctor can perform a blood test to check for the antibodies. If you are not immune, you can receive the chickenpox vaccine. After vaccination, you should wait one month before attempting to conceive.

If you are already pregnant, not immune to chickenpox, and are exposed to someone with the virus, contact your doctor immediately so you can receive a shot called varicella zoster immunoglobulin (VZIG), which can greatly reduce your chance of getting the infection.

Fifth disease is caused by parvovirus B19 and produces a red rash on the face that resembles a slapped cheek. Sixty percent of adults have been exposed to parvovirus and are immune. If a nonimmune woman is infected during pregnancy, she may develop mild body and joint aches. In most cases, there will be no effect to the fetus. However, in 5 percent of babies, especially those exposed during the first twelve weeks, a severe anemia can develop.

If you have been exposed to parvovirus during pregnancy, contact your doctor to have a blood test to see whether you are immune. If you are not immune and the blood test reveals you developed a recent infection, your doctor may monitor your baby with ultrasounds to check for signs of anemia in the fetus. There is no vaccine or medicine to treat fifth disease. Its spread can be prevented through good hygiene practices.

Hand-foot-mouth disease is caused by a variety of viruses; the most common is coxsackie virus. The disease is usually seen in children less than twelve and causes fevers, sores in the mouth, and a skin rash. This illness rarely affects adults. If a pregnant woman is exposed to the virus, there are no known consequences for her fetus.

Cytomegalovirus (CMV) is one of the viruses that causes mononucleosis (mono), an infection with sore throat, fever, and swollen lymph nodes in the neck. Often, adult patients do not have any symptoms. About half of adults have been exposed earlier in life and are immune.

If you are exposed to CMV during pregnancy, tell your doctor so you can have a blood test to see whether you are immune or have contracted the infection. If you have CMV while pregnant, especially during the third trimester, your fetus has a 10 percent chance of developing congenital CMV, which is characterized by hearing loss and vision problems. There is no treatment for CMV while pregnant. Prevention is through good personal hygiene.

Genital herpes, or herpes simplex virus (HSV), is a sexually transmitted disease affecting one out of six adults in the United States. It causes blisters or ulcers on the skin around the vagina or rectum about two weeks after exposure (primary infection). The symptoms can return (recurrent infection) throughout your life.

Outbreaks of genital herpes during pregnancy can be safely treated with herpes medication. The virus does not affect your fetus unless the outbreak occurs at the time of delivery. For this reason, if you have symptoms of herpes when you go into labor, you should have a cesarean to prevent passing the infection to your baby. For infants who are exposed through childbirth, especially with the primary infection, the disease can be severe, with inflammation of the brain or death.

If you have a history of herpes and want to deliver vaginally, you can take a herpes medication such as acyclovir during the last month of pregnancy to decrease the chance of an outbreak during delivery. This treatment is effective and safe for you and your baby.

Influenza (the flu) is a respiratory virus that causes body aches, fever, a dry cough, and fatigue. The symptoms of influenza are much more severe than the common cold. Although influenza doesn't affect a fetus, pregnant women who are infected can become very sick, sometimes requiring hospitalization.
According to the CDC, all pregnant women should be vaccinated for influenza. If you are exposed to someone with the flu and haven't been vaccinated, you can safely take Tamiflu or Relenza to prevent the infection.

Human papilloma virus (HPV) is a family of sexually transmitted viruses that cause genital warts (condyloma) and cervical cancer. After you are sexually active, you have a 75 to 90 percent chance of being exposed to this virus during your lifetime. Some strains of the virus cause genital warts, some cause precancerous cells on the cervix (which can be detected on a Pap), and some have no consequence.

HPV does not affect your ability to get pregnant, carry a baby, or give birth. It also does not cause birth defects in the fetus. Rarely, if a woman has extensive genital warts at the time of delivery, the baby can be infected with the virus. In most cases, however, HPV does not harm the baby, but there are reports of babies who have developed throat infections. Nonetheless, because these infections are so rare, women with genital warts can have a vaginal birth.

Two vaccines—Gardasil and Cervarix—can prevent infection with some of the most common strains of HPV. These vaccines are Category B in pregnancy. However, because safety data is still limited, most doctors recommend waiting until after delivery to receive the vaccine. If you received a dose of the vaccine when you didn't know you were pregnant, don't worry because no birth defects have been linked to the vaccine.

Sleep Positions

myth: You have to sleep on your left side while pregnant or you'll harm the baby.

FACT: We'd like you to, but please don't lose any sleep over it. You should sleep in the most comfortable position for you.

Most books will warn women against sleeping on their backs while pregnant, often to the point of inducing fear. We've received panicked phone calls at 3 in the morning from moms who went to sleep on their side and woke up on their back, terrified that they have hurt their babies. In our years of experience, we have never seen a baby injured because a mother slept on her back.

Why do we recommend that you sleep on your left side? A large blood vessel called the inferior vena cava runs along the right side of your spine and returns all the blood from the lower part of your body to your heart. Theoretically, the weight of the baby along with your uterus could press on the vena cava and compromise blood supply to your heart, the rest of the body, and the uterus.

In the first and second trimesters, though, the fetus is still small, weighing less than two pounds, so any position is safe. What normally happens is that as you grow, lying flat on your back with a really big belly is not comfortable and can make you feel short of breath as the uterus presses up into the lungs. So most women naturally tend to lean to one side or another or to sleep propped up with pillows or in a chair.

So do we want you to sleep on your left side as much as you can? Sure we do. But if lying flatter is more comfortable, do so. Your body will tell you if you should move by making you short of breath or dizzy. And if you wake up in the middle of the night and find yourself on your back or your right side, don't worry. You haven't harmed your baby. Remember, during labor and delivery, when the baby is at its largest, a mom may be lying on her back for hours at a time; we monitor the baby the entire time so we know the baby is fine.

●   ●   ●

This chapter has presented a lot of information, but we believe knowledge is power. We want you to know what is real and what is a myth when it comes to the vast world of pregnancy lore so you will spend less time worrying and more time enjoying the experience of your pregnancy. We talk more about those experiences in the following chapters!

chapter three

THE FIRST TRIMESTER:
0 TO 14 WEEKS

▶ ▶ ▶ **READING THE TEST**

With short but neatly manicured nails on her trembling hands, the woman struggled to tear open the cellophane wrapper for the over-the-counter pregnancy test box. "Why the CIA-level security around these things?" she grumbled to herself, becoming more agitated and frantic at every attempt. After several tries, she couldn't get a good hold, so knocking over toothbrushes and mouthwash bottles, she groped around on her bathroom counter for something sharp. Yes! There they were: a pair of tweezers! Digging violently into the cellophane with the tweezers, she managed to get the wrapping off and then, in one fluid motion, ripped open the box and shook loose the plastic stick inside it.

She didn't need to read the instructions. Two other completed tests already lay on the bathroom counter. Within sixty seconds after urinating, she watched a faint purple line start to materialize in the window of the test stick. As it darkened, the woman held it up higher, toward the overhead light, adjusting the angle and squinting. She picked up the other two sticks from the counter and compared them. Yes, this one was definitely looking darker than the one from two days ago. She knew her pregnancy hormone should be going up, not down, so the purple line should be darker each day.

But what if the artificial light was playing tricks on her? She crashed through the bathroom door, all three pregnancy tests in hand, and stumbled toward her home's best east-facing window to compare purple lines in the streaming morning light. She laid each test in front of her, in the order that she had taken them. Wait! Why did the first test from four days earlier look darker than today's? Or did it? Oh no! Had she mixed up the order?

All three pregnancy tests showed the result she'd wanted to get—yes, the woman was definitely pregnant. Yet here she was, obsessing over the darkness of a purple line on a plastic stick!

The woman in this story could have been any of a number of our patients. But I'm coming clean here: It was me. When I first discovered I was pregnant with my son Luke, I bought three home pregnancy tests and, despite all my training and experience, didn't trust any of them! Of course, they were all correct. I still have those tests in a drawer somewhere.

—Allison ◀ ◀ ◀

Congratulations, You're Pregnant!

When any woman does a home pregnancy test and the little window lights up with a positive result, the first thing she'll want to do is rush over to her ob-gyn's office. This event often happens at the time of her missed period, about four weeks in. Some patients have spotting during this time, which can cause anxiety that may lead to an early office visit. Unfortunately, between four to six weeks, we can't tell you anything definite about the health of the pregnancy. Therefore, we recommend that most women see their doctors about two weeks after their first missed period, which will make them about six weeks pregnant.

When we enter the exam room to meet you for your very first OB appointment, we, too, are excited. During this important first visit, we will review your medical and past obstetrical history, and perform a physical examination, ultrasound, and blood tests.

If a mom-to-be hasn't had any preconceptional counseling, we will start her on prenatal vitamins right away (see page 13 for more about prenatal vitamins). In our practice, we also give new patients a packet of general lists and guidelines that offer our basic suggestions for diet and exercise, along with suggestions for certain medicines that are safe to take if they get sick.

Visiting Your Doctor

At each prenatal appointment in the first trimester, you can expect the following tests or procedures to take place:

- Blood pressure evaluation
- Weight recording
- Urine dip for protein and glucose
- Determination of fetal heart activity by ultrasound or Doppler
- Review of your symptoms and questions

A pregnancy is forty weeks long. If everything is proceeding smoothly, your doctor will likely want to see you every four weeks between the time you first come in until about the twenty-eighth week of pregnancy, then every two weeks between the twenty-eighth to the thirty-sixth week, and then every week after that until you deliver your baby.

In some cases, very early in the pregnancy, you may need to come in more often than once a month. After we have confirmed that the fetus is growing well and we see a strong heartbeat, we can spread out the visits. If you have a high-risk pregnancy (see Chapter 9), you may need more visits with your doctor and your specialists.

Pregnancy Hormone

Human chorionic gonadotropin is a mouthful, so we usually refer to it as *hCG*. A unique hormone manufactured by the fetal tissue, this is the hormonal clue that those home pregnancy tests are looking for to give you a plus or minus answer on the little plastic stick that analyzes your urine. hCG has two subunits: alpha and beta. The pregnancy test senses the beta subunit. Usually, beta hCG can be detected in blood or urine samples as soon as eight to ten days after fertilization,[1] or about four weeks after the last period started. During the first trimester, hCG levels double every two to three days and peak at ten weeks. HCG plays a huge role in the myriad of physical symptoms pregnant moms-to-be may experience, especially during the first trimester.

The main purpose of hCG is to maintain the corpus luteum in the ovary, which produces progesterone. Progesterone is the hormone that supports the pregnancy by thickening the uterine lining and nourishing the developing embryo.

Ultrasound

Ultrasound allows your physician to monitor the growth of the fetus, as shown in Figure 3-1. Developments in radar and sonar led to the invention of the ultrasound machine, which was first used with a pregnant woman in 1957.[2] This technology, which utilizes high-frequency sound waves, not radiation, is considered safe and has revolutionized obstetric medicine.

All three of us have used ultrasounds since we began our training. We couldn't envision not using one during the first trimester. During the first twelve weeks, the ultrasound is done vaginally. The ultrasound works with a long thin probe (called a transducer) that we insert into a patient's vagina the same way we do a speculum for a Pap smear. It is not painful but you may feel pressure. This method is the best way to visualize the fetus when it is small.

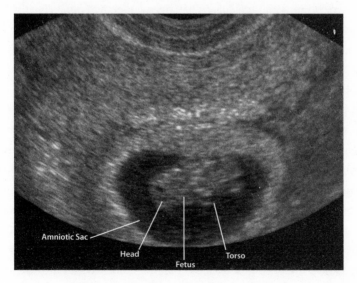

Figure 3-1: Ultrasound of an Eight-week Fetus

Ultrasound in the first trimester can answer everyone's foremost question: "Am I really pregnant?" Around five weeks, we can see the first evidence of pregnancy on ultrasound: the amniotic sac. At the six-week milestone, we can see the embryo and the first heartbeat. The ultrasound also allows us to answer the next most asked question, which is: "Do I have twins or triplets?" The ultrasound confirms how many babies there are, as well as the location of the embryo. We want to make sure the embryo is in the uterus and not an ectopic pregnancy, a potentially dangerous situation in which the fertilized embryo implants somewhere outside the uterus (see page 368).

At the point when we can see the heart beating, even if the fetus is only six weeks old, the chance of a woman losing the pregnancy drops dramatically *to less than 5 percent*. So if you get to that heartbeat stage, the odds are that you're on your way to a successful pregnancy. This finding is probably the most reassuring piece of information for our newly pregnant patients.

▶ ▶ ▶ FIBROIDS WITH A HEARTBEAT

We always knew when Juliana was in our office because we'd recognize her infectious laughter as it filled the waiting room. A university professor with an unfailingly positive attitude, Juliana had been our patient during her first pregnancy several years earlier, until she moved to South Carolina to be near her family. Now that she was back in Los Angeles with her husband and two children, we were thrilled to have her back in our lives again when she came in for a routine gynecological exam.

As I performed the checkup, Juliana mentioned she'd been exercising a lot lately, trying to get back into shape. "I don't know what's going on, but no matter how much abdominal work I'm doing, I cannot get rid of this pooch," she said, pointing to her lower abdomen. When I began to examine her, feeling an enlarged uterus, I wondered whether perhaps Juliana had some benign uterine fibroid tumors. I asked Juliana to move to the ultrasound room to confirm the fibroids, but instead, I saw something quite different going on inside her uterus—a baby! Jokingly, I said, "Oh, look, your fibroids have a heartbeat!"

I reassured a very confused Juliana that her "pooch" was actually her growing uterus with a healthy baby inside. Juliana was about twelve weeks pregnant at the time, and she and her husband were both ecstatic—as well as completely surprised—over the appearance of their third child. They ultimately gave birth to a beautiful baby daughter.

—Alane ◀ ◀ ◀

Your Due Date

myth: A pregnancy is nine months long.

FACT: Pregnancy lasts for 280 days, or 40 weeks, counting from the first day of your cycle on the month you became pregnant. Using "months" to describe your pregnancy only creates confusion. Pregnancy has three trimesters lasting 1 to 14 weeks, 14 to 28 weeks, and 28 weeks to delivery.

Having an accurate estimated date of confinement (EDC), also known as your due date, is very important as the pregnancy progresses. In the event that there are complications, such as a possibility that the baby is not growing well, we need to know exactly how far along the pregnancy is. In addition, if you go past your due date, we need to know how long it is safe for you to stay pregnant.

Your doctor determines the due date by two methods: your last menstrual period and first ultrasound. The EDC is 280 days from the first day of your last period. However, some women have irregular cycles and may not ovulate exactly at the time we would have predicted. For this reason, we confirm the due date with an ultrasound. The earlier the ultrasound, the more accurate it is. If the due date calculated by the last period and by first trimester ultrasound are within seven days of each other, we use the date based on the period. If they are more than seven days apart, we re-date the pregnancy based on the ultrasound.

If a woman does not come for her first prenatal visit until the second or third trimester, the due date will not be as accurate. This is because the accuracy of ultrasound to date the pregnancy is reduced as the baby gets bigger.

After your due date has been assigned, it will not be changed. The most accurate dating we have is at your earliest visit. However, your due date is just an estimate. Only 5 percent of babies arrive exactly on their scheduled day. We tell patients to think of the due date as the peak of a bell curve. Most of the babies will deliver around that date, but there will always be outliers—delivering on both slopes of the curve. A full-term baby will come anywhere between thirty-seven and forty-two weeks.

Telling People You're Pregnant

When to spread the good news about your pregnancy is a personal decision. Traditionally, the recommendation was to wait until a woman completes her first trimester before she starts announcing to the world that she's pregnant. However, with the advent of early and more accurate ultrasounds, we can generally know the well-being of the fetus by about eight weeks. That said, women can miscarry after the eight-week mark, although the risk is low.

Some women choose to wait to reveal their news until after they have completed their genetic screening tests. Which tests to do and what a woman does with the results is another individual decision. Everybody has their own—and often very strong—opinions about these sensitive issues, and people can be hurtful or judgmental, even if they care about you. We recommend that you wait until you're over those screening hurdles before you start telling anybody who isn't in your most intimate circle.

On the other hand, we've seen situations where a woman gets pregnant, doesn't tell anyone, and then has a miscarriage. She feels very alone in her grief. In these cases, it may be helpful to tell close friends and family so they can lend their support. We've noticed that some women don't tell a soul, and then after they have a miscarriage and open up about it, they find that friends or colleagues have also lost pregnancies and are extremely sympathetic. Sharing your very personal pain with another who has had the same experience can be the most healing thing you can do in this situation.

What You Can't Control

We always tell our first-trimester patients that *a healthy pregnancy is going to grow, practically no matter what you do.* And conversely, an unhealthy pregnancy is not going to grow, no matter what you do. If the fetus is not healthy at the beginning of a pregnancy, the cause is usually genetic, which you can't change.

◆ ◆ ◆ **THE WAITING GAME**

When I became pregnant with my second son, Max, I checked my beta hCG hormone level and it was quite high. Based on that level, I should have been able to see a fetus with a heartbeat on the ultrasound, but there was no sign of either. The doctor taking care of me was concerned that perhaps this meant I didn't have a normal pregnancy. I was going out of town the following week and seriously thinking about taking a medication to induce miscarriage because both my doctor and I feared the pregnancy wasn't normal.

Then another colleague stepped in and asked me, "What are you doing? Let nature take its course. You should go on your trip because it's way too early for you to say that this is not a normal pregnancy. If you have a miscarriage while you're out of town, then you have a miscarriage." So I followed his advice, went on my trip, came back, did a scan . . . and there was Max.

This experience taught me a lesson that I try to pass on to my patients: When in doubt during these first weeks, it's best to let go and let nature take its course. If it would make you feel better to come in every week and check your blood tests and ultrasounds, we'll gladly accommodate you. But usually if you just sit tight and wait, you'll see a good healthy pregnancy if it was meant to be or nature will do its proper job and let this one go.

—Alane ◀ ◀ ◀

First Trimester Development of Your Baby

The changes that take place in the growing fetus during the first trimester are nothing short of remarkable. Seeing the look on a mother's face when she first recognizes her baby's heartbeat on the ultrasound reminds us just how fortunate we are to be obstetricians. We are in the presence of miracles every day of our lives.

Some people say that the first trimester ends when you start your fourteenth week of pregnancy. Others will assert that it continues until the end of your fourteenth week. But in our practice and for this book, we consider the first trimester to be ninety-eight days, or fourteen *full* weeks.

By four weeks into pregnancy—just two weeks after fertilization—the embryo has burrowed its way into the uterine wall, establishing a connection to its life source, its mother. As Figure 3-2 indicates, during the next two weeks, the brain becomes prominent, arm and leg buds form, and the heart begins to beat, even though the embryo is only two to three millimeters in size. At eight weeks of pregnancy, essentially all the organs are formed. There are fingers, toes, and ears. The embryo is now about twenty-two millimeters, or one inch long.

Starting at ten weeks, we refer to the embryo as a fetus. The eyes can open and close and fingernails begin to develop. The fetus can move spontaneously, opening its mouth and squinting. All the organs that were formed in the embryo stage begin to grow and mature. By the end of the first trimester, the fetus is almost nine centimeters (almost four inches) and weighs forty-five grams.

Considering the enormity and complexity of the many biological processes taking place inside the uterus, it is no wonder that many women feel completely exhausted during the first trimester. We tell our patients it is like they have a major construction project going on inside them, 24/7.

First Trimester Symptoms

▶ ▶ ▶ WHERE IS THE GLOW?

We all have patients who can lift our spirits just by smiling at us from the waiting room. Natalie, whom I had known since I started practice, was such a patient. She and her husband had been together for six years and finally decided to take the leap into parenthood. Natalie stopped taking her birth control pills and, within one month, she had the good news. She came to the office about two weeks later, overflowing with anticipation. As soon as I walked in the room, I could see and feel her elation. We viewed her baby on the ultrasound and she cried tears of joy when she saw the heartbeat. We went through her list of questions, I gave her my words of wisdom, and she went on her way.

I saw her again four weeks later—and I couldn't believe this was the lovely woman I had known for so many years. She looked haggard, exhausted, and miserable: a Jekyll-and-Hyde transformation. She had practically floated out of my office at the last visit, but after that she had battled horrible nausea, fatigue, and bloating. On top of that, she was filled with fear and dread, and was in a constant ill-temper. She told me she wasn't able to keep up with the extra stresses at work and had been fighting with her boss. With desperation, she

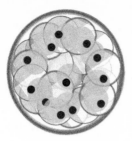

Three Days

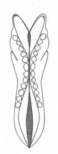

Three Weeks

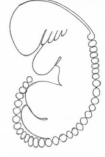

Five Weeks

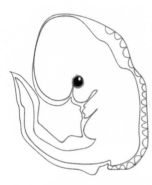

Six Weeks

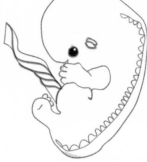

Seven Weeks

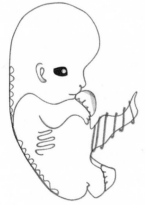

Nine Weeks

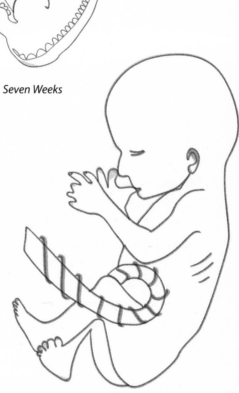

Twelve Weeks

Figure 3-2: Fetal Development

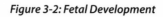

asked me, "Aren't I supposed to look and feel beautiful when I'm pregnant? What happened to that healthy glow I am supposed to have? I feel like I've been run over by a truck."

We laughed together as I told her my opinion about that old wives' tale about the healthy glow: It's all a ruse to convince us to have children. Otherwise, no one would ever do it! Her symptoms finally subsided a few weeks later, and she did become one of those beautiful glowing mothers.

—Allison ◀ ◀ ◀

The first trimester is practically infamous for all the unpleasant physical sensations associated with it. Many of these are directly or indirectly caused by rising hCG levels in a woman's body. The hCG causes the corpus luteal cyst in the ovary to continue to produce progesterone. Think of progesterone as meaning "pro" gestation—in other words, critical for fetal development. During our patients' first visit, we always want to alert them to the range of possible symptoms they might experience:

Morning sickness (nausea)   Cramping
Fatigue   Dizziness
Breast tenderness   Headaches
Forgetfulness   Spotting

Morning Sickness

Morning sickness is thought to be caused by rising hCG and estrogen levels, and may be an evolutionary adaptation to protect women from foods that may be dangerous. Morning sickness can start as soon as two to three weeks after conception. The nausea and vomiting experienced by women in their early weeks can become afternoon sickness, night sickness, or all-day sickness as well. Picture yourself during rush hour, stranded in the backseat of a careening taxi that will never stop to let you out. This is how many pregnant women feel for the first twelve weeks. About 75 percent of pregnant patients will experience some degree of these symptoms. Most women feel much better by fourteen to sixteen weeks, a small group may feel sick until twenty to twenty-two weeks, and a few unlucky moms may feel sick the entire pregnancy. About 20 percent of women who suffer from severe nausea and vomiting will experience it in their next pregnancies as well.[3]

We have no guaranteed fixes for the symptoms of morning sickness. We're fighting against a strong hormone that's eliciting all these symptoms, so even some of the strongest drugs, including antinausea medications for cancer patients, aren't necessarily effective, although they may provide relief for some women. At this time, you should listen to your body. If you are really nauseous and have no appetite, it is okay to skip a meal—you are not going to harm your growing baby by missing one lunch or dinner. However, make sure you stay well hydrated.

During this time, nausea and vomiting can be treated in a few ways. One is to make dietary changes, which include eating smaller meals (little snacks) frequently during the day. Another is to avoid triggers, which are certain smells or even thoughts that make you feel nauseated. Your ob-gyn can prescribe some safe antinausea medications for you. Some patients have also used acupuncture or special herbs to help reduce nausea, but before taking even "natural" herbs, run them past your doctor to make sure there are no interactions with any other medications you are taking.

It helps to get lots of rest, and put soda crackers by your bed to munch on before you even start moving. You can also take ginger supplements. One of our patients says the only thing that helped her morning sickness was crystallized ginger slices. Ginger and vitamin B6 supplementation have been scientifically proven to decrease nausea and vomiting in pregnancy.[4] Gatorade or low-sugar energy drinks can be used to replace lost fluids, which, in itself, can help with the nausea. Following are some nonprescription remedies for nausea that you might like to try:

Powdered ginger capsules (250mg) twice per day

Pressure at the P6 point inside the wrist through acupuncture, acupressure, or sea sickness bands

Vitamin B6 (25mg) three times per day

Doxylamine (12.5mg) four times per day (available in over-the-counter sleep aids)

Scopolamine (sea-sickness patch)

◗ ◗ ◗ MY NAUSEA . . . AD NAUSEUM

No, being an ob-gyn does not make you magically resistant to morning sickness! In my case, it was just the opposite. During my pregnancy with my son Luke, I was vomiting until about twenty weeks, stretching the limits of when most people get relief, which is usually around fourteen to sixteen weeks. During that time, I didn't gain any weight.

My morning sickness started almost immediately, and I was truly miserable. I had planned a trip to the Kentucky Derby during that time, and ended up staying in my hotel room the entire weekend. I didn't see a single horse.

The morning sickness wasn't constant. Instead, I would experience waves that seemed to come out of nowhere. I would be in an exam room with a patient, one of the waves would roll in, and I would have to run out of the room, get sick, return to my patient, and get back to business. After a while, I became so accustomed to throwing up that I didn't even think about it.

Unfortunately for me, none of the usual remedies helped. I tried the normal antinausea medicines, sea-sickness medications, ginger, vitamin B6, and vitamin B12. The only thing that gave me any relief was acupuncture. As a Western medicine–trained doctor, I can't explain exactly how the acupuncture worked, but my attitude was, "If it helps me, I'm just going to go with it. I'm not going to ask any questions."

—Allison ◖ ◖ ◖

Fatigue

The most universal symptom that our patients experience in the first trimester is probably fatigue. Some people feel as if they have been thrown under a bus. Women are exhausted and want to nap all the time. Again, the culprit is hCG. It's a myth that you need more sleep when you're pregnant; your sleep needs are probably about the same. However, most people are sleep deprived to begin with, and now their bodies are ruled by a hormone that won't let them get away with it anymore. We tell our moms that they need to listen to their bodies. If you feel really tired, you probably need to nap.

Breast Tenderness

Breast tenderness is often one of the earliest symptoms of pregnancy. By eight weeks, many women will notice an increase in the size of their breasts as well as extreme tenderness. Many hormones cause these changes, including estrogen, hCG, prolactin, and progesterone. There is not a cure for the tenderness, but wearing an extra supportive bra and avoiding underwires can help.

Forgetfulness

Forgetfulness is one of the strange phenomena of the first trimester. Women come to their prenatal appointments complaining that they can't remember what they were going to say, where they put their car keys, or what they needed to pick up at the grocery store. Although we have no scientific explanation for this phenomenon of absentmindedness, we attribute it to the pregnancy hormone beta hCG, and have jokingly dubbed it the "beta brain." Women will make up for their beta brains by writing down everything. We make the diagnosis when we see a woman at her prenatal visit pulling out lists of questions scribbled on cash register receipts, dry cleaning stubs, and napkins! Somehow, by the time the pregnancy ends, the beta brain disappears.

Cramping

Cramping occurs in most pregnancies during the first trimester. Many women say they feel like they are about to get their period. In the short time of about three months, the uterus goes from the size of a fist to the size of a cantaloupe. This rapid muscular stretching is what causes the crampy sensation or pain. No treatment exists for cramping, but it may improve if you rest a little more and increase your fluids.

Dizziness

Dizziness is also common in the first trimester, but can wax and wane up to the delivery day. Many women become nervous about this sensation, especially if they have never felt it before. The dizziness starts with a little lightheadedness and may progress to a cold, clammy feeling with nausea, visual changes, and sometimes even passing out.

Of the number of causes for dizziness in pregnancy, the most common is that the veins in the legs dilate (influenced by the pregnancy hormones), blood pools in the feet, and not enough oxygen gets to the brain. In addition, your expanding uterus places pressure on your pelvic blood vessels and slows down the blood returning to your heart. Dizziness occurs especially when you are lying or sitting and then stand quickly. However, you can also get dizzy when standing still, such as when you are in line at the grocery store. Other causes of dizziness are anemia (due to low iron), low blood sugar (due to long periods of time between meals), and dehydration.

If you start to feel dizzy, you should lie down or sit with your head between your knees. Drink some fluids and eat a small snack. The sensation usually passes within a few minutes. To prevent dizziness, eat frequent snacks to keep your blood sugar levels stable, drink lots of fluids during the day, and stand up slowly from a seated position.

Headaches

Headaches occur most frequently in the first and third trimesters. Dull achy pain, throbbing, or neck tightness—unfortunately all of these headache symptoms are part of normal pregnancy. In the first trimester, the pregnancy hormone itself can contribute to headaches, as well as the increase in blood flow and congestion of the arteries and veins in the head. Later in the pregnancy, we see the effects of poor posture and weight changes on the muscles of the neck and upper back, leading to tension headaches.

The treatment for these headaches is the same, regardless of their cause. We recommend that you increase fluid intake, relax in a cool dark room, or get a massage. In addition, you can take acetaminophen. In severe cases, narcotics can also be prescribed. Because there is a link between headaches and preeclampsia, you should always notify your doctor if a headache doesn't go away with these simple steps.

Spotting

Spotting occurs in as many as 30 percent of women during the first trimester. However, when a pregnant woman sees any sort of bloody discharge, she naturally imagines the worst. Usually, spotting is due to implantation bleeding, which is a natural by-product of the embryo burrowing into the wall of the uterus. When this occurs, delicate, new blood vessels can break apart, resulting in bleeding. As long as you don't experience heavy bleeding, blood clotting, or a lot of cramping, there is usually nothing to worry about.

Many women are understandably concerned when they see bleeding and ask, "If I'm not miscarrying, why am I bleeding?" The truth is that, sometimes, we don't know. But we see many situations where women who've had a significant amount of bleeding in their first trimester go on to have perfectly normal pregnancies.

We understand that at this early juncture, it's hard to distinguish what is normal from what is not without getting an ultrasound. A small amount of spotting is usually not a problem, but occasionally it can signal complications. If you are in doubt, don't hesitate to call your doctor.

▶ ▶ ▶ THE BIRTHDAY PRESENT

I remember a patient named Tamara from the early days of our practice. She was seeing me for her second pregnancy. At her eight-week visit, we saw a normal embryo with a heartbeat, so I happily sent her out to share the good news at her thirtieth birthday party that night. Later that evening, I got an emergency call from Tamara at my home. In a breathless voice, she told me her guests were still in the other room, but she was having bright red bleeding. "I've told my guests to leave because I know I'm having a miscarriage," she said, choking back sobs. I tried my best to console her and asked her to come to the office first thing in the morning. When she arrived, I did another ultrasound. Much to our surprise, a completely normal fetus, with a strong heartbeat, was in her uterus. She was elated. While she continued to have some bleeding over the next few weeks, she went on to deliver a healthy baby girl. Ultimately, my experience with Tamara taught me that first trimester bleeding can put patients and their doctors on an emotional roller coaster—but often, everything works out perfectly.

—Allison ◀ ◀ ◀

Stopping Work

Some women find they need to take time off from work during the first trimester. If a woman is having excessive bleeding or is struggling with severe nausea and vomiting, she may need to take a leave from her job. In some cases of persistent vomiting (hyperemesis), we'll want to hospitalize a patient to get her on IV fluids until she stabilizes. Most women will qualify for medical disability in these severe cases.

Emotional Symptoms

Truthfully, we haven't seen any good scientific studies that confirm exactly how much pregnancy hormones dictate a woman's emotional state. Anecdotally, however, we'd agree that some women do seem to become more emotional from the hormones generated by pregnancy.

Emotionally, our pregnant patients run the gamut. We've seen women euphoric, depressed, easy to anger, filled with Zen-like calm, or riddled with anxieties. We've also seen women cycle through every emotion on the spectrum within one trimester. What determines this range of emotions is hard to say.

If someone tells you, "You're feeling this way because you're pregnant," take it with a grain of salt. There is no one universal emotion that every pregnant woman feels. We believe our job as physicians is to advise people what to expect, validate the experiences they are having, and help them get through the rough times. We have to keep reminding our patients that it will get better soon. One good thing about the worst physical symptoms happening in the first three months is that the initial excitement of the pregnancy can be the bright light that helps women get through some miserable days.

In our experience, the emotions that a pregnancy brings out in a woman are as much driven by her life situation, past experiences, and coping skills as they are by the pregnancy itself.

▶ ▶ ▶ INVASION OF THE BODY SNATCHER

Deanna is thirty-seven years old and has a fairly high-pressure job that she has always loved, working at the concierge desk of a busy and prestigious Los Angeles hotel. I delivered her last two children and knew both she and her husband to be enthusiastic, dedicated parents.

For the first OB visit of her third pregnancy, Deanna came to see me in tears. She said that ever since she found out that she was pregnant, she had been crying nonstop. She had been feeling nauseous and hadn't been able to keep up at work. Her boss was upset with her for not taking care of the hotel guests in her usual, unflappable manner. She was coming home from her job to two demanding children and a house full of chores. She confessed that she didn't know if she could handle the stress of another baby while being a full-time working mom. And then on top of it, she felt guilty for not being more excited about the new baby. She told me her husband was worried about her and wanted to know what happened to his normally joyful wife.

I told Deanna that her feelings were normal. Feeling scared, sad, overwhelmed, and guilty are all part of the roller coaster of early pregnancy. She decided to talk to her husband and her boss openly about how she was feeling and ultimately took a short leave of absence from work to get her head together. By the four-month mark, she was back to her old self. In retrospect, she said she felt like something had taken over her body, and she was more than happy when it was gone.

—Allison ◀ ◀ ◀

The Pregnant Woman's Partner

We love to see husbands and other partners who are involved and excited about the pregnancy. What we usually tell the significant other is this: Your partner may feel lousy during the first trimester, so try to be as understanding as possible. Offering to help her around the house, taking the initiative in planning some meals, and allowing her some quiet time to rest are just a few of the ways to help her through the discomfort of this phase of pregnancy. But we also discourage the mom-to-be from using her hormones as an excuse to be demanding and disrespectful to her partner. Respect and support should go both ways.

▶ ▶ ▶ **THE SECRET SYMPTOM**

Trinh, a quiet, conservative woman from a large Vietnamese family, was a first-time mother-to-be who came to see me for her ten-week visit. I checked her baby on the ultrasound, went through her test results from the last visit, and asked if she had any questions. She told me that there was something bothering her that she wanted to talk to me about, but she felt embarrassed. I reassured her that I had heard it all and that she should just ask.

Trinh cleared her throat and then proceeded to tell me that for the last month, she has been having difficulty sleeping. I told her that was normal—especially in early pregnancy. Trinh nodded, looked away, and then dropped her voice to just above a whisper. "The reason I'm not sleeping well is because of the dreams I'm having." It turns out she was experiencing erotic dreams almost every night, and she wanted to know how to make them stop. I explained to her that this is a common symptom of pregnant women, that her hormones are fluctuating, and that there isn't anything we could do about it from our end.

Reassured that she wasn't the only one who'd experienced this, Trinh laughed as she admitted it was a better first trimester symptom to have than morning sickness.

—Alane ◀ ◀ ◀

Accept the Inevitable

We advise our patients to accept the fact that the first trimester of their pregnancy may not be the best period of their lives. Some women may experience nausea and vomiting to the point that they need to be hospitalized and given IV feeding because of severe dehydration. Spotting is normal, but it can trigger powerful fears; many moms imagine that they are losing the pregnancy. In addition to being an anxiety-filled time, they might also feel just plain lousy.

We can't tell who will suffer which symptoms. It's amazing to us how some women seem to sail through their first three months with ease, while so many others drag through those days as if they have an endless hangover. We've also had patients who will have miserable symptoms in one pregnancy and then no problems in the next. Fortunately, as your pregnancy progresses and the hCG levels finally peak at ten weeks and then drop by fourteen weeks, these symptoms eventually pass.

On the other hand, if you suffer from severe pregnancy symptoms but suddenly wake up symptom-free before ten weeks, notify your doctor because the change can be a warning sign. Most of the time, however, this means you have weathered the worst part of the storm.

First Trimester Tests

On your first prenatal visit, expect to have a number of tests performed in the office, including a check of your blood pressure, weight, and urine. You will also have a full physical exam including a breast exam, and a pelvic exam including a Pap smear, chlamydia and gonorrhea screenings, and also, in some cases, vaginal cultures for bacteria and yeast. Finally, you will have a number of blood tests taken: complete blood cell count to check for anemia, blood type and Rh, rubella immunity, syphilis, hepatitis B, cystic fibrosis screen, and HIV.

Cervical and Vaginal Cultures

During the first trimester, we screen for cervical and vaginal infections such as chlamydia and gonorrhea, which are sexually transmitted infections. If any tests return positive, we prescribe antibiotics for the patient as well as her partner. These diseases can cause eye infections and even blindness in the newborn if left untreated, although these outcomes are rare.

Urine Culture

Urinary tract infections (UTIs) are the most common bacterial infections in pregnancy. The traditional symptoms of a UTI—urgency and frequency of urination—are normal side effects of pregnancy, so women may not be aware when they have an infection in their urine. Hence, we screen all pregnant moms with a urine culture during their first visit.

Even if you have no symptoms, if your culture returns positive, you should be treated with antibiotics. If left untreated, a proportion of women with a UTI will develop a kidney infection (pyelonephritis). This more serious condition usually requires hospitalization with IV antibiotic treatment. Although urinary infections don't cause birth defects in the baby, they place a woman at risk for preterm labor or loss of the pregnancy if left untreated. Thankfully, UTIs can be treated easily if detected and caught early, and a healthy pregnancy can continue.

Urine Dip for Glucose and Protein

At each visit, your urine will be checked for the presence of sugar and protein. Sugar, or glucose, in the urine can signify underlying diabetes, and protein in the urine is a sign of kidney diseases or preeclampsia.

Blood Type, Rh, and Antibody Status

We will determine your blood type during your first visit. Often patients will ask if they have "good" or "bad" blood. The answer to this question is that there is no such thing as a good or bad blood type. This test is performed specifically to determine whether you are Rh positive or Rh negative. The blood group (A, B, O or AB) is not relevant.

The Rh factor is a protein that 93 percent of people have on their red blood cells, making them Rh positive. About 7 percent of the population does not have this protein and is Rh negative. If a fetus is Rh positive and the mother is Rh negative, the mother will form antibodies to attack the Rh protein on the fetal red blood cells, causing a condition called hydrops fetalis, which will eventually lead to fetal death. Because of this potential problem, all mothers who are Rh negative are given a shot called RhoGAM during their pregnancy if their partner is Rh positive. A mom can have her partner tested to see if RhoGAM is necessary. RhoGAM stops the formation of these antibodies by the mother and eliminates the risk of this condition. If properly administered, RhoGAM will protect the babies almost 100 percent of the time. There is no risk to using RhoGAM.

Rubella (German Measles)

We screen for the presence of immunity to the rubella virus in the first trimester. Most people were vaccinated against rubella as children, but the effectiveness of the vaccine may have worn off in some cases. If we find that a woman is not immune to rubella, we'll instruct her to avoid contact with people with rubella infections during her pregnancy. If a woman were to contract rubella while pregnant, this virus can cause many severe birth defects. Because the vaccine contains a live virus, a woman cannot be vaccinated during pregnancy but can receive it after she gives birth. For the same reason, if a woman has recently been vaccinated, we recommend that she wait three months before attempting to conceive.

Hepatitis B

All women are screened to see if they are chronic carriers of the hepatitis B virus. If a woman is found to be a carrier, her newborn will receive hepatitis B immunoglobulin and vaccine immediately after birth to prevent transmission to the newborn. We also encourage moms who are carriers to seek continued care with their general doctor or liver specialist after their baby is born, to monitor their liver function and screen for liver cancer.

Syphilis

Screening for syphilis is performed in the first trimester. Women found to have syphilis are treated with penicillin during the pregnancy. If left untreated, this infection can cause severe infection and death of the fetus.

HIV

In the United States, every pregnant woman is offered HIV testing. If a mother has HIV while she's pregnant, she can safely take antiviral medication, reducing the risk of infection to the baby. Happily, the rate of fetal infection improves every year because the retroviral medications are more and more effective. In addition, if a woman is HIV positive, giving birth by cesarean delivery greatly decreases the risk of transmission to the baby. Without these treatments, approximately 25 percent of babies will become infected with HIV. With medication and cesarean delivery, this risk is reduced to 1 percent.

Cystic Fibrosis Screening

Please refer to Chapter 1 for details on screening for cystic fibrosis.

First Trimester Screening for Genetic Diseases

"Is my baby normal?" is one of the most common questions we hear in the first trimester. We explain to patients that birth defects are uncommon, occurring in 3 to 4 percent of all pregnancies. We can screen for some of these defects but definitely not all of them. Current screening methods include blood tests on the mother, ultrasounds, and direct chromosome analysis of the fetus.

Don't Freak Out

When we set out to write this book, we wanted to reassure women about their pregnancies, not scare them silly like so much current information in print and in the blogosphere does. Yet we're about to devote several pages talking about a slew of genetic diseases and some fairly scary worst-case scenarios. When you read about these genetic issues, it can seem as though you have plenty of things to be worried about. And if you are looking for all the things that could possibly go wrong, the prospect of pregnancy can seem overwhelming.

But even though there is an abundance of testing for these problems (see Table 3-1 on pages 120-121), remember that *the vast majority of pregnancies are completely normal*. We remind all our patients that most of the diseases we test for are very rare. For example, we cumulatively have had more than forty-five years of practice and not one of us has had two parents who are both carriers of the same single gene defect. So your chances of a healthy pregnancy are far greater than your chances of carrying a baby with a rare disease or genetic disorder.

Single Gene Defects

During the past decade, advances in DNA technology have allowed us to identify the cause of many genetic diseases. We offer blood tests to pregnant patients to see whether they are carriers of some of the more common defects, such as cystic fibrosis, Tay-Sachs, Canavan disease, and sickle-cell anemia. Which tests you will be offered depends on your ethnic background and family history. You can discuss these tests with your doctor at your first visit. Please see Chapter 1 (pages 27 to 32) for more details and information about these diseases and the testing that we can do. If a test shows that you are a carrier of one of these single gene defects, your partner will also be screened. If he too is positive, the baby can be checked.

Numerical Genetic Abnormalities

Some genetic disorders occur because of an extra or a missing chromosome. Normally a fetus receives one set—or twenty-three—chromosomes from the mother and one set from the father, for a total of forty-six chromosomes. Sometimes, an egg mistakenly has an extra chromosome, and then the resulting fetus has forty-seven chromosomes. Two examples of this are Trisomy 21, when the fetus has an extra copy of chromosome #21, also known as Down syndrome (see Figure 3-3), and Trisomy 18.

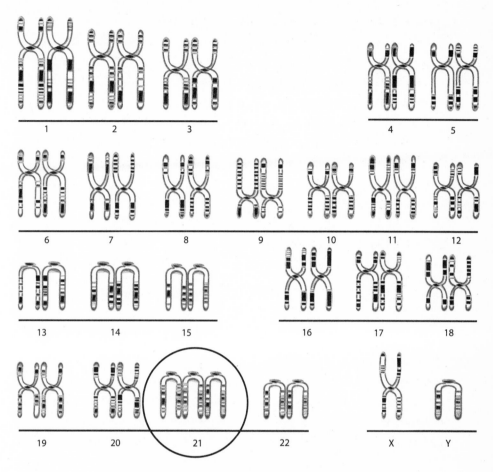

Figure 3-3: Down Syndrome Chromosome

These numeric genetic abnormalities occur more frequently in women who are over 35 because their older eggs are more likely to have the wrong number of chromosomes. Unlike other birth defects such as holes in the heart, cleft lip, and spina bifida, which occur at the same rate regardless of the mother's age, the incidence of numeric genetic disorders increases as the mom gets older. Some fetuses with these disorders will not survive through the pregnancy, while others may survive until shortly after birth, and still others may live a full life.

Testing for these genetic diseases involves two methods: screening tests and diagnostic tests. Screening tests are noninvasive (blood tests and ultrasounds) and will tell you the odds, or the likelihood,

Table 3-1: Tests for Genetic Defects and Birth Defects

Test	Tests For	When
First trimester blood test	T21 (trisomy 21, or Down's), T18 (trisomy 18)	10 weeks to 13 weeks, 6 days
Nuchal translucency	T21	11 weeks, 2 days to 14 weeks, 2 days
Quad screen	T21, T18, NTD (neural tube defect) AWD (abdominal wall defect) SLOS (Smith-Lemli-Opitz syndrome)	15 weeks to 20 weeks
Fully integrated screen	T21, T18, NTD, AWD, SLOS	First trimester, Nuchal translucency and quad screen combined
Chronic villus sampling (CVS)	T21, T18, and other chromosomal abnormalities	10–14 weeks
Amniocentesis	Same as CVS, NTD, and AWD	15–20 weeks
Structural ultrasound	Anatomic defects such as holes in the heart, brain abnormalities, cleft lip	18–22 weeks
Single gene mutation test	Cystic fibrosis, Tay-Sachs, Canavan disease, etc.	Prepregnancy or first visit

that your baby could be born with one of these disorders. Diagnostic tests are invasive, meaning material from the pregnancy is directly analyzed, and will give you a "yes" or "no" answer. Examples of diagnostic tests are chorionic villus sampling (CVS) and amniocentesis.

Down syndrome

Down syndrome is the most common of these numerical genetic diseases, and we can identify it only after a woman is pregnant. According to the National Institutes of Health, Down syndrome occurs in 1

How	Detection Rate	Pros	Cons
Blood test on the mother checks for PAPP-A and hCG	Accuracy is not reported	Performed early in the pregnancy and no risk to the fetus	False positives and negatives
Abdominal ultrasound measures thickness of skin behind the neck	65%		
Blood test on mother checks HCG, estriol, inhibin-A, and AFP	T21: 80%, T18: 67%, NTD: 80% AWD: 85% SLOS: 60%	No risk to the fetus	
First trimester, Nuchal translucency and quad screen combined	T21: 90%, T18: 81%		
Small piece of placenta is removed either through cervix or abdomen, and cells are grown in the lab	>99%	Early and accurate	Risk of miscarriage is 1:100
Amniotic fluid is sampled with a needle through abdomen, and fetal cells are grown in the lab		Accurate	Risk of miscarriage is 1:500
Abdominal ultrasound	60–70%	Can detect defects that can make a difference in delivery	Doesn't check genetics; doesn't detect all birth defects
Blood test on mother to isolate specific gene mutations	98–99%	Easy to perform	Numerous tests are expensive; all diseases are rare

out of every 740 live births in the United States, across all ethnic and economic groups.

Although we think of Down syndrome babies as a phenomenon of the trend of older mothers, more babies with Down syndrome are born to moms under the age of thirty-five, simply because more women in that age category have babies. In fact, 55 percent of all babies with Down syndrome were born to moms under age thirty-five (see Table 3-2). Because of this, all pregnant women are offered screening tests for Down syndrome.

Table 3-2: Down Syndrome in Relation to Mother's Age[5]

Mother's Age	Incidence of Down Syndrome
25 and under	Less than 1 in 1,000
30	1 in 720
35	1 in 272
36	1 in 205
37	1 in 153
38	1 in 114
39	1 in 85
40	1 in 65
42	1 in 42
45	1 in 27

Individuals with Down syndrome can have learning disabilities, congenital heart disease, hearing loss, congenital hypothyroidism, intestinal problems, as well as vision problems and seizure disorders. The babies have a characteristic appearance that includes a short stature, a flat nose, slanted eyes, a squarish face, and a single transverse crease in their palm. A child can be affected by this syndrome in a wide spectrum of ways that vary in severity. Many people have seen Chris Burke, the actor with Down syndrome who played the character of Corky in the TV series *Life Goes On*. He was obviously highly functional. Children on the other end of the spectrum cannot feed themselves and have multiple medical problems.

At this time, we cannot predict how a child with Down's will be affected. Previously, children with Down syndrome were institutionalized and didn't live into adulthood. Now, with medical treatments, physical and occupational therapy, and advances in education techniques, many people with Down's will live well into adulthood with productive, healthy lives. Whether or not to keep a baby with Down syndrome can be an agonizing decision for parents because it's not a lethal disease, but it brings with it the possibility of a future that they may not have imagined for themselves. Some people will gladly take on the challenge of raising their Down syndrome child, while other parents feel very strongly that they just couldn't handle it. In addition, because Down's children can live into adulthood, another sibling or family member could be left with the caretaking duties of that child after you and your partner have passed on. This is another element that can factor into a couple's decision.

▶ ▶ ▶ DOING WHAT IT TAKES

My patients Claudia and Lorenz were both attorneys, a high-achieving, loving couple of German descent in their late twenties. Claudia had placed her career on hold to raise a family. They had a healthy daughter with their first pregnancy. We had the privilege of taking care of them for their second pregnancy, which was uncomplicated and going smoothly. Claudia was a compliant patient who took great care of herself and came to all of her prenatal visits. She had negative blood screening tests for chromosomal problems and normal ultrasounds. To everyone's surprise, when she delivered, we were suspicious that her son had Down syndrome. We had our confirmation after a blood test that checked his chromosomes.

Claudia and Lorenz didn't waste a moment feeling sorry for themselves or their child. They faced the fire and decided to take on the role of being parents to a Down's baby as their next big life achievement. Claudia jumped headfirst into the challenge of raising a Down syndrome child and put her career on hold longer to do physical therapy, occupational therapy, and special education at school with her son, making it her full-time job. These parents had both the financial resources and the determination to get the best available care and to raise their son to be as highly functioning as possible. They then chose to have a third child, a healthy daughter without Down's.

This story has the happiest possible ending but also illustrates the reality of Down syndrome: It can be a life-changing situation.

—Alane ◀ ◀ ◀

Trisomy 18

Trisomy 18 is the second most common numeric genetic disorder. It occurs in 1 of 6,500 pregnancies. This disorder, like Down syndrome, is the result of an extra chromosome, but in this case it is an extra #18. Trisomy 18 occurs more frequently in women over thirty-five. (As stated, note that although the risk of Down's and trisomy 18 is higher for women over thirty-five, the total *number* of babies born with

Down's is higher in women under thirty-five simply because more women in that age group have babies.) Trisomy 18 is associated with severe mental retardation and multiple physical problems such as heart defects and small brains, both of which can be life-threatening birth defects. There is also an increased risk of stillbirth and neonatal death. About 40 percent of children with trisomy 18 will survive to their first birthday, but it is rare for these children to survive beyond childhood.

Screening Tests

Each state in the United States has its own prenatal screening program, and the tests may vary slightly from state to state. In this section, we describe the tests available in California. You should check with your doctor about variations in your state.

In California, the screening test has three components: a blood test in the first trimester, an ultrasound in the first trimester, and a blood test in the second trimester.

> The first trimester blood test can be drawn between ten weeks and thirteen weeks and six days. It tests for two hormones made during pregnancy: PAPP-A (pregnancy associated plasma protein) and hCG (human chorionic gonadatropin).

> The ultrasound in the first trimester is called the nuchal translucency and can be performed between eleven weeks and two days and fourteen weeks and two days. The doctor measures the thickness of the skin behind the neck of the fetus. Increased thickness can be associated with Down syndrome.

> The second trimester blood test is performed between fifteen weeks and twenty weeks of pregnancy and is often called the quad screen because it tests the levels of four hormones made by the pregnancy: hCG, estriol, inhibin, and alpha-fetoprotein (AFP).

The results of these three tests are combined to give a risk assessment for the presence of trisomy 21 and 18. With this combination, 90 percent of babies with Down syndrome and 81 percent of babies with trisomy 18 are detected. When the result arrives from the lab, it will say "The risk of Down syndrome is 1 out of *x*, with *x* any number from 5 to 100,000. The state of California considers a positive result to be any risk higher than 1 out of 200. When the screening test is positive, the patient is referred to a specialist for genetic counseling, ultrasound, and possible diagnostic testing.

The third portion of the test—the quad screen—will also screen for neural tube defects (spina bifida and anencephaly), abdominal wall defects (gastroschisis and omphalocele), and Smith-Lemli-Opitz syndrome. These disorders are not related to the age of the mother and involve multiple genes as well as environmental factors.

The screening test, unlike the diagnostic test, does not carry any risk. It is noninvasive and does not affect the baby. Diagnostic tests, on the other hand, carry the risk of miscarriage by introducing infection or causing the water to break as the fetal cells are removed. The disadvantage to the screening test is that it is not perfect. About 5 percent of patients will receive a false positive result, meaning that the screening test was positive but the baby is completely healthy. Remember, the test isn't telling you whether or not your baby is *going to* have Down's; the test is telling you *what your chances are* of having a baby with Down's. For example, if the test says the risk of Down's is one in fifty, the chances are forty-nine out of fifty that you're *not* going to have a baby with Down's.

▶ ▶ ▶ PROBABILITY ISN'T INEVITABILITY

We treated a woman named Catherine and her husband, Ted. A supportive, hard-working couple, they had a beautiful daughter and were excited to add a second child to their family. Catherine was thirty-five and chose to do the quad screen instead of going straight to amniocentesis. We got the message from the genetic counselor that her screening test showed an increased risk for Down's. Alane called Catherine with the troubling news that her screening test was positive, that is, there was a chance her baby could have Down's. Alane went through the details and outlined the next steps.

A few hours later, Alane got a call back from Catherine's husband, Ted. Catherine had told him that Alane had explained everything, but she could not remember a single thing she said after the words "the test was screen positive." Alane went through the details with Ted and explained that there was a greater chance than not that their baby would have normal chromosomes.

Catherine and her husband had to wait a few days to see the perinatologist for the ultrasound and amniocentesis. During the two weeks they had to stand by for the results, they went through a roller coaster of emotions but ultimately settled on the idea that if anyone could care for a baby with special needs, it was them.

They received the results—no Down's—and were overjoyed to be having a healthy baby boy they named Jonathan.

◀ ◀ ◀

Diagnostic Tests

Diagnostic tests for genetic disorders, including chorionic villus sampling (CVS) and amniocentesis, directly remove fetal cells for chromosome analysis. In this chapter, we cover CVS because it occurs in the first trimester. You can find information on amniocentesis in Chapter 4 (page 159). Diagnostic tests are offered to women thirty-five and older because they are at a higher risk of having a genetic problem. However, women of any age have the option to do these tests.

The magic age of 35

Many patients ask, why age thirty-five? The reason age thirty-five was selected as the age to offer diagnostic tests has to do with the risk of having a baby with Down syndrome at that age. Years ago, having an amniocentesis to detect Down syndrome carried a risk of miscarriage of one out of two hundred. At age thirty-five, the risk of having a baby with Down's is also about one out of two hundred. Because the risk associated with the test was equal to the risk of having the disorder, thirty-five was selected as the age to offer this form of testing. (The risk of miscarriage after amnio has since decreased to about one out of five hundred.)

Chorionic villus sampling

Chorionic villus sampling is a genetic test that can be performed between ten and thirteen weeks of pregnancy. An instrument is placed

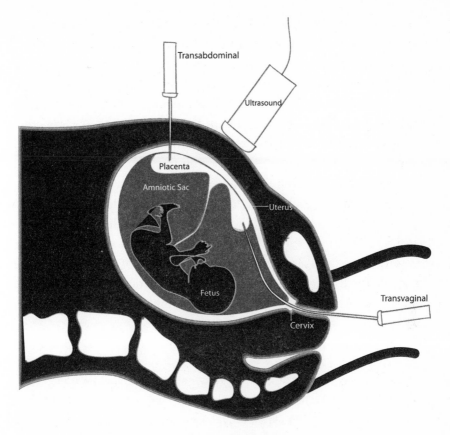

Transabdominal

Ultrasound

Placenta

Amniotic Sac

Uterus

Fetus

Transvaginal

Cervix

Figure 3-4: CVS Procedure

into the uterus and a small piece of the placenta is removed and ana-lyzed for its genetic makeup (see Figure 3-4). With CVS, we can see if there is an extra chromosome, as in the case of Down syndrome, or a missing chromosome. The accuracy of CVS is more than 99 percent.

The CVS procedure can be performed two ways. With ultrasound guidance, a catheter is passed vaginally through the cervix or a nee-dle is placed through the abdominal wall. Doctors make that decision based on the location of the placenta. The placental cells are removed and grown in a laboratory for ten to twelve days. Then the analysis of the chromosomes, or karyotype, is performed. The procedure feels like a long pap smear with mild cramping and takes about five min-utes. We recommend that patients do not exercise or do any strenu-ous activity for forty-eight hours after the procedure.

The advantage to CVS is timing: You get results at the end of the first trimester, so if you decide to terminate your pregnancy, the medical procedure is safer and easier. In addition, CVS is highly accurate. The downside is that the risk of miscarriage is one out of a hundred but can vary amongst different doctors. Because the risk of miscarriage with an amniocentesis is one out of five hundred, CVS is not as popular as amniocentesis. Signs of complications with CVS include excessive bleeding, fever, or severe cramping.

An additional phenomenon that previously had been linked to CVS in the past is called limb reduction defect. The incidence of this birth defect is one out of two thousand. Years ago, some doctors believed it could be caused by CVS performed before ten weeks. However, after reviewing more than six hundred thousand cases of CVS, an increased risk of this birth defect has not been proven. Nonetheless, we still recommend that all CVS procedures be performed after ten weeks.

▶ ▶ ▶ MY CVS EXPERIENCE

With both of my pregnancies, I knew from the beginning that I was going to take the CVS test. Even though I was only thirty-three with my first and just thirty-five with my second, I knew I could not enjoy or embrace my pregnancy until I had that information. Perhaps I was more paranoid than an average person because of what I do for a living and what I see on a regular basis.

Physically, the procedure wasn't bad. It took only five minutes, and I was slightly crampy and uncomfortable afterward for about twenty-four hours. I received my results a few weeks later, and so by about twelve weeks, I knew that both of my kids were genetically normal. To me, the risk of the CVS was low and was outweighed by my desire to get accurate results as quickly as possible.

—Allison ◀ ◀ ◀

▶ ▶ ▶ MY FIRST TRIMESTER SCREENING TEST

I was forty-one when I had Kylie. I had her three weeks before I turned forty-two, so I had a high risk of having a baby with Down's: about a one in forty chance. I had two previous miscarriages, so I was too nervous to accept the higher miscarriage risk associated with CVS. I knew I was eventually going to have an amniocentesis, but I did the first trimester screening test because I wanted to have an idea of my risk while I waited for my amniocentesis appoint-

Table 4-1: The Development of the Fetus during the Second Trimester[1]

Age	Length (CRL)*	Weight	Events
12 weeks	6 cm (2.4 in)	14 gm (about 0.03 lb)	
14 weeks	8–9 cm (3.4 in)	45 gm (about 0.1 lb)	The genitalia of your baby has formed
16 weeks	12 cm (4.8 in)	110 gm (about 0.24 lb)	The legs of your baby are well formed.
18 weeks	14 cm (7 in)	200 gm (0.44 lb)	Your baby's ears are sticking out from the sides of his or her head.
20 to 22 weeks	16 cm (6.4 in)	320 gm (about 0.7 lb)	Your baby now moves more regularly. Your baby will also have some hair on his or her head and hair throughout the body.
24 weeks	21 cm (8.4 in)	630 gm (1.4 lb)	The skin is red and wrinkled.
26 weeks	23 cm (9.1 in)	820 gm (1.8 lb)	Your baby now has fingernails!
28 weeks	25 cm (9.8 in)	1,000 gm (2.2 lb)	Your baby begins to open his or her eyes with those beautiful eyelashes.

*Crown-rump length measurement.

Table 4-1 shows the progression of the baby's development during the second trimester. At twelve weeks, a baby is only six centimeters (about two-and-a-half inches) in length and weighs just fourteen grams, as shown in Figure 4-2. By the end of the second trimester, a baby will weigh about 1,000 grams (a little over two pounds). The length from head to toe is thirty centimeters (a little less than twelve inches). Of course, your baby could vary a bit in either direction. By the end of this trimester, your baby will be kicking, sleeping, waking, swallowing, urinating, and sucking its thumb.

The Placenta and Amniotic Sac

Shortly after conception, the fertilized egg becomes a fluid-filled ball of three layers of cells called the blastocyst. The inner two layers eventually become parts of the baby, and the outer layer of cells becomes the placenta and amniotic sac. The placenta is fully formed and functioning by twelve weeks of gestation.

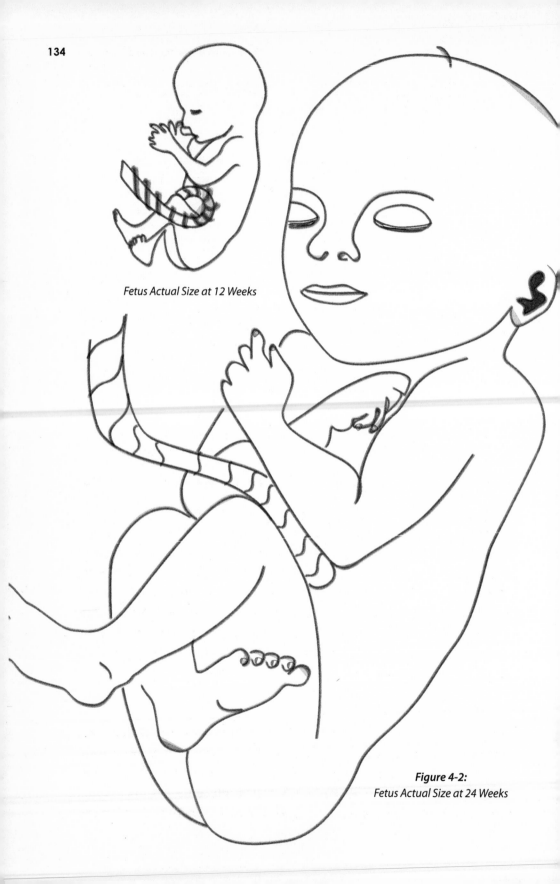

Fetus Actual Size at 12 Weeks

Figure 4-2:
Fetus Actual Size at 24 Weeks

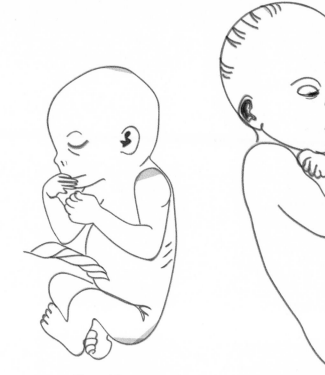

Figure 4-3:
Fetal Development at 20 Weeks   *Figure 4-4: Fetal Development at 28 Weeks*

Alane's son, Matt, has a children's dictionary that defines an organ as "a part of the body that does a particular job." The placenta is truly an amazing organ, and it definitely has an important job: It is the direct connection between the mother and baby. Without maternal and fetal blood ever mixing, it provides oxygen and nutrients to the fetus, and transports waste and carbon dioxide to the mother. It also produces many hormones that are essential to keeping the baby and pregnancy healthy.

Umbilical cord

The umbilical cord connects the baby to the placenta, which then connects to the mother. One side of the placenta attaches to the uterus, and the other side, the smooth side with the umbilical cord in the center, goes directly to the baby's belly button. At term, the umbilical cord is fifty-five centimeters (about twenty-two inches) in length.

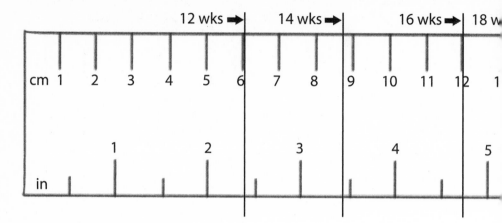

Figure 4-5: Fetal Growth-Second Trimester (measurements from crown to rump)

The umbilical cord contains two arteries and one vein, as shown in Figure 4-6, and they function in the opposite direction of the normal circulation in your body. The vein transports oxygen and nutrients from the mother to the baby, and the two arteries carry waste materials and carbon dioxide from the baby to the placenta, where they are filtered away to the mother.

It is important to have free flow of blood to the fetus through the umbilical cord. If we see that a baby is not growing well, we can do an ultrasound to check the blood flow through the cord.

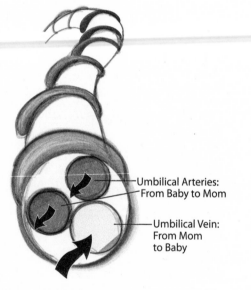

Figure 4-6: Umbilical Cord

Amniotic fluid

Did you know that after twenty weeks, the amniotic fluid is primarily made up of the baby's urine? Among other things, baby's urine con-

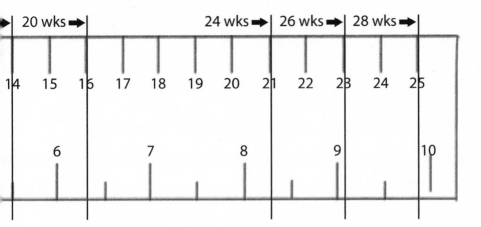

tains elements that are essential to the development and maturation of the baby's lungs. The amniotic fluid also serves several other critical functions. It provides a cushioning effect, becoming the protective pool that gives your baby a safe place to develop, and also helps to maintain a constant temperature for the baby.

The Doppler

At approximately eleven to twelve weeks, we can hear the baby's heartbeat with an electronic handheld instrument called a Doppler. Your health care provider will place the Doppler on your abdomen over the uterus at each visit to hear the baby's heartbeat. The Doppler uses sound waves to measure the heart rate, so it is not harmful to the baby.

The normal heart rate of a fetus ranges from 110 to 160 beats per minute. Fetal heart rates less than 110 beats per minute may indicate that the baby is not receiving enough oxygen. We also listen for the regularity of the beats. A pattern of skipping beats may indicate that the baby has a heart condition called an arrhythmia. However, from listening to the heartbeat alone, we cannot determine if your baby has any birth defects or if he or she is growing normally. Whether the heartbeat sounds loud or faint is related to how far the heart is from the skin surface, not how strong or healthy the baby is.

myth: If you have an active baby inside you, you will have an active child.

FACT: Alane believes this myth! But as doctors, we've searched high and low for any reliable studies that confirm or deny it and found nothing. So as it stands, it's safe to say that there's no documented correlation between how active your baby is in utero and how high energy your child will be when it's out in the world.

Fundal Height

Fundal height is the measurement, in centimeters, from the top of the mom's pubic bone to the *fundus*, or top of her uterus. Between twenty to thirty-four weeks, the fundal height almost always equals the number of weeks she's been pregnant. For example, at twenty weeks, the fundal height is twenty centimeters; at twenty-four weeks, it should reach twenty-four centimeters. Each consecutive week, it should grow by another centimeter. (Nature is pretty terrific.) We are not sure who figured out this trick, but it gives us a simple, quick way of determining if the baby's growth is normal.

Keep in mind, however, that fundal height measurement is not an exact science. For example, in women who are overweight, the fundal height may measure larger because they have an extra fat layer around their belly. If the fundal height doesn't precisely equal a woman's pregnancy weeks, we still need to make sure it is increasing properly from week to week. If, for example, a woman's uterus measures twenty centimeters at twenty weeks and then a month later it still measures twenty centimeters, this may be a sign of growth problems. In contrast, if a woman is thirty weeks, but her fundal height is measuring thirty-four centimeters, this could be a sign of a large baby. In either scenario, we would investigate further by using an ultrasound, which is more accurate.

Feeling the Baby Kick

Quickening is the term we use for the first time that a mother feels her baby move, and it's an emotional moment for any woman and her partner. In general, first-time moms will feel the baby's movements at eighteen to twenty weeks. In subsequent pregnancies, you may feel the baby move about two weeks earlier, or at about sixteen to eighteen weeks, simply because you now know how to identify this unique sensation.

It's hard to describe exactly what a baby's movement feels like. Quickening can feel like a distinct shifting, like a gentle thump or an internal tap or flick. The taps are tiny in the beginning but get stronger as the baby grows. Some women have described it as feeling like flutters or bubbles.

▶ ▶ ▶ MY FIRST FLUTTERS

During the first trimester, many of our patients remain anxious and uncertain until the moment they begin to feel their baby move inside them. I know, because I was that same mom, looking down at my belly for all those weeks, saying, "Hey? Are you okay in there?" Then it finally happened. Was that gas? Was I imagining it? No, it really was Matt's movement that I felt for the first time.

—Alane ◀ ◀ ◀

If you haven't felt the baby moving at sixteen to eighteen weeks, don't be nervous. However, if you're at twenty weeks and still aren't feeling anything, report this to your doctor. Most likely, you simply are not sensitive to the movements yet.

So why do some women not feel their baby move? They may have their placenta on the anterior, or front, part of their uterus. In this situation, another layer of tissue is between the fetus and the mother, making perception of the movements more difficult. In the same way, women who are overweight may not be as sensitive to their baby's movements because their abdominal fat layer is thicker—yet another layer of tissue between the baby and mother's abdominal wall.

Second Trimester Symptoms

▶ ▶ ▶ MY NIGHTLY RITUAL

After a long day at work, my bed looks heavenly and inviting. And I'm not on call, which means I may get some overdue uninterrupted sleep tonight. But wait—it's 4:00 a.m. and I feel myself waking up. I have to pee again! Didn't I just do this at 2:00 a.m.?

—Yvonne ◀ ◀ ◀

Bladder Pressure

Urinary frequency and incontinence are consequences of the growing uterus. Anatomically, the bladder sits directly in front of the uterus. As the uterus enlarges, it pushes against the bladder, so naturally, you'll have the sensation that you need to urinate more frequently. Most women will get up a few extra times during the night to empty the bladder. In addition, with a cough or sneeze, some women may suffer from incontinence (inability to hold the urine in) and may lose bladder control.

As inconvenient as it may seem for many active women, we urge our patients not to hold their urine for long periods of time because it may cause urinary tract or kidney infections. Kidney infections, also known as pyelonephritis, can cause tremendous pain and, in extreme cases, even send you to the hospital with preterm labor if left untreated. The best thing to do is to drink lots of fluids to help flush out the kidney and the bladder. If you have to go, you have to go.

Cravings

▶ ▶ ▶ **MY ICE CREAM DREAMS**

Okay, I admit it. In my first trimester, fruits and vegetables kept my nausea at bay. But as I entered the second trimester of my second pregnancy, with Max, I could not have enough of those yummy Häagen-Dazs Coffee Almond Crunch bars. My husband kept boxes of them in the freezer because I loved them so much. My lower belly and bottom will never forgive me for those ice cream bars!

—Alane ◀ ◀ ◀

We've observed that more than half our moms-to-be start to crave different types of foods around the second trimester. Now that they finally have an appetite again, they may start to go a little bit overboard, and the weight begins to creep up.

If this describes you, go back to page 56 and reread our assessment of how much weight you should actually be gaining in pregnancy. Remember, you need only about 300 extra *healthy* calories a day to provide the nutrients your growing baby needs. We're not saying that you can't indulge in your favorite treat once in a while, but use your common sense and remind yourself to eat healthy.

Pica

One morning in the bustling OB clinic at USC, Alane saw a quiet, petite young woman for her routine prenatal care visit. Alane did all the routine checks—blood pressure, fundal height, and baby's heartbeat—and everything was normal. She ended the visit with the usual, "Do you have any questions for me today?" Looking worried and embarrassed, the patient took a deep breath and then piped up: "Dr. Park, I've been craving dirt and eating it. Is this okay? I'm worried."

Pica is a condition in which pregnant women experience strange cravings for non-foodstuffs, most often for starch, clay, stones, ice, or dirt. It occurs in 8 percent of pregnant women, but in some ethnic groups, it may be as high as 30 percent. Some believe that this condition is caused by the body's attempt to replace iron or other minerals that are not present in regular food. When a woman reports symptoms of pica, we usually check her blood count and often recommend supplemental iron tablets. Eating these substances can be dangerous because they may contain toxins such as lead or interfere with the patient's ability to absorb regular food.

Ptyalism

Ptyalism is an overproduction of saliva. Some of our more unfortunate patients suffering with this condition carry around a cup—what we call the spit cup—to collect the extra saliva. Either there is too much saliva to swallow, or swallowing the saliva causes nausea. Scientists do not know the exact cause of this inconvenient condition, which affects 1 percent of pregnancies, but it may be related to overstimulation of the salivary glands by starch. Luckily, it does no harm to the baby or the mom, and we have yet to see a mom continue to have this problem postpartum. We have suggested to some women that they try chewing gum or decrease their starch intake, but most just resort to keeping a cup on hand.

Leg Cramps

Many women suffer from leg cramps during pregnancy, especially at night. As far as we know, no cause has yet been determined for these painful cramps. Doctors and scientists have been searching for causes, researching theories such as low potassium, magnesium, or calcium levels. None of these ideas have thus far been proven, and it is just as likely that the cramping occurs simply from muscle fatigue from carrying around the extra pregnancy weight. These cramps most often occur in your calves, but they can affect your feet and thighs as well. If you get leg cramps, try the following:

- Stretch the affected calf by flexing at the ankle so that your toes are pointed toward your head. Do not point your toes as this may aggravate your cramp.
- Wear support hose.
- Stretch your legs and calves before going to bed.
- Drink plenty of fluids throughout the day and evening.
- Massage the affected muscle.
- Apply local heat.
- While holding on to something for support, such as a counter-top, squat down to the floor.

▶ ▶ ▶ MY KILLER CRAMPS

I had terrible leg cramps in my first pregnancy. I woke up one night in excruciating pain, with my calf clenched in a tight ball. I couldn't even move my leg. I woke up my husband who, after desperately trying to massage it out, finally asked me, "Should I take you to the emergency room?" The thought of my ER colleagues massaging cramps out of my calf made me laugh through my pain. No, I did not want to go to the ER! That killer cramp eventually disappeared with stretching and massage.

After I started wearing support hose during the day and while I slept, the leg cramps never returned. I don't know that there's any scientific proof for the effectiveness of support hose, but they definitely worked for me.

—Alane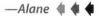

Heart Palpitations

When you can feel your heart beating in your chest, you are experiencing heart palpitations. These are common in pregnancy due to the physiologic changes in your cardiovascular system. Because your blood volume increases by 50 percent, your heart has to pump harder to move the blood around. In some people, the symptoms range from a hyperawareness of the heart beating more strongly or more rapidly than usual, to the feeling that the heart is skipping beats or stopping. Other women describe a sensation of their heart rolling around in their chest.

Such sensations can be uncomfortable and often worrisome, but most cases of palpitations are harmless and usually last for a few seconds to a few minutes. However, if heart palpitations occur frequently or are associated with chest pain, shortness of breath, or lightheadedness, you should contact your doctor because these symptoms may indicate a possible cardiac arrhythmia.

Round Ligament Pain

Certain aches and pains are unique to pregnancy. On each side of the uterus, you have ligaments called *round ligaments* that travel from the top of the uterus to the sides of your pelvis near the groin. As the baby gets bigger and the uterus expands, these ligaments lengthen, leading to a pulling sensation down your side and into your groin. How women experience this sensation—and how painful it may be— varies from woman to woman. Some of our patients describe round ligament pain as a stabbing pain; others say that it is so uncomfortable that it hurts whenever they stand, walk, or change position in bed. Alane had it in her third trimester. "I would be walking," says Alane, "then all of a sudden I would have to stop. I would take the time to stretch out the groin and the pain would disappear."

There is no explanation as to why some women suffer from this and others don't. The good news is, round ligament pains are just side effects of pregnancy and don't harm the baby in any way. Unfortunately there's not much you can do to alleviate the discomfort other than resting and avoiding sudden movements. You can also try stretching and massaging the area. On occasion, we've had to admit patients to the hospital because their pain was so severe, and we had to be certain that it was just round ligament pain and not a more serious problem such as appendicitis or cervical insufficiency. It's always better to err on the side of caution when it comes to abdominal pain in pregnancy. When in doubt, see a doctor.

◗ ◗ ◗ MY LIGAMENT PAIN RECKONING

When I was eighteen weeks pregnant with my daughter Kate, I got out of bed one morning with the most horrible pain on my lower right side. I was doubled over, couldn't walk, and felt nauseous because of the pain's severity. I started to wonder whether I had appendicitis. I knew that appendicitis symptoms would worsen over time, so I decided to see what would transpire. I lay back down, drank some water, and within a few hours, the pain subsided. It was then that it hit me that I'd experienced round ligament pain. Truly, I had no idea how bad it could be. I was ready to go to the emergency room and demand that they work me up for a ruptured appendix. It was a sobering moment and I finally understood what my patients have been complaining about for all these years.

—Allison ◀ ◀ ◀

Allison herself almost mistook her round ligament pain for appendicitis, which illustrates how similar these conditions can feel. Appendicitis results in intense pain on the right side of your body, which can be in the same general area where you might feel round ligament pain. The difference is that appendicitis can affect your pregnancy by causing preterm labor. And if not diagnosed in a timely fashion, it can cause the mother to become extremely ill. Diagnosing appendicitis during pregnancy can be tricky because the uterus pushes the appendix from its normal position in the right-lower abdomen into the right-upper abdomen. Symptoms of appendicitis may include right-sided abdominal pain, decreased appetite, fever, diarrhea, nausea, and vomiting. In general, these symptoms worsen over time. If you are experiencing any of these symptoms, don't just assume that it's round ligament pain. Call your doctor or go to the emergency room to make sure it isn't appendicitis.

Your Skin

Many pregnant women will start to notice changes in their skin by the second trimester. Beyond that glow everybody talks about, many of these changes may not make them so happy.

Dark spots

A whopping 90 percent of women will develop dark spots on their skin. These occur mostly on the breasts and face but may be seen in the genital areas, in the armpits, and on inner thighs. These spots are due to the increased production of a pigment called melanin. When they occur around the eyes and nose and on the cheeks, the condition is called melasma, which is also known as the "mask of pregnancy."

In addition, preexisting moles will often darken and some women will develop a line down the middle of their belly called the *linea nigra,* as shown in Figure 4-7. Women with darker skin are more prone to getting these dark spots. All these darkening changes are worsened with sun exposure, so we recommend using sunscreen or wearing a hat when outside throughout pregnancy and postpartum. Most of the spots fade within six months of delivery, but some never go away completely.

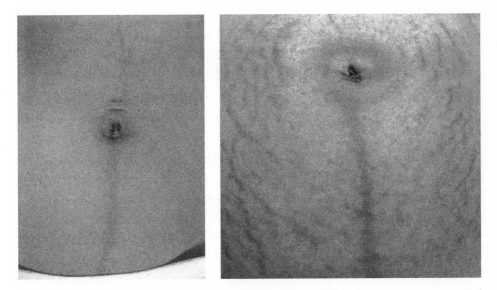

Figure 4-7: Linea Nigra, Stretch Marks

Stretch marks

About 80 to 90 percent of pregnant women will develop stretch marks, also known as *striae gravidarum*. They occur when the second layer of skin, the dermis, tears due to extreme stretching, and they are most commonly seen in the late second trimester and into the third trimester. You'll most commonly find them on your abdomen and breasts, but they may also crop up your buttocks or thighs. Having a large baby can increase your chance for stretch marks. Genetically, some women just have the type of skin that predisposes them to stretch marks.

Contrary to myths and modern marketing claims, there currently are no reliable ways for a woman to prevent stretch marks! Many expensive creams and lotions are on the market, but most have never been proven to decrease the rate of stretch mark formation. Creams are absorbed into the epidermis, the top layer of skin, not the lower dermis where stretch marks occur. The red-purple color of the marks will fade with time to a paler color. After pregnancy, a dermatologist can perform laser treatment or dermabrasion to attempt to remove them.

Acne

myth: If you have acne during your pregnancy, you are having a boy because of all the testosterone coursing through your system.

FACT: The condition of your skin has nothing to do with the gender of your child.

Acne is another skin disorder that may affect some pregnant women. It is most likely due to hormonal changes. This acne can occur on the face but may spread to the chest and back. Over-the-counter medications, such as those containing benzoyl peroxide or salicylic acid, appear safe. Your doctor may also prescribe a topical antibiotic solution such as erythromycin or clindamycin, which may be used during pregnancy. However, isotretinoin should never be used during pregnancy because it is one of the rare medications that can cause birth defects (see section on medications in Chapter 1, pages 26 and 28).

Tiny, itchy bumps

Itchy little bumps, called *prurigo*, can occur anywhere and anytime. They usually break out in patches on the trunk, arms, and legs. We don't know what causes them, but they can be treated with oral anti- histamines such as Benadryl or topical steroid creams.

Varicose veins

As your baby and uterus grow, they place pressure on your pelvic vessels, slowing down the blood flow from your legs to your heart and causing veins to swell in your legs, vulva, and anus. These are called varicose veins, and when they form around your anus, they are called *hemorrhoids*. They do not affect the baby but may cause pain, discom- fort, and swelling in the mother. Although you may not be able to pre- vent them completely, try the following to help alleviate some of the symptoms:

- Wear support stockings. We know they are tight and can make you hot, but they can really work for swelling and leg cramps.
- Avoid sitting or standing for prolonged periods. Move around intermittently to get the blood circulation going.
- Elevate your legs.
- Exercise regularly.

Increased hair growth

myth: If you cut your hair while you are pregnant, you baby will have vision problems.

FACT: We hope that it is obvious that there is no relationship between cutting your hair and the development of your baby's eyes.

During pregnancy, estrogen and androgen hormones change the nor- mal pattern of hair growth by shifting more hairs into the growth phase and out of the shedding phase. The hair on your head may sud- denly become the longer, thicker mane of your dreams, but you may also notice increased hair growth on parts of your body where you really don't want it: on your face, chest, abdomen, and arms. You may wax, shave, use electrolysis, and tweeze, but remember to use clean supplies. Luckily, these changes will return to normal within about six months after you deliver your baby.

Leukorrhea (Vaginal Discharge)

One of the most common complaints of pregnant women is an increase in vaginal discharge, or *leukorrhea*. You may notice that your underwear is constantly a little damp, necessitating frequent underwear or panty liner changes throughout the day. The elevated estrogen levels of pregnancy increase cervical mucus production. Leukorrhea is not associated with itching or an odor. The discharge may be white, yellow, or clear. Although vaginal discharge may be uncomfortable, it is normal and doesn't indicate that anything is wrong with the pregnancy.

Vaginal infections are also common in pregnancy due to the changes in hormonal levels and pH balance. Some of the following require treatment.

Bacterial vaginosis (BV) occurs when there is an imbalance in the normal bacterial flora of the vagina, resulting in an overgrowth of the bacteria Gardnerella. Patients will often complain of a fishy odor. BV is not transmitted sexually and can be treated with oral or vaginal antibiotics. Although BV has been loosely associated with preterm births, we do not routinely screen for BV in asymptomatic pregnant women because treating it has not been shown to definitively prevent preterm births.[2]

Candidiasis (yeast) is caused by a yeast called *Candida albicans*. It may cause itching, burning, and swelling of the vagina or vulva or both along with a thick, white-yellow vaginal discharge. If the yeast does not cause any symptoms, you do not need to treat it. Symptomatic pregnant women may use antifungal vaginal creams or suppositories. Aside from the irritation and discomfort for the mom, Candidiasis does not cause any harm to the baby.

Trichomonas may cause a foamy vaginal discharge causing itching and irritation. It is easily treated with oral antibiotics. Because trichomonas can be passed sexually, your partner should be treated as well.

Constipation and Heartburn

myth: If you have a lot of heartburn during your pregnancy, your baby will be born with a lot of hair.

FACT: We would have written this one off as an old wives' tale right off the bat, until we read an interesting recent study that followed sixty-four pregnant women. In that very small sample, the results tentatively found the heartburn-hair connection to be true![3] In our combined experience, however, there hasn't been much of a correlation. Alane had terrible heartburn with her first son, Matthew. She had Tums in her bag at all times. And Matthew was practically bald for the first two years of his life! Yvonne had horrible heartburn when pregnant with both of her children, Ryan and Kylie, and neither one had an abundance of hair. After reading the study, we've each been taking our own unofficial survey whenever we see a baby with a lot of hair, and so far, none of those mothers remembers having much heartburn.

Constipation and heartburn are common symptoms related to the production of the hormone progesterone. Progesterone relaxes smooth muscle cells so that everything happening inside your body happens a lot slower. Constipation and bloating occur because the small and large intestines move more slowly, resulting in more water absorption and therefore firmer stools. Constipation can be treated with dietary changes such as increasing your intake of water, eating fresh fruits and vegetables, and eating more high-fiber foods. In addition, stool softeners, fiber additives, and laxatives can be used. In severe cases, an enema may be necessary.

Heartburn, or acid reflux, occurs due to relaxation of the smooth muscle sphincter that separates the esophagus from the stomach. As this sphincter loosens, the acid from your stomach goes back up the esophagus, which leads to the classic burning sensation and bad taste.

Try the following to alleviate your symptoms of heartburn:

- Eat small, frequent meals.
- Avoid lying flat or bending over after eating for at least three hours.
- Don't eat two to three hours before bedtime.
- Use over-the-counter antacids (Tums, Maalox, or Mylanta). Consult your doctor before taking any medicines, and ask him or her what to do if these remedies don't relieve your heartburn. Prescription medications may be needed.

Braxton Hicks Contractions

Back in 1872, an obstetrician named J. Braxton Hicks observed that the uterine muscle contracts painlessly beginning in the first trimester. By the second trimester, these contractions can be felt through the skin, and by the third trimester, they can become quite frequent.

If you have Braxton Hicks contractions, you may feel them as early as your second trimester. These contractions feel like a tightening or balling up of the uterus that is irregular and nonrhythmic. They are not painful. Not everyone will experience these contractions, but some women will have them regularly. The presence of Braxton Hicks does not mean that you will deliver early.

If Braxton Hicks contractions occur more than five to six times per hour, you should hydrate with a few glasses of water and then lie down to rest. If the tightening of the uterus persists and becomes regular and painful, you should contact your doctor.

How do you distinguish Braxton Hicks contractions from true labor contractions? True labor contractions are regular, rhythmic, and grow stronger in intensity over time. They generally will not go away despite drinking fluids and resting. And most importantly, unlike Braxton Hicks contractions, true labor contractions will cause a change in your cervix.

▶ ▶ ▶ THE OVERLY EAGER UTERUS

An experienced labor and delivery RN, our patient April was well versed in identifying uterine contractions. When she was pregnant with her first baby, she began having regular Braxton Hicks contractions at twenty-two weeks. We did every possible test to ensure that these contractions were not preterm labor. First, we measured April's cervical length and monitored her cervix for dilation, which never happened. Then we placed her on bed rest, and she ended up delivering after her due date. With her second pregnancy, April started contracting again, but this time we were aware that she just happens to have a uterus that is prone to contractions, not one that dilates early. April's story illustrates a few things: Although most people experience Braxton Hicks contractions later in their pregnancies, these false contractions can start early. And having Braxton Hicks contractions doesn't mean you won't go on to have a term delivery.

—Yvonne ◀ ◀ ◀

Changing Doctors

myth: After you're into your eighth month of pregnancy, it's too late to change doctors.

FACT: We don't recommend it, but sometimes a woman is better off changing doctors, right up until delivery.

All three of us have experienced pregnancy from both sides of the operating theater—as doctors and as patients. We take seriously a woman's need to be happy with the doctor she's chosen. We've all had patients who have come to us when they weren't happy with their previous doctors, and conversely, we've all been "rejected" by a few patients and replaced by other doctors they liked better. We've come to the shared realization that, if a patient truly isn't happy with a doctor, she probably is better off seeing someone else.

Obviously, your goal is to get the right doctor from the start. Research carefully and do your part to keep the lines of communication open between you and your health care provider. We don't recommend changing doctors during a pregnancy, but there are times when it can't be avoided. If you decide to change doctors, the process is not difficult. You need to sign a release of medical records to transfer your file to a new provider. Some women don't want to confront their previous doctors face to face, and are relieved to learn that they can easily transfer their records without interacting with him or her. You can have your new doctor's office process the release, or you can simply ask the front office staff at the old office to send the records over to your new doctor.

Of course, you have the option of telling your doctor that you are leaving and why. We advise patients that it doesn't hurt to say something and give the reasons. If you're upset with a doctor or a person on the staff or the doctor did something that you didn't like, how would the person ever know there was a problem unless you spoke up? Who knows—maybe in the future that doctor or staff member might change that policy or behavior. All three of us would prefer to understand if there is a way we can serve our patients better, rather than be left scratching our heads over why a patient switched.

Adjusting Your Activities

▶ ▶ ▶ MY EXERCISE ROUTINES

Of the three of us, I am admittedly the worst about regular exercise. Despite the fact that I played a lot of competitive sports when I was younger, work and family obligations made it hard for me to keep up with a regular exercise routine—except when I am pregnant. It must be some sort of mothering guilt that overtakes me. I can be lazy for myself but not for my babies!

I became a huge fan of prenatal yoga. It was a rare hour of quiet, meditative "me and baby" time, and a chance to stretch and be in tune with my changing body. Also, it was an opportunity to be with other women going through the same experiences as I was and learn from their joy and concerns.

Prenatal yoga is great for your hips, lower back, and pelvis. I am convinced that it helps you during labor and helps ease the pushing process. Whatever exercise you choose, make sure you do it—for you and your baby. I recently resumed my yoga practice (despite the fact that I am not pregnant), and still enjoy it very much. It makes me happy to see my two small boys imitate me in some of the poses, saying "Om."

—Alane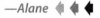

By the midpoint of the second trimester, which is around twenty weeks, the uterus has increased in size so much that the top of it is now at the level of your belly button.

As your belly grows bigger, it may be more difficult to do the kinds of exercises that involve twisting movements. Activities such as tennis, golf, and even some yoga moves might prove to be a little more challenging. You may also find it is harder to jog or run because it will feel like you're bouncing a cantaloupe on your bladder. In addition, you may actually lose urine as you bounce up and down.

As this trimester progresses, you may need to make some adjustments to your fitness routine. However, low-impact activities such as swimming, walking, and riding a stationary bike are effective ways to get a cardiovascular workout. And our favorite, prenatal yoga, can be both a means of gentle exercise and an aid to keeping the body limber for the hard work of childbirth that lies ahead.

Second Trimester Tests

Sometimes, we have the privilege of having our patients' mothers or mothers-in-law present at routine OB visits. It's interesting and fun for us whenever grandmothers are present. We always feel that we learn something from their wisdom and experiences. Having multiple generations of moms in one room is also a good reminder of how far modern obstetrics has progressed through the decades, or even in recent years. When grandparents see their future grandchild on that ultrasound screen, they'll often gasp in amazement and tell us that they never imagined it would be possible to see a baby before birth. They also remember their own experiences of uncertainty and fear, and express awe at the number of tests that their daughters can take to reassure them that their pregnancy is a healthy one.

Indeed, a myriad of tests are now available to pregnant moms. The goal of any prenatal test is to gain information that will reassure you that your baby is healthy. The odds are unlikely that your baby may have some medical issues, but if it does, test results can then help guide both you and your medical team to be better prepared for the outcome. Remember, all these tests are optional, and you have the right to decline any and all tests offered to you.

"Can you tell yet if it's a boy or a girl?" is one of the first questions many parents-to-be want us to answer. Sometimes, they even ask it at their first visit, at six or seven weeks. The second trimester is the soonest you can find out the sex of your baby through ultrasound (see Figures 4-8 and 4-9) or amniocentesis, if you didn't find out through CVS in the first trimester.

Do you see a penis or the "hamburger sign?" It may sound strange, but many things in medicine are described in terms of food. And interestingly enough, on the ultrasound, the vulva of a baby girl looks like a hamburger. The two labia on either side looks like the two buns on a hamburger!

Structural Ultrasound

▶ ▶ ▶ TO KNOW OR NOT TO KNOW?

A charming young couple came in for their routine OB visit, filled with enthusiasm and wide-eyed excitement for the journey on which they were embarking. They were planning on having their structural ultrasound the following week. My patient was excited and wanted to know the baby's gender as soon as possible. Her partner, on the other hand, explained that it had always been his family's tradition to wait until the birth. After quite a debate, I suggested that on the date of the ultrasound, the gender of the baby be written on a piece of paper enclosed in an envelope to be taken home. And should they decide to find out, they would have the opportunity to find out together. The parents-to-be breathed a sigh of relief and agreed on this compromise solution.

—Alane ◀ ◀ ◀

We obtain a structural ultrasound at eighteen to twenty weeks of pregnancy. At this time, parents who want to know the gender of their baby can discover whether they're having a boy or a girl. Now you know why many patients are excited when it's time for their structural ultrasound. But as doctors, we are more interested in whether the baby is formed normally. We want to evaluate the details of the major parts of the brain, heart, kidneys, bladder, and stomach; the insertion of the umbilical cord into the abdomen; and the spinal cord, arms, legs, and face. In addition, we assess the location of the placenta, amniotic fluid, and baby's position.

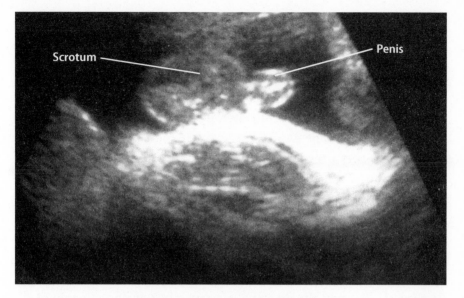

Figure 4-8: Ultrasound of Male Anatomy

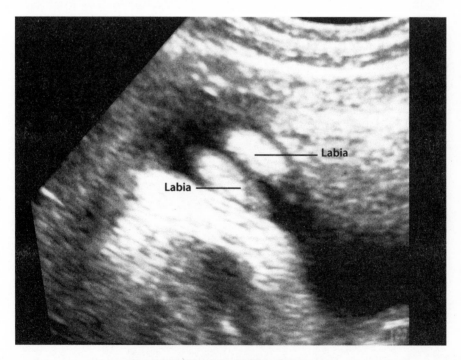

Figure 4-9: Ultrasound of Female Anatomy

We also have the ability to evaluate the blood flow through the umbilical cord so we can determine whether the baby is receiving all the nutrients it needs. Lastly, by measuring the baby's head, abdomen, and femur (thigh bone) length, we can estimate the size and weight of the baby. These measurements not only allow us to confirm proper dating for the pregnancy but also give us information about the baby's growth.

But does every pregnancy require such an ultrasound? If a medical complication is affecting your pregnancy, you usually will receive a structural ultrasound, and potentially quite a few more to monitor the baby throughout the duration. But if you are considered a low-risk mom, you may not be offered one of these ultrasounds because studies have shown that pregnancy outcome is not significantly improved by the routine use of structural ultrasounds in low-risk pregnant women.[4] Ultimately, the decision as to whether or not you should receive a structural ultrasound should be made between you and your doctor.

Our opinion is that the structural ultrasound has many advantages. It is true that birth defects are rare, even in our busy practice located in Los Angeles. But knowing about the presence of fetal abnormalities before birth gives everyone time to figure out what special preparations may be necessary in the delivery room. This information also gives parents a chance to mentally, emotionally, and financially make themselves ready for whatever changes those complications might require. And having seen our own children on that ultrasound screen well before their birthdays, all three of us agree—you can't help but feel more bonded to your pregnancy when face to face with the little person growing inside you.

▶ ▶ ▶ KNOWLEDGE IS POWER

We can think of only one word to describe our operating room tech nurse, Isabella: "Awesome!" Isabella is always on top of things and can anticipate anything that can or might happen in a surgical setting.

When Isabella was in the middle of her second pregnancy, she began working at our hospital. At her structural ultrasound, she found out that her baby had *gastroschisis*, a condition where the fetal abdominal wall fails to close properly, and parts of the baby's abdominal organs, such as the intestines or liver, are found outside the baby's body, floating in the amniotic fluid. Because we were aware of this abnormality before the baby's birth, we were able to make special plans for the delivery. In addition, Isabella received predelivery counseling from pediatricians about what to expect after the birth.

On the scheduled delivery date, we had arranged to have a team of specialists—nurses, pediatric surgeons, and a transport team—standing by. We safely delivered her beautiful baby girl by cesarean and transported her just moments after birth to the Children's Hospital, where a pediatric surgical team was waiting for her arrival. She underwent a successful surgery to correct the defect that same day. She is four years old now and healthy as can be. And Isabella continues to amaze us in the operating room on a daily basis.　◀ ◀ ◀

As much as we are advocates of structural ultrasounds, keep in mind that even when such an ultrasound is performed by a highly skilled ultrasonographer, physicians can identify only 60 to 70 percent of structural birth defects.

3D and 4D ultrasounds

The standard ultrasound in obstetrics is two-dimensional, measuring objects in length and width using sound waves to bounce off tissues like echoes. As the echoes return to the transducer, they are converted into pictures. Two-dimensional (2D) ultrasounds can be used to evaluate almost all fetal parts with great accuracy. In recent years, 3D and 4D ultrasounds have been developed. In 3D, thousands of images are collected at once and made into pictures that include the third dimension, depth. In 4D, the 3D image also shows movement. Both types of ultrasound can be performed by a doctor or an ultrasound technician.

No clear evidence exists about the consequences of using these ultrasounds. They appear safe, but they are a new technology so we cannot evaluate any long-term effects that repeated exposure may have on fetal tissues. Medically, most fetal abnormalities can be diagnosed with the standard 2D method. Although some fetal conditions may be better visualized with 3D and 4D images, most 3D and 4D ultrasounds are performed to generate mementos for the parents, not to determine if your baby is healthy.

The Quad Test

The quad test is the third part of the genetic screening program discussed in Chapter 3. The quad test is a blood test taken between fifteen weeks and twenty weeks of pregnancy. It screens for Down syndrome (trisomy 21), trisomy 18, neural tube defects, abdominal wall defects, and a rare cholesterol defect in the baby called Smith-Lemli-Opitz Syndrome (SLOS).

As with all genetic tests, the quad test is optional. Patients often ask us whether or not this test is recommended. There is no right or wrong choice; your decision is between you, your family and your doctor.

The quad test measures four substances in the woman's blood:

- Human chorionic gonadotropin (hCG): a hormone made by the placenta
- Unconjugated estriol: a hormone made by the fetal adrenal glands, fetal liver, and placenta
- Inhibin A: a protein made by the ovaries and placenta
- Alpha feto-protein (AFP): a protein made by the fetal liver

The accuracy of the quad test follows:

- Down syndrome: 80 percent of cases will be detected
- Trisomy 18: 67 percent of cases will be detected
- Neural tube defects:

    Spina bifida: 80 percent of cases will be detected
    Anencephaly: 97 percent of cases will be detected
    Abdominal wall defects (gastroschisis, omphalocele):
      85 percent of cases will be detected

- SLOS: 60 percent of cases will be detected

Note that detection rates of the integrated screen, which is a combination of the first trimester test and the quad test, are 90 percent for

Down syndrome and 81 percent for trisomy 18 (see Chapter 3, Table 3-1, pages 120–121).

Remember that the quad test is only a screening test, which is different from a diagnostic test. A screening test will tell you your chance of having a baby with one of these disorders but does not give you a definite answer. A positive screening test does not mean that your baby has the affected condition; it means that you have a higher risk of having a baby with one of the conditions. You will be referred for formal genetic counseling and a structural ultrasound, and be offered amniocentesis, a diagnostic test that has a 99 percent accuracy. The vast majority of patients have screen negative results. However, remember that a negative test does not mean that your baby will not have the condition. Unfortunately, yours could be that one baby out of ten thousand that has Down syndrome.

The quad test has a 5 percent false positive rate, which means there is a 5 percent chance that the blood test will screen positive for a defect when the baby is normal.

Amniocentesis

▶ ▶ ▶ MY AMNIO APPOINTMENT

I'm at my perinatologist's office. On most days, we'd be here discussing the status of one of our shared patients, but this time, it's my turn to be the patient. His assistant greets my husband and me and ushers us inside for our amniocentesis counseling appointment. Several weeks ago, my husband asked me briefly about what the test was for. Today, however, he grabs my arm and asks me, "Do you *have* to get this done?"

I tell him, "No, we do not *have* to get this done," but it will give us more information about the health of the baby—I'm thirty-five and have a higher chance of birth defects. We go through the counseling, sign the consent form, and are led to the room where the amniocentesis will be performed. The doctor places the abdominal probe over my belly, and we can see little seventeen-week-old Matthew swimming around, content as can be. The doctor then looks for a nice pocket of fluid where the needle will be placed. I am looking intently at the screen the entire time. He cleans my lower belly and then there's a quick sharp sensation on my skin, much the same as when you get your blood drawn. As the needle enters my uterine wall, I feel mild cramping at the insertion site. I can see the glimmer of the needle in the pocket of amniotic fluid on the ultrasound, and about ten seconds later, I hear the words, "Finished." The doctor shows me Matthew again to reassure me that he is just fine.

—*Alane*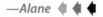

Amniocentesis (see Figure 4-10) is a second trimester diagnostic test usually performed between fifteen to twenty weeks of pregnancy. It gives you a definitive answer to the question "Does my baby have normal chromosomes?" It will also tell you the gender and whether or not your baby has a neural tube defect or an abdominal wall defect. Amniocentesis is 99 percent accurate.

Because the long needle we use can look intimidating, amniocentesis has a scary reputation, but it's a relatively easy and quick proce-

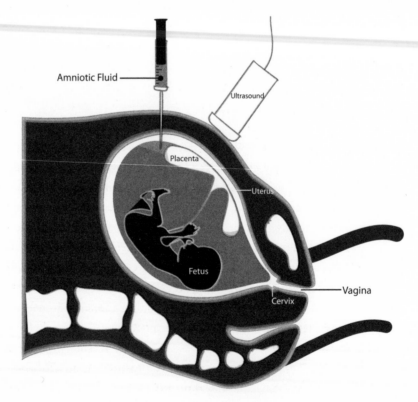

Figure 4-10: Amniocentesis

dure. A *perinatologist,* an obstetrician who specializes in high-risk obstetrics, usually performs the procedure. With the patient lying on her back, the doctor uses an ultrasound to look at the fetus, measure its size, and examine the gross structure of the baby to check for any obvious anomalies.

Next, a nurse or an assistant holds the transducer (the ultrasound device that we put on the abdomen) over a pocket of amniotic fluid, while the doctor cleans the skin where the needle will be placed with an antibacterial solution. An anesthetic is usually not necessary. The ultrasound is used to guide the placement of the needle into the pocket of fluid, so the doctor can see at all times precisely where the needle is going and where it is placed in relation to the baby. Approximately 20 milliliters (one-half ounce) of amniotic fluid is obtained.

After the doctor removes the needle, he or she checks the baby one more time to make sure the heart is beating well. The mom is instructed to rest for the remainder of the day, to avoid exercise and sexual intercourse for twenty-four hours, and to take it easy for a day or two following. We also generally will advise patients not to travel somewhere far for about two weeks after the procedure in case a problem occurs.

Complications related to amniocentesis are small and rare. The procedure may cause some cramping and spotting and a small leakage of amniotic fluid through the vagina. However, if you notice severe abdominal pain, a large amount of fluid leakage through your vagina, or a fever of 100.4 Fahrenheit or greater, call your doctor immediately for an evaluation.

In the past, the risk of miscarriage due to amniocentesis was one in two hundred. In recent years, however, the rate is now one in five hundred. The complications from amniocentesis are not usually from the needle "poking," or injuring, the baby. As described, the perinatologist has a visual on the baby and the needle at all times. It is true that on very rare occasions the needle can contact the baby, usually from the baby moving into the needle rather than the doctor hitting the baby, but the likelihood of this happening is quite small. Instead, the likeliest risk of this procedure that can lead to losing the baby is related to infection. Despite the fact that the abdominal skin is cleaned and a sterile needle is used, there is always a small risk that an infection will occur. Also, if the small hole in the amniotic sac made by the needle does not reseal and instead ruptures, the baby will be exposed to all the germs in the vagina and the outside world, which can lead to infection and miscarriage.

So in which situations are patients offered amniocentesis?

- If a woman requests it. In the past, we offered amniocentesis to women who were thirty-five years or older at their due date. Current recommendations are that no matter what the maternal age, the mother should be allowed to have the procedure if she wants it.
- If the results of the first or second trimester blood screening tests return positive.
- If the mother had a previous baby with a chromosomal abnormality.
- If the patient or partner has a chromosomal abnormality.
- If a major birth defect is discovered on structural ultrasound.
- If both parents are carriers of an autosomal recessive genetic disorder (see Chapter 1).

Some patients ask us, "What should I do?" We can only give them the relevant information and statistics and share our own personal experiences with amnios. In the end, it's your choice.

Another common question women ask is "Why should I have an amniocentesis if I'm going to continue the pregnancy regardless of the results?" In that case, you certainly don't have to do an amniocentesis. On the other hand, the procedure can provide you with valuable information, allowing you to prepare for any special needs your child may have.

Gestational Diabetes Screening and Diagnostic Tests

Gestational diabetes (diabetes that develops during pregnancy) and pregestational diabetes are discussed in detail in Chapter 9. Screening for gestational diabetes takes place between twenty-four and twenty-eight weeks of pregnancy. If you have additional risk factors for diabetes, such as having had gestational diabetes with a previous pregnancy, your doctor may recommend that you do the screening test earlier in the pregnancy. Based on a recent conference on gestational diabetes, some doctors may choose not to screen every pregnant woman but to screen based on whether the patient belongs in the low-, average-, or high-risk category.

In our practice, we screen everyone between twenty-four and twenty-eight weeks.

50-gram oral glucose test

In this test, you drink 50 grams of a glucose solution, and take a blood test one hour later. You do not need to be fasting, and the test can be performed at any time of day. If your blood glucose level is more than 130 to 140 mg/dL, your test is positive. About 20 percent of women will test positive and will need to complete the second part of the test (the 100-gram test) to make the diagnosis of gestational diabetes.

Many women dread the one-hour test because they have been warned by other moms that the drink tastes terrible and causes nausea or the jitters. Rest assured: Although you may not enjoy the drink, it is flavored, carbonated, and easily consumed in five minutes. In addition, the amount of sugar in the drink will raise your blood sugar about as much as one slice of white bread, so you should not feel abnormally hyped up on sugar.

100-gram oral glucose tolerance test

In the second phase of the test, you follow a high carbohydrate diet for three days (meaning you should consume a diet rich in items such as whole-wheat bread, pasta, rice, and fruit). Then you fast overnight for eight to fourteen hours and have your first blood test in the morning. Following the fasting glucose test, you drink a 100-gram glucose solution. Blood is then drawn at one hour, two hours, and three hours after the glucose solution is taken. The diagnosis of gestational diabetes is made if two or more of the four values meet or exceed the cutoffs. If only one of the four values is high, you do not have gestational diabetes. Following are the cutoffs:

Fasting	$\geq$ 95 mg/dL
One hour	$\geq$ 180 mg/dL
Two hours	$\geq$ 155 mg/dL
Three hours	$\geq$ 140 mg/dL

Ultimately, 15 to 20 percent of women who undergo the 100-gram test will be diagnosed with gestational diabetes.

Complete blood cell (CBC) count

In the second trimester, we will often recheck your blood count to see if you have developed anemia. In the same test, we are also able to check your platelet count.

The most common cause of anemia is low iron levels. Because your iron stores are being utilized rapidly to create blood for you and the baby, you may develop anemia as the pregnancy progresses. If we find you to be anemic, you will be asked to take iron supplements in addition to your daily prenatal vitamin.

Platelets are blood cells that act as a kind of glue to stop bleeding. If your doctor tells you that you have a low platelet count, known as thrombocytopenia, try not to worry. Most likely, it is caused by the pregnancy itself. We call this gestational thrombocytopenia. It is usually mild, will not harm the baby, and will resolve after delivery. However, if your platelet count dips too low, your obstetrician may refer you to a hematologist—a blood specialist—to make sure there aren't more serious problems with your platelets. If you develop significant thrombocytopenia, you may not be able to receive an epidural for pain management in labor because it requires placement of a needle near the spinal cord, and complications from bleeding in this area could occur.

Thyroid stimulating hormone (TSH)

Your doctor may also check your thyroid stimulating hormone (TSH) to make sure you do not have undiagnosed thyroid disease.

Potential Complications in the Second Trimester

The following is a list of potential complications that can occur in the second trimester. We have committed an entire chapter (Chapter 9) to address these topics. Remember, the majority of pregnancies progress normally! Most of these conditions are relatively rare, so you may skip this section and Chapter 9 unless you think that they apply to you:

- Preterm labor or premature rupture of membranes: When contractions occur or the water breaks before thirty-seven weeks.
- Preeclampsia: High blood pressure caused by pregnancy (see page 374).
- Gestational diabetes: Elevated blood sugar levels resulting from pregnancy (see page 380).
- Intrauterine growth restriction: When the baby doesn't grow well (see page 415).
- Cervical insufficiency: When the cervix is weak and opens well before term (see page 383).
- Vaginal bleeding from placenta previa: When the placenta implants over the cervix (see page 388).

Our goal in explaining these topics is not to scare you or elicit unnecessary fear but to educate you about what to expect if you are diagnosed with a complication. In the chapter on high-risk pregnancies, Chapter 9, we will talk about the frequency of these problems and their diagnoses, symptoms, and management. We also share real-life stories of women—including ourselves—who have not only survived these conditions but thrived. For every complication just listed, we have seen positive outcomes. Even if diagnosed with a pregnancy complication, with good care and treatment, you can remain healthy and deliver a healthy baby.

Childbirth Classes

At this point, you're probably wondering, "What will the experience of birth be like?" The second trimester is the perfect time to start thinking about the impending birth day. Following are a few of the questions and concerns that our patients most often express:

- "I'm not sure what to expect from the experience. I'd like to give birth as naturally as possible, but I'd like to be open to all possibilities. What are these possibilities?"

- "I'm determined to do this without pain meds or epidural. It's very important for me to experience everything."
- "As soon as I walk on to the labor and delivery floor, I'd like to be sure there will be an anesthesiologist to place my epidural. Can I reserve the epidural now, please?"
- "Do I need an episiotomy? Do you do one on everyone? How do you know you need one?"
- "Do you use vacuums or forceps?"
- "How do I know when to come into the hospital?"
- "I'd like to breastfeed. What do I do?"
- "I've never changed a diaper in my life."
- "Can I have a tour of the hospital?"

It's not always possible to get all these answers from your busy obstetrician, so we strongly urge our patients to take childbirth classes if they're available. Most parents should sign up for these classes by the end of the second trimester. If you're a first-time mother, childbirth classes can give you a better idea of what's going to happen on the other side of those hospital doors after you go into labor. A good childbirth class presents an overview of the entire process: from the IV setup, to the fetal monitoring, to the actual labor bed. Women and their partners can familiarize themselves with the various procedures and terminologies involved, and feel like they're in a safe place where they can ask any questions, such as "What's an episiotomy?" and "What happens with an epidural?" Getting on top of this information goes a long way toward making the childbirth experience less frightening.

Taking these classes requires a time commitment, and often patients don't feel that they can sacrifice so many hours. Some women or couples will be able to commit to a two-hour, once-a-week childbirth class that lasts eight or ten weeks, while others prefer a one-day crash course. If your time is limited, you can always check out a DVD at the library to view at your leisure in the comfort of your home.

We feel that anything parents can do to prepare will be helpful when the big day arrives. Here's a comparison that the three of us like to use: When we were in medical school, we wanted to be as familiar as possible with every surgical procedure we'd have to do, before we actually performed the operation hands-on. So before we entered an operating room to hold the instruments ourselves, we had read everything there was to read about, say, cesarean deliveries, asked our professors many questions, and observed other doctors performing the procedure. Because we were so well prepared beforehand, we felt a lot more comfortable when it came time to do the operation ourselves. Similarly, while childbirth and breastfeeding classes obviously can't totally prepare you for the real deal, you'll remove a lot of anxiety and stress if you can familiarize yourself with the process ahead of time.

In these classes, some childbirth instructors teach relaxation techniques that can be incredibly effective for pain management. But be warned: The perception of pain is a very individual experience. All the classes in the world cannot predict the level of pain you will have to deal with and how you will cope with it when it happens.

Some classes also offer a section on breastfeeding as well as basic childcare. They may also teach infant CPR. These classes provide both knowledge and reassurance to make parents more comfortable with how to care for their new infant.

Most people who take birthing classes are first-time moms. Other moms might want to take refresher courses, especially when it's been a long time since they had their last baby.

Classes may be offered by the hospital where you will deliver your baby or at local community centers. Ask your health care provider for recommendations.

The Second Trimester Comes to an End

By the time you near the end of the second trimester, you begin to develop that pregnant woman waddle, or wider stance, caused by your center of gravity shifting as your belly grows. Suddenly, it's harder to get up from your bed or get out of that chair. "I can't see what's down on the floor by my feet!" is a frequent complaint. Even your loosest pair of regular blue jeans becomes impossible to button. Now, you finally need to buy some maternity clothes.

We are always happy as our moms pass the twenty-eight-week mark. Should the baby need to be delivered for some reason, he or she has an excellent chance of survival after this point, with continued care in the NICU (neonatal intensive care unit). Of course, we don't want you to have your baby quite yet—not at least until you pass thirty-seven weeks when the child is considered term.

As you enter your third trimester, everything begins to get harder with your growing belly and increased swelling. We tell our patients that, through any growing discomfort, they should keep their eyes on the prize. At the end of this odyssey, you will hold your own child in your arms—and the day that will happen is coming up sooner than you think. Congratulations on finishing your second trimester!

chapter five

THE THIRD TRIMESTER:
29 TO 42 WEEKS

▶ ▶ ▶ **THE END IN SIGHT**

The third trimester is the end of the long road. I spent the first trimester bent over the toilet and even made a few trips to the hospital for dehydration. The second trimester was a breeze. I ate a lot and felt almost, dare I say, sexy? My hair was thick, my nails were lovely, my cleavage was amazing, and I honestly felt like I had a glow.

By the time the third trimester began, I had forgotten the troubles of the first and was enjoying the highs of the second, but then all of a sudden things changed. I can no longer see my feet, and to be honest I really don't want to since they are so swollen. That sexy feeling is gone, only to be replaced with feeling like a beached whale. It takes an awful lot of work to turn over at night!

—Linda, Allison's patient ◀ ◀ ◀

The Final Haul

The third trimester extends from twenty-nine to forty-two weeks. A baby born in the third trimester, even prematurely, has an excellent shot at surviving in the outside world. When a baby makes it to twenty-eight weeks, we breathe a sigh of relief, because even if the baby comes early, he or she has more than a 90 percent chance of surviving with good NICU care. (See Chapter 9, page 397, on preterm labor and the survivability of preemies.)

During this final leg of your pregnancy, you can continue all your normal daily activities as long as you feel up to them and haven't encountered any complications. Women can continue to work, drive, exercise, and, if they are in school or college, continue their studies— unless they have been advised by their doctors not to do so. You can even have sex right up to delivery day, as long as you're healthy, although you may not always feel like it.

Visiting Your Doctor

Visits to the doctor will be much more frequent during this trimester. This is the time when most complications occur, so we need to monitor your blood pressure and baby's growth more closely. Generally, you will be seen every two to three weeks, and then weekly during the last month. You can expect the following to occur at each visit:

- Blood pressure evaluation
- Weight recording
- Urine dip for protein and glucose
- Doppler assessment of fetal heart rate
- Fundal height measurement
- Evaluation for bleeding, pain, leakage of amniotic fluid, and fetal movements
- Cervical exam beginning at 37 weeks (see below)
- Review of any questions/concerns

During the last month of pregnancy, when you have weekly doctor's visits, you may undergo your first cervical exam. Your doctor or midwife will feel your cervix to see if it has begun to prepare for birth by dilating and effacing (more on this on page 222 in Chapter 6). Although we cannot predict the exact day you will deliver, the exam gives us an idea whether birth is impending or if you have more time. In addition, we can confirm that the baby has his or her head down and assess if the baby has descended into the pelvis. The cervical exam can be mildly uncomfortable. In addition, you may encounter some light, bright red bleeding after the exam or later when you use the bathroom. Don't worry. The blood isn't coming from your baby; instead, the soft cervix bleeds easily when touched. This bleeding or spotting can last for one to three days.

Your Third Trimester Experiences

For moms-to-be, the realization that something momentous is pending—that they're about to usher a new human life into the world—usually hits home during the early part of the third trimester. By this stage, a mother should clearly feel her baby moving and actually be able to see the baby's movement through her belly.

At this turning point, the experience of being pregnant becomes decidedly more exaggerated, as well as more challenging. At twenty weeks, a lot of our patients can still fit into their jeans. They can camouflage their pregnancy and their mobility isn't too impaired. By the third trimester, though, things have changed. For moms who have succeeded so far in hiding their condition from coworkers, the jig is up. The day a woman realizes that she's not going to disguise her pregnancy with a big dress or a loose pair of pants can be a transitional milestone.

▶ ▶ ▶ FEEL FREE TO COMMENT

I often look down to see if I am wearing some sort of sign that reads, "Everyone, please tell me exactly what you are thinking!" By the time I made it to the third trimester I thought I had heard every woman's story of her painful, long, hard-fought deliveries. When people see a pregnant woman, I believe that it automatically triggers this need to share their experience and then comment on how I look. So now I have really heard it all. "Oh my God! You are huge!" "You look exhausted." "You poor thing." "Mommy look, she has a pumpkin in her shirt!" My personal favorite is "What's your due date? Oh honey, you won't make it." I usually respond with a half smile and an "Okay, thank you?"

—Bethany, Allison's patient ◀ ◀ ◀

As the weeks wear on and your baby gets heavier, you're going to experience the physical discomforts of being pregnant. You may feel more pain in your lower back and hips, and pressure in your pelvis. You're more likely to have heartburn, and you may need to eat smaller meals. You definitely shouldn't eat right before bedtime, unless you want to pay for it all night long. Finding a comfortable sleeping position—and sleep in general—becomes more difficult. All these conditions progressively exacerbate until your baby is delivered.

Group B Streptococcus Screening

In the third trimester, no routine blood tests are performed. You may receive an ultrasound to document the position of the baby and to estimate the fetal weight. All women undergo testing for a bacteria called Group B streptococcus.

Group B streptococcus (GBS) isn't a disease you catch from a dirty restaurant fork or a toilet seat. The truth is, the human body is filled with various strains of bacteria, both good and bad, that help us carry out basic functions like digestion and elimination. GBS happens to be one of those bacteria; one that takes up housekeeping in a woman's vaginal and/or gastrointestinal tracts. There are no symptoms or consequences for the mom herself if she has Group B strep, nor is it something that she can pass to her sexual partner.

However, GBS is the most common bacterial infection causing newborn death in the United States. If a mother is a GBS carrier, there is a one in two hundred chance that her baby will become infected with the bacteria during a vaginal delivery.[1] The infection manifests in meningitis, sepsis, or pneumonia. Of the term babies who get infected, about 5 percent will die.[2]

Because of the severity of illness in the newborn, we screen all women for GBS between thirty-five and thirty-seven weeks of pregnancy. The test involves taking a swab from the woman's vagina and rectum. If a mother tests positive—20 to 30 percent do—we give her IV antibiotics when she's in labor to prevent transmission of GBS to the baby. With antibiotics, the chance the baby will get a GBS infection decreases from one in two hundred to one in four thousand. The reason we use an IV drip instead of an oral form of the antibiotic is because labor slows the digestion process, potentially rendering the drug ineffective. In addition, the IV-delivered antibiotic will get into your system more quickly to eradicate the bacteria from your vagina. Women who are planning cesareans don't need to take this precaution because the baby doesn't come through the birth canal where the bacteria lives. We still screen for GBS in women who have planned cesarean deliveries, however, just in case the patient goes into labor and there is a delay in the cesarean.

Third Trimester Development of Your Baby

As you approach your due date, your baby's development is also preparing him or her for the grand entrance into the new world (see Table 5-1). After thirty-four weeks, all your baby's working parts are technically functional. His or her fingers and toes will be wiggling, heart will be beating, and brain will be continuing its rapid development. The final organ to mature, the lungs, does so at the thirty-four-week mark. Between thirty-four weeks and forty weeks, the baby will gain fifteen hundred grams (about three-and-a-half pounds).

Table 5-1: The Development of Your Baby in the Third Trimester[3]

Age (weeks)	Length*	Weight	Events
30	40 cm (15.7 in)	1,300 gm (2.9 lb)	Your baby's eyes can fully open. The skin is still slightly wrinkled.
32	42.4 cm (16.7 in)	1,700 gm (3.7 lb)	All ten toenails are present, and if you're having a little boy, his testes are descending.
34	45 cm (17.7 in)	2,100gm (4.6 lb)	Your baby's fingernails are now long enough to reach the finger tips. The skin has smoothed out and is pink.
38	47.4 cm (18.6 in)	2,900 gm (6.4 lb)	The toenails now reach the tip of each toe, and your baby is now plumped up.
40	51.2 cm (20.1 in)	3,400 gm (7.5 lb)	The fingernails have grown long enough to reach beyond the fingertips. Your little boy's testes are now in his scrotum.

*Crown to heel measurement

At the twenty-eight-week mark, the baby is about fifteen inches long and weighs just over two pounds. By the end of this trimester, however, the average baby weighs just over seven pounds. That means your baby is going to gain at least five pounds in a matter of twelve weeks! This acceleration of growth explains why, practically overnight, a mom-to-be suddenly appears to be more pregnant. The rapid growth rate steps up even more as she approaches her last six weeks of pregnancy.

Fetal Movement

Moms-to-be should start to feel their babies moving around twenty weeks of gestation. Especially after twenty-four weeks, you should feel the baby move every day. Some moms will ask if the baby can move too much. The answer to this question is no. When a baby is moving, it means that the baby is getting lots of oxygen and nutrition. Therefore, movement is one of the simplest ways for us to assess fetal well-being. Fetuses have sleep cycles just like newborns. Usually they will be asleep for an hour and then awaken for an hour. If you are trying to feel your baby move during a sleep cycle, you may get worried that something is wrong. Usually, if you give it time, the baby will wake up and start moving around again.

"I feel my baby moving all the time at night, but not during the day." Many moms will tell us that the baby is more active at night. The truth is that the baby doesn't know if it is day or night, and moves the same throughout the twenty-four-hour period. Instead, moms are more perceptive of the baby's movements at night because it is quiet and there are fewer distractions.

Measuring Fetal Kick Counts

How much movement is normal? We have devised a way for you to monitor the baby's movements so you can tell how the baby is doing. This method, called fetal kick counts, helps you learn about your baby's unique daily routine: how your baby moves, when it is active, how long it likes to rest. By familiarizing yourself with your baby's habits, you will know when something seems different. You don't have to strictly record the kick counts unless your doctor instructs you to do so; usually, this is necessary only when a mom has a high-risk condition such as high blood pressure, diabetes, or fetal growth problems, or if she is significantly past her due date.

To perform fetal kick counts, we recommend that you lie down in a quiet place—no TV, no radio, no cell phone. Have something to eat or drink something sweet such as orange juice and then try to feel the baby moving. The baby should move ten times within an hour. Every little flick counts as a movement. Most women—if they are really paying attention—will feel ten movements within ten to fifteen minutes. If you don't feel ten movements within an hour, your baby might be asleep, so count for a second hour. If you still don't feel ten movements, you should call your doctor.

You may feel your baby moving less for several reasons: You may be distracted, the baby could be in the breech position, your placenta may be on the front wall of the uterus, you might have a lot of fat covering the abdominal wall, the amniotic fluid may be low, or the baby may not be getting enough oxygen. Most of these explanations don't indicate anything serious, except the last two. That's why, if you notice a measureable change in your baby's habits, you need to call your doctor to make sure low amniotic fluid or lack of oxygen aren't causing decreased movement. It's unlikely, but it's possible.

So what happens if you feel your baby moving less? First, you will go to your doctor's office or to the hospital, where you will be placed on a fetal monitor to check the baby's heart rate and your uterine activity over a period of time. This is a called a nonstress test, or NST. We will check for certain patterns of the baby's heart rate that could indicate that he or she is not getting enough oxygen. In addition, we will perform an ultrasound to check the amniotic fluid levels. If both evaluations are normal, we can reassure you that your baby is doing fine.

Do the baby's movements slow down closer to the due date? No—babies continue to move as frequently as they did earlier in the pregnancy. However, because the baby is bigger and has less room to move inside the uterus, the sensations may seem more subtle. They may feel like a rolling motion instead of the punches you experienced in the past. You may have to pay closer attention to notice them, but they should still be there.

Every year, we have one or two patients who *never* feel their baby moving. We check the baby's heart rate, monitor the amniotic fluid, and even have the mother look at the ultrasound to visualize the baby moving. But the mother does not feel it at all. We don't have an explanation for this phenomenon, other than the possibility that the nerves in her uterus are not as sensitive.

We also have moms who worry that the baby is moving too much, or are worried that the baby is having a seizure. A baby's movement is the sign that the placenta is working well and the baby is receiving normal amounts of oxygen. The baby may be wiggling because its arm or leg is stuck; this can feel like erratic behavior to the mom. Another possibility is that the baby may be having hiccups, which feel rhythmic, and happen quite frequently toward the end of the pregnancy. Hiccups occur because the baby's phrenic nerve near the diaphragm is stimulated. So don't worry, your baby is not in distress when he or she is having the hiccups.

Normal Fetal Growth

"Is my baby growing normally?" Women often wonder if their baby is big enough . . . or if he or she is too big. As soon as a mom is big enough to be showing, it seems that every person on the street has an opinion about the size of her belly and what it signifies—opinions that are almost always wrong. People will tell a pregnant mom that she's too small for someone in her eighth month or wonder aloud if her baby is growing normally. On the other hand, they may blurt out "God, you're huge!" or ask her if she's carrying multiples. None of these "helpful" opinions coming from a family member, coworker—or especially a total stranger—are usually very comforting—or accurate.

By the time you reach your third trimester, your physician or midwife should be well aware of the general size and growth patterns of your baby. As we mentioned, starting at twenty weeks in the second trimester, we begin to monitor your baby's growth by measuring the fundal height, which stretches from the pubic bone to the top of the uterus. We may also perform periodic ultrasounds that confirm the growth of the baby. So although it's understandable that a mom would be worried about her own or her baby's size—especially if she's been hearing lots of unsolicited comments about it—let your doctor, not your overreactive Aunt Bessy, decide if you should be concerned.

▶ ▶ ▶ YOGA CLASS CRITICS

Stasia was a first-time mom who found a great deal of physical and mental relief in her prenatal yoga classes. Having gone to these classes myself during my own pregnancies, I can attest to the fact that it's impossible not to compare yourself to the other women who are at the same stage as you are in your pregnancy. This was true for Stasia, whose class included several women whom she knew were about the same gestational age as herself. All of these women had bigger bellies than she did, and she found herself barraged by comments like, "You don't even look like you're pregnant!" When Stasia came in for her next visit, she was concerned. "Is my baby growing okay?" I measured her fundal height, which was normal, and explained to her that nothing was wrong. Some women have taut abdomens, are in really good shape, or have a longer torso and consequently don't show as much. Just because other women stick out a lot more doesn't mean that your baby isn't growing well. If you are ever concerned, don't listen to the yoga critics. Listen to your obstetrician or midwife.

—Alane ◀ ◀ ◀

If patients come into our office saying that a well-meaning friend has just told them that they are too big (or too small), we suggest that they let their friend know that they've been measured by the doctor and the baby's growing just fine.

Third Trimester Symptoms

You are now in the home stretch of your pregnancy. For many of us, the third trimester is the most difficult because of our enormous bellies. There is literally just no way of getting around them! These are the days when it's hard to get up from that chair and even harder to turn over in your bed. You can't quite see what's on the floor in front of you, and you've now got that adorable third trimester waddle because your center of gravity is seriously off-kilter. You are probably feeling tired, anxious, and impatient.

On the other hand, this is also a time when you can revel in your sense of excitement and anticipation. You can have fun shopping, checking out different car seats and strollers, not to mention the cute booties and onesies. Then there's the traditional baby shower and all the preparations that entails. So despite the uncomfortable symptoms, keep your eyes on the prize. Your baby is coming soon!

Clumsiness and Falls

By the thirty-sixth week, the baby's rapid growth starts to make the end of the third trimester a lot more uncomfortable. This period is when the extra weight kicks in, taking its toll on your joints and your veins. Just about every part of your body cries out for relief.

Have you ever had the experience of driving a compact car and then switching to a minivan in the same day? You temporarily lose perspective about how much clearance to give your side mirrors, and how far you can back up into a parking space without touching bumpers with the car behind you. In the late third trimester, some women can lose a similar sense of perspective about their body size. We've had patients who burned their bellies when cooking at the stove—so be careful.

As the ligaments and joints in the pelvis loosen to allow for the impending birth, a woman's hips become unstable, leading to more frequent stumbling or even falling. If you slip on your hands, knees, or buttocks, you will most likely not injure the baby. However, if you fall and hit your abdomen, you could cause injury to the placenta or fetus. If such a fall occurs, call your doctor or go to the hospital to be monitored.

Back Pain

Imagine that you have a backpack full of rocks, weighing thirty pounds. You have to carry this backpack around all day, every day, and you can never put it down. No wonder many pregnant women complain of exhaustion, with back and joint discomfort. Lower back pain is one of the most common complaints in the third trimester, occurring in nearly 75 percent of moms. It is more pronounced in women who are overweight or have had poor fitness before their pregnancy.

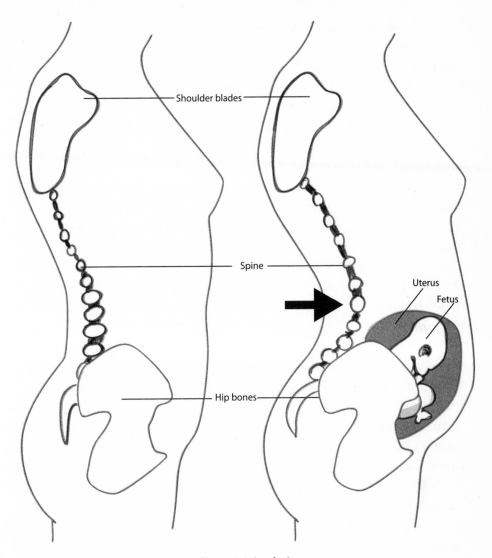

Figure 5-1: Lordosis

The chronic excess weight in the belly pulls the lower spine forward, causing the back muscles to constantly strain as they work to straighten the spine. This new curvature to the lower spine, called *lordosis* (see Figure 5-1), contributes to the dull, achy feeling our patients describe to us. In addition, loss of tone in the abdominal wall muscles puts more pressure on the low back. We often see this in women who do not have good core strength or in women who have had several babies, one after the other.

A simple remedy for back pain is an old-fashioned heating pad, which relaxes the muscles near the spine. First, make sure the pad is not too hot so it doesn't injure the skin. Lie on the heating pad with your legs elevated or your knees bent, taking the pressure off both your lower back and the sciatic nerves. A support belt, like a maternity girdle, can take some of the pressure off as well, and also help realign the back. Uncomfortable moms-to-be can also see a chiropractor or a physical therapist, or use pain relievers such as acetaminophen or creams such as Bengay or Capsaicin.

All three of us, as well as many of our patients, have found prenatal yoga to be a lifesaver. Prenatal yoga stretches the back and the pelvic core while working the inner thighs and hips. By strengthening the core abdominal muscles, yoga both prevents and helps to ease back pain.

Finally, we always advise our patients' partners to massage their long-suffering mom-to-be, as frequently as possible. It's a helpful way to show support, especially during this final stretch of pregnancy.

Neuropathies

When a nerve is injured or compromised, a peripheral *neuropathy* can occur, resulting in pain, tingling, burning, or numbness along the course of the nerve, or dermatome. Neuropathies are common in pregnancy because increased swelling in surrounding tissues causes nerve compression. Also, direct pressure from the uterus can pinch the nerves. The most common types of neuropathy are carpal tunnel syndrome and sciatica.

Carpal tunnel syndrome affects 30 percent of pregnant women. Compression on the median nerve that runs through the wrist causes tingling or burning on the thumb side of the hand. It can also cause weakness or numbness in the fingers and make grasping objects difficult. Carpal tunnel can be worse in women who do jobs that involve repetitive wrist work, such as typing on a computer all day. The treatment for carpal tunnel is to rest the hand in a neutral position with a wrist splint. This allows excess fluids that have accumulated in the wrist joint to flow back up to the heart, relieving nerve compression.

Sciatica is caused by the uterus exerting pressure on the sciatic nerve, which runs down the lower back, through the middle of the buttocks, to the back of the leg. Sciatica can also be caused by swelling near the nerve root as it comes out of the spine. Symptoms include shooting pain down the back of the leg and buttocks, weakness in the leg, and tingling. The treatment includes sessions with a chiropractor or physical therapist.

Other Neuropathies

Similarly, women can get hot spots or numb areas on their abdomen. They will complain that one specific area on their skin feels hot, burning, or numb. This symptom is also due to nerve compression, either from uterine pressure or tissue swelling. As the baby grows and moves out of the way, the compression will be relieved and the symptom will disappear.

Hemorrhoids

Hemorrhoids are enlarged veins, similar to varicose veins, that occur in the rectum and are caused by the increased pressure inside the abdomen from the growing uterus. This pressure causes the surrounding veins to swell. Hemorrhoids are usually just a nuisance but can become more serious. We've even had a patient who had to forgo a vaginal delivery for a cesarean because of severe hemorrhoids. Her hemorrhoid had developed a blood clot within it and became so painful that there was no possibility of her pushing the baby out.

Hemorrhoids can be prevented in some cases by avoiding constipation through increased water and fiber in the diet. After they have formed, you can treat them with over-the-counter hemorrhoid creams, witch hazel, or Tucks pads. Also, soaking the area in warm water in the bathtub, commonly known as a sitz bath, can help. We also encourage women to avoid prolonged periods of sitting. For women who must sit for their jobs, a doughnut-shaped air cushion can be helpful. Hemorrhoids developed during pregnancy will usually go away after delivery but may not disappear completely. In fact, some patients will encounter their first hemorrhoid after delivery. If our patients are still having troubles postpartum, we may refer them to a colorectal surgeon for further treatment.

Bleeding Gums and Bloody Noses

Many women will notice bleeding from their gums when they brush or floss. In addition, they may also be caught completely off guard by spontaneous, unexpected nosebleeds. Increased maternal blood volume is the culprit in both cases. As your total blood content expands from five liters to seven-and-a-half liters, all the blood vessels in your body are going to swell, particularly at the end of your pregnancy. The delicate blood vessels in the mouth and nose also become enlarged and can bleed with very little stimulation. Pregnant women should see a dentist during pregnancy if they have significant gum bleeding. To prevent nosebleeds, you can try keeping your nasal passage moist with over-the-counter saline spray.

Stuffy Nose

About 30 percent of pregnant women will notice an increase in nasal congestion, called *pregnancy rhinitis*. This congestion is due to increased blood volume as well as high estrogen levels. Estrogen causes an increase in mucous production and swelling of the nasal passages. The condition is not dangerous but can definitely become annoying. You can treat rhinitis with saline nasal sprays and antihistamines.

Shortness of Breath

The rapidly growing uterus pushes up on a woman's diaphragm—the muscle that separates the abdominal cavity from the chest cavity and lungs. This growth compromises the amount of space that a woman has for respiratory exchange and reduces her overall lung capacity. Add this to the fact that women who are in their third trimester are bigger, heavier, and perhaps not in the same cardiovascular shape as they were six months before, and you often end up with a frequently winded mom-to-be who does a lot more huffing and puffing. Shortness of breath is a common complaint that has no cure—until we deliver your baby. Some women will find that reclining makes the symptoms worse, so sleeping propped on pillows or in a chair may be helpful.

Breast Changes

Pregnant women experience the first round of breast changes in the first trimester, with both tenderness and appreciable growth. The glands and ducts of the breast, however, continue to mature until delivery.

Think of the breast's structure as a tree: a trunk containing different branches and leaves (see Figure 7-1 on page 300). Milk is made in the leaves, or glands, and travels down the branches, or ducts, and out into the trunk, or nipple. Under the influence of the various pregnancy hormones—estrogen, progesterone, and prolactin—all of those structures grow and multiply.

Most women will go up one to two cup sizes during their pregnancy and gain one or two pounds in their breasts. The discomfort from the increase in size can be distressing. You can mitigate your discomfort by wearing a comfortable pregnancy bra with support.

In the third trimester and sometimes even earlier, women may begin to leak a white or yellow substance from the breast. This is the first sign of *colostrum,* or premilk. About half of women will have leakage as they massage the breast tissue out toward the nipple. However, the presence or absence of leakage does not determine whether you will make a lot of breast milk after delivery. Women with and without leakage can be equally successful at nursing.

Costochondritis (Bad Rib Pain)

Costochondritis is the fancy name for an inflammation between the ribs, especially in the rib joints. As the rib cage expands during pregnancy, the muscles between the ribs are stretched out of place. The result can be a horrible pain in the rib cage that increases when you take a deep breath. Usually a mom will feel a particular spot that is incredibly tender. When not pregnant, the treatment for costochondritis is a nonsteroidal anti-inflammatory (such as ibuprofen), which unfortunately can't be taken during pregnancy. However, you *can* take Tylenol. You can also try a heating pad or therapy from a chiropractor or an acupuncturist.

▶ ▶ ▶ MY PAIN IN THE RIBS

I had costochondritis when I was pregnant with Luke. It was one of the worst and most annoying pains I have ever experienced. One spot on the left side of my back drove me crazy. Every position was uncomfortable. I suffered with the pain for more than two months. When I finally went to deliver Luke, I got an epidural—and the pain was instantly gone. At that moment, I wished I would have had the epidural for the last few months of my pregnancy! After my delivery, the pain never returned.

—Allison ◀ ◀ ◀

Umbilical Hernias

Most people walk around for the majority of their lives rarely thinking about their belly buttons. Pregnant women, however, become acutely aware of their navels. The navel—or umbilicus—is the scar where your umbilical cord was attached when you were a fetus. The scar usually pushes in (an "innie"). But during pregnancy, the pressure from the uterus pushing out from the inside can cause a previous innie to become an "outie." This change is just cosmetic and nothing to worry about.

However, in some cases, the muscle in this area gets so stretched that there is now an opening for the abdominal contents—the intestines—to push through. When this happens, an *umbilical hernia* develops, which means that a portion of small intestine is coming through the weakening in the umbilical area, as shown in Figure 5-2. The woman's outie becomes even larger, and she'll notice it pushes out even more when she's straining, lifting, or coughing. Most umbilical hernias will resolve after delivery. However, if the hernia is very large or painful, it will need to be surgically closed either during pregnancy or postpartum.

Swelling

How much a woman's tissues swell during her pregnancy depends on the individual. A few of our luckier patients have little or no swelling; others suffer incessantly from it. We have a lot of moms who can wear only flip-flops and sandals toward the end of their pregnancies because they can no longer fit into any of their regular shoes.

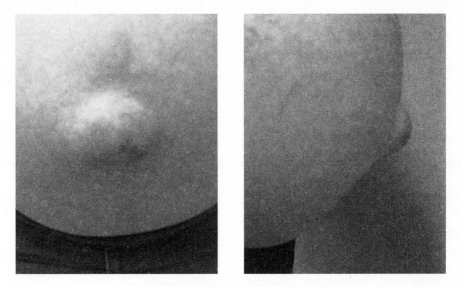

Figure 5-2: Umbilical Hernia

Swelling is a sign that water is leaving the vascular space—the blood vessels—and is being absorbed by the surrounding tissues. We can see this fluid shift as early as the first trimester, but it's more exaggerated by the third, especially in women who are prone to it. Swelling usually occurs in the legs, feet, and hands but can even occur on the abdominal skin—causing the skin to have the texture of an orange peel, called *peau d'orange*.

If you're one of those women who are destined to retain large amounts of fluids in your tissues, don't worry. Most of the time, swelling is merely an annoyance and doesn't indicate that anything is wrong with you or your pregnancy. In some cases, however, excessive swelling has been associated with preeclampsia (discussed in Chapter 9). For this reason, if a patient reports a new onset of swelling, we always check her blood pressure. In addition, if the swelling occurs in only one leg and not the other, you should immediately call your doctor, as this can be the sign of *deep venous thrombosis,* or DVT (a blood clot).

Many moms will notice a shift in their fluids during the day. When a woman lies down to go to sleep at night, the fluids will accumulate in her hands. Upon waking, she finds it hard to make a fist, or she may feel numbness and tingling in her fingertips—a form of carpal tunnel syndrome. As the day goes on and she spends more time upright, the fluids will follow the pull of gravity and move down to her legs and feet. That often means swollen and achy feet at the end of a long day.

To relieve this discomfort, a woman can wear support hose during the day and use wrist splints at night. Taking a swim or a lukewarm bath may also give symptomatic relief. Going for light, brief walks can stimulate circulation and increase the blood return from the legs. However, some pregnant moms who are very large or are retaining an inordinate amount of fluid find even walking unpleasant. We tell our patients with extremely uncomfortable swelling to elevate their legs, lifting them above the level of their heart, to help the swelling go down.

Potential Complications in the Third Trimester

Many of the symptoms we've discussed in this chapter are just common side effects during this last phase of pregnancy. However, more troubling medical conditions may also develop in the third trimester.

Anemia

Anemia is a blood disorder in which a person does not have enough healthy red blood cells, leading to lack of oxygen in tissues. During pregnancy, iron, which is an essential part of hemoglobin in red blood cells, is being used rapidly, both to make fetal blood and to increase maternal blood volume by more than 50 percent. This increase makes enough blood available to nourish the baby through the placenta as well as to protect the woman from becoming anemic after the impending blood loss of delivery. Remember, a nonpregnant woman has about five liters of blood in her body, but in pregnancy, with her expanded blood volume, she'll have about seven-and-a-half liters. About 50 percent of women will become anemic even if they've been taking their prenatal vitamins.

When a mom becomes anemic, she feels unusually tired and dizzy. In severe cases, there is not enough iron for the fetus, and he or she can also become anemic, which can lead to serious consequences such as heart failure. We check for anemia at the beginning of the third trimester. If our tests alert us to the condition, we ask the patient to increase her dietary iron or take additional supplements on an empty stomach with vitamin C, which helps to increase the absorption of iron through the intestines.

PUPPP Skin Rash

PUPPP stands for *pruritic urticarial papules and plaques of pregnancy.* It's a mouthful—and also a nightmare—occurring in one out of two hundred pregnancies. PUPPP is an extremely itchy red rash that starts on the belly, as shown in Figure 5-3. It can spread all over the body but usually spares the umbilicus, face, palms, and soles. This condition is more common in Caucasian patients, first-time moms-to-be, and those with multiples (twins or more). For unknown reasons, 70 percent of moms with PUPPP are carrying boys. PUPPP usually starts in the third trimester, but 15 percent of cases begin after delivery. The rash typically lasts for six weeks. The treatment consists of topical steroid creams, oatmeal baths, and oral antihistamines for symptomatic relief. Oral steroids may also be used. For most patients, the rash eventually subsides as the pregnancy hormone levels decline after delivery. We even had one mom who had to be induced a little early because she was ready to scratch her skin off with PUPPP!

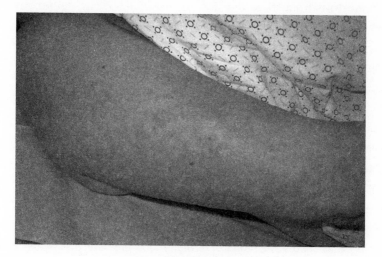

Figure 5-3: PUPPP Skin Rash

Our poor patients with this skin condition suffer from the intense itching, but luckily, the baby is not affected in any way. This condition is unrelated to other skin complications during pregnancy. Although we do not know what causes this condition, it usually does not affect subsequent pregnancies.

Cholestasis

Cholestasis is characterized by itching all over the body, but unlike PUPPP, no visible rash appears on the skin. This disorder is caused by the slow movement of bile through the liver. Interestingly, the incidence of this condition varies by population. For example, it is not very common in North America, affecting one in five hundred to one thousand pregnancies. But in Chile, one in twenty-five pregnant women may be affected. The itching usually begins in the third trimester, and occasionally late in the second trimester. The soles of the feet and palms of the hands may be especially itchy. Cholestasis is diagnosed by measuring the level of bile acids in the blood. Treatments for the itching may include oral antihistamines and oral medications called cholestyramine or ursodeoxycholic acid.

Does this condition have a negative effect on the baby? The studies are conflicting.[4] Because some studies show increased risk of sudden fetal deaths, we observe the babies closely with fetal monitoring and ultrasound evaluation of amniotic fluid levels. Your doctor also may recommend early delivery at thirty-seven to thirty-eight weeks.

Activities in the Third Trimester

▶ ▶ ▶ HOW LONG SHOULD YOU STILL WORK?

It's hard to know just how much activity you are able to do in this last stretch. When I was pregnant with my first son, Matthew, I was able to work right up until I went into labor without too much difficulty. I was filled with energy and felt great. Not so with my second child, Max. I was a lot more fatigued and had a much more difficult time performing my daily activities. This was on top of the fact that I had some issues with high blood pressure. Remember, every pregnancy is different. Listen to your body. Respect your instincts.

—Alane ◀ ◀ ◀

Up until the third trimester, many moms have been minimally affected by their pregnancies and are able to go about most of their usual activities with only minor adjustments. They may have been managing to work long, hectic schedules, to make it to the gym, and even to have sex. Now, all of a sudden, these ordinary tasks and daily pleasures may become much more difficult or even impossible, due to an enlarging uterus and growing baby. This may be the first time when the mom feels a need to slow down her life for the sake of her baby, and the loss of independence may be a bit of a shock.

Sleeping

It gets increasingly harder to sleep as you get closer to delivery day. Following is a list of reasons for your sleepless nights:

- The baby is moving a lot.
- You are having Braxton Hicks contractions.
- You have to urinate frequently because there's so much pressure on the bladder from the baby's head.
- You have heartburn.
- You can't find a comfortable position.

For women who are truly suffering from insomnia, we recommend an over-the-counter sleep aid, such as an antihistamine (Benadryl). Sleeping pills are used only in severe cases because there are no studies to document their safety. Your doctor can give recommendations.

We encourage our moms to look at it this way: This is a dress rehearsal for life with a newborn, when you're going to have to wake up to tend to your new child every two to three hours. If you were to go straight from getting a sound eight hours a night to weeks of constantly interrupted sleep, it would be a shock to the system. Maybe predelivery sleep patterns are our bodies' way of easing us into this strange and new way of life that's just around the corner.

Nesting

No matter how civilized we may think we are, our evolutionary biology still kicks in from time to time. In the second and third trimesters, many pregnant women will feel the uncontrollable urge to organize their lives, a phenomenon we call *nesting*. Nesting isn't a myth; it's a primal instinct among all mammals and birds that directs them to prepare a sheltered, safe place in which to give birth. As humans, we still carry the seeds of this instinct deep in our genes. A mom-to-be may find herself cleaning the house, sorting clothes, or organizing the garage, which is what Alane did, with a vengeance. Many couples find themselves making a major move right before birth because they need more space before the baby comes. Yvonne had to move into an apartment two weeks before Kylie was born so she and her husband could start remodeling their home to make room for a new little one. She undertook the move, the remodel, and all their related tasks with an unusual burst of energy. If this describes you—or your partner— relax, you're not going crazy. You're just following the time-honored directions of Mother Nature.

Traveling

As we explained in Chapter 3, the act of flying in an airplane itself is not going to hurt your baby. However, you need to take into consideration many other serious issues if you are thinking about traveling after the twenty-fourth week of your pregnancy.

Prior to twenty-four weeks, traveling locally or even internationally is fine. If something unexpected—such as preterm labor—should occur, causing the baby to be born prematurely, nothing could be done, no matter where you are. However, at twenty-four weeks, the baby becomes viable—meaning it can live outside the mom with intensive care support. So after twenty-four weeks, we want our patients to be in a place where they are always within easy reach of good medical care. We tell our moms that we don't want them going to remote places—or to anyplace where it may be difficult getting to a hospital—after their twenty-fourth week.

▶ ▶ ▶ HOLIDAY SURPRISE

A young first-time mom named Lucy wanted to visit her family in Cleveland for Christmas. The holiday fell around the twenty-eight-week mark, and because her pregnancy had been uncomplicated thus far, she didn't think twice about flying from Los Angeles to Ohio. The visit went smoothly until the day after Christmas, when Lucy suddenly went into labor. Her family rushed her to their local hospital, where the doctors tried to stop her labor but ultimately failed. They delivered a healthy, but small baby girl weighing only two pounds. The baby was put on a ventilator and transferred to another hospital with a NICU. A traumatized Lucy was relieved to learn that her daughter would eventually be all right, but was then told that she would have to remain in the NICU for three more months. Suddenly, Lucy was faced with the reality of having a job and home in Los Angeles and a preemie baby on a ventilator in Cleveland. She was forced to take a leave of absence from her job and move in with her family so she could be near her child. After three months away from home, the baby was finally discharged and everyone came back to Los Angeles. Lucy's story illustrates that you can never know exactly what surprise turns your pregnancy might take.

We recommend that all our moms think very critically of any trips that they take after twenty-four weeks. Is this trip absolutely necessary? Do you really want to risk being on a twelve-hour flight to Singapore when your water breaks or you begin experiencing strong contractions?

What would *you* do in case of an emergency?

Driving

Women can continue to drive during their pregnancy all the way to the delivery day. You should always use a lap and shoulder belt with the lower portion of the belt placed under the baby. If you are in a car accident, even the slightest jolt or pull of the belt on the uterus should warrant a call to your doctor, and a possible trip to the hospital for fetal monitoring.

Your Baby's Changing Positions

Many patients come to us around the thirty-sixth week of their pregnancy to ask us what position their baby is in. "Which way is my baby?" they'll ask nervously. "Is it . . . you know . . . the right way?" By thirty-six weeks, whether a baby will enter the birth canal head-first or butt-first has most likely been determined. However, we often cannot predict the position of the head (face-down or face-up) until you are in labor. So don't stress about the position—most babies will find the path of least resistance just in time.

We describe the baby's orientation within the uterus as its lie, position, and presentation. Let's look at these terms in more detail:

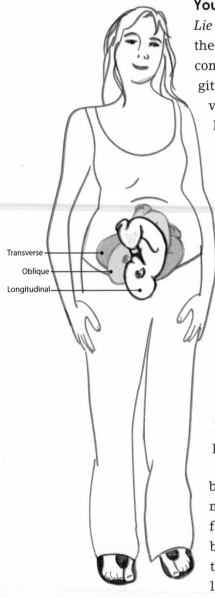

Your Baby's Lie

Lie refers to the angle of the baby's body in the uterus (see Figure 5-4). The baby can come out vaginally only if he or she is longitudinal (straight up and down). Transverse (sideways) and oblique (diagonal) lies require a cesarean delivery or an attempt at external cephalic version (ECV), which is described later in this section.

Your Baby's Position

Position refers to the rotation of the baby's head in the birth canal. When the back of the head is under the mother's pubic bone, the baby is in *occiput anterior (OA) position*. A baby born OA will be facing the floor. This is easiest position for a baby to deliver because it allows the baby to tuck its chin to minimize the diameter of the head that needs to pass through the pelvis.

In *occiput posterior (OP) position,* the back of the baby's head is near the mother's spine, and the baby comes out facing the ceiling, or sunny-side-up. OP babies cannot flex their neck as well, so the diameter of the head as it descends is larger. Just a few millimeters difference

Transverse
Oblique
Longitudinal

Figure 5-4: Your Baby's Lie

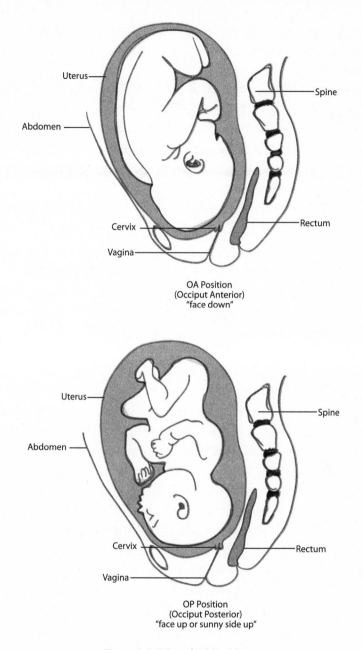

OA Position
(Occiput Anterior)
"face down"

OP Position
(Occiput Posterior)
"face up or sunny side up"

Figure 5-5: OA and OP Positions

from OA to OP can make a much more difficult delivery. Both positions are shown in Figure 5–5.

---

myth: If you have "back labor" or feel the contractions more in your back, it means your baby will come out of the birth canal facing upward.

FACT: We've had just as many people with back labor whose babies are facing downward as facing upward. Some women simply feel their labor pain in different parts of their bodies.

Your Baby's Presentation

Presentation describes which part of the baby—in longitudinal lie—is coming out first. In a vertex presentation, the baby's head is down. A breech baby, shown in Figure 5-6, has its buttocks or feet down instead of the head. While 25 percent of babies are breech at twenty-eight weeks, only 3 to 4 percent of babies will be breech at term.

We confirm if your baby is breech by manual palpation or by an ultrasound. The most common reason that a baby is breech is simply that its head has become wedged between the mother's ribs and its buttocks are stuck in the pelvis. Although the risk of birth defects is slightly higher in breech babies, it usually does not mean that something is wrong with your baby. The birth defects associated with breech presentation are obvious on ultrasound, so they would have been diagnosed earlier in your pregnancy.

Most breech babies are born by cesarean. A serious complication, head entrapment can occur in vaginal breech delivery. If the cervix dilates to allow passage of the smaller buttocks or feet, the larger head may get stuck. This condition is an obstetrical emergency that can lead to lack of oxygen to the baby. If we find that the baby is breech at term, we offer our patients two options: an elective cesarean delivery or an attempt to turn the baby by a procedure called *external cephalic version (ECV)*. There are physicians in the United States and other parts of the world who perform vaginal breech deliveries successfully. If you are planning to attempt a vaginal breech delivery, please be certain that you are in a facility where you have an

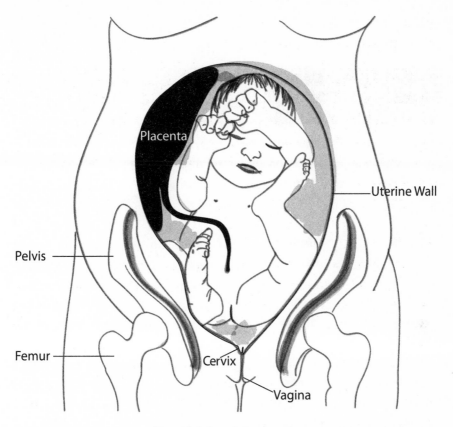

Figure 5-6: Breech Presentation

experienced obstetrician and a team ready to handle emergencies. *Do not attempt a vaginal breech delivery at home or in a facility without adequate support.*

External Cephalic Version (ECV)

In an *external cephalic version,* or *ECV,* your doctor will attempt to turn your baby manually to the head-down position. Studies have shown that ECV is successful in 35 to 86 percent of cases (the range is broad because so many variables are involved with each case). If your obstetrician is successful in turning your baby to a head-down position, it will usually stay down.

So what variables affect this success rate? You will have better success if your baby is average size, if you've had babies before, if there is plenty of amniotic fluid, and if the baby is not wedged into your pelvis. However, if your placenta is on the front side of your uterus or you are overweight, your success rate may be lower.

ECV is performed in a hospital setting because both mom and baby need to be monitored, during and after the procedure. ECV can cause fetal distress and the need for an emergency cesarean. Because many babies will find their own way to the vertex position by thirty-six weeks, the ECV procedure is usually performed around thirty-seven weeks. If the ECV necessitates an emergency cesarean because of fetal distress, most babies will have sufficient respiratory development to prevent an admission to the NICU.

Before an ECV, we administer a medication to relax the uterine muscle. Then, under ultrasound guidance, we attempt to rotate the baby to a head-down position by pushing on the baby's head and buttocks. In this way, we try to get the baby to do a somersault. A moderate amount of force is needed to move the baby, and some moms are not able to tolerate the procedure because of discomfort.

Risks of ECV include breaking the water bag, tangling the fetus in its umbilical cord, or *placental abruption,* where the placenta shears off the uterus. If any of these complications occur, we perform an emergency cesarean.

Many patients ask if there is anything they can do to encourage a breech baby to turn. Before attempting ECV, we will often refer our patients to an acupuncturist to try *moxibustion*. This is a traditional Chinese treatment in which an herb is burned next to the small toe to stimulate an acupuncture point related to the uterus in order to flip the baby into a head-down position. Limited studies have been conducted, but they do show an increased rate of breech-to-vertex movement.[5] We feel this procedure is not harmful to the mother or to the baby, and is something she can try before an ECV.

Planning for the Delivery

As the countdown to your due date continues, you can control some things but not others. We recommend that you begin making a few practical plans for how you will approach the big day and the many life changes that will come afterward, such as taking a leave of absence from your job, preparing your home for the baby, and creating a birth plan that will help you and your doctor communicate more efficiently when labor begins.

Taking Time Off from Work

It's true what they say: Having a baby does change your life. Many of our patients, especially those in their first pregnancy, don't have a sense of what's coming their way after they deliver—the lack of sleep and relentless demands of being a new mom. (See Chapter 7 for more about how to prepare for this.) You will have very few breaks. So why not grab some time for yourself before the birth day arrives? We recommend that our patients try to take some time off from work at the end of their pregnancies, even if they are feeling fine.

Some moms resist taking full days or weeks off and want to keep on going right until delivery. Ultimately, this is a personal choice. If a mom feels that she'll be bored at home all day, we suggest she try a half-day schedule instead. This will still give her a chance to relax the other part of the day and finish last-minute preparations. From our own experiences as well as our patients', this time can be invaluable.

▶ ▶ ▶ FROM DOCTOR TO MOM IN ONE SHORT NIGHT

I learned the hard way about taking time off. During my first pregnancy with Matthew, I lucked out and had a very smooth, easy time of it. I worked full force with few problems except leg swelling. I can still hear our office nurse, Silvia, scolding me while I was running out the door from our office to the hospital to deliver a baby, "Dr. Park, slow down! Don't run! You might fall and hurt yourself!" I thought I had everything all planned. I was supposed to be induced on a Wednesday, so I was going to take off Monday and Tuesday. I was on call the weekend before, and had an unusually busy time, delivering three babies on Saturday and two babies on Sunday. By the time I arrived home Sunday night, I was exhausted. But I thought to myself, "Finally, I can enjoy a few days off, relax, go on some walks, and run my last errands before the baby arrives."

My Matthew had other ideas. At 2:00 a.m. that same night, I broke my bag of water! My planned two days off turned into a few short hours. So much for planning! I did fine, but looking back, it would have been nice to have personal time because once Matthew arrived, my life changed—for the better but much busier. For those moms reading this who have never had babies before, you will one day wonder, "What was I doing on Saturdays and Sundays before my baby?" Those moms who already have children know exactly what I'm talking about.

—*Alane* ◀ ◀ ◀

Disability

As a pregnant mom, you may be eligible for a paid medical disability for part of your pregnancy and postpartum period. Check your state's laws about what is allowed. For example, the state of California permits women to receive disability payments for four weeks before their due date in a normal, uncomplicated pregnancy. In other states, the day you go into labor is the day you qualify for benefits. If medical complications arise during the pregnancy, you may get more time.

In California, if a portion of your salary goes to the State Disability Insurance (SDI) program, you can get paid a percentage of your salary, with a monthly maximum. If you are self-employed and don't pay into California's disability system, you may not be eligible.[6]

In addition to disability, a federal program called the Family Medical Leave Act (FMLA) allows moms—and dads—to take an additional twelve weeks off work to care for a newborn. However, this leave is unpaid. FMLA is available only to people who work in big companies, usually with fifty employees or more. Please check with the Web site www.dol.gov/whd/fmla for more details.

▶ ▶ ▶ **LAST-MINUTE MOM**

When I was pregnant with my first son, Ryan, I worked for a university practice in California that offered good maternity benefits, allowing eight weeks of paid leave. I had a choice—take either two weeks off before and six weeks off after the baby is born, or take the eight weeks at once, after delivery. I wanted to have as much time at home with my baby as possible, so I chose the second option. I planned to work right up to my delivery day.

The practice was a busy one. I was on call for twenty-four hour shifts and was on my feet all day, delivering babies and teaching residents. The night I went into labor, preterm at thirty-six weeks, I had a gynecological surgery scheduled in the morning and was also supposed to give a lecture to the nursing staff later that day. As I was huffing and puffing on the way to the hospital, I had to call a colleague to cover my surgery. I also asked her to give my lecture.

Because we'd left everything to the last minute, my husband and I were unprepared for an early labor. We hadn't even bought a car seat yet! The day after I delivered Ryan, I was going over my lecture notes with my colleague while my husband was at the store trying to find a car seat. The problem with working right up until delivery is that you aren't able to rest or get prepared before your life completely changes. We learned with Ryan that it's better to be ready and organized and have a few quiet moments with your spouse to talk, see a movie, or have a nice dinner before your baby comes into your life.

—Yvonne ◀ ◀ ◀

Growing Belly, Growing Concerns

As the delivery date approaches, many of our patients start to voice new fears, especially about their upcoming labor. This makes sense because not many women who have experienced labor have come back raving about the process; most of what pregnant women hear are the horror stories.

We always make sure to spend extra time with our patients during the last months of their pregnancies, not just to monitor their medical conditions but also to help maintain their emotional equilibrium. We feel it's important to address a woman's hopes and fears well before delivery day. On the birth day itself, you can control very little, so being armed with information and reassurance ahead of time goes a long way toward making that event as stress-free as possible.

Big Head, Small Opening

A lot of moms have a difficult time visualizing how their baby's head and body will make it through the small opening of their vagina. The concept can be frightening if a woman doesn't understand the mechanics.

One of Alane's third trimester patients, Jeri, had come in for a consultation and had asked to look at herself with a handheld mirror. "Dr. Park," Jeri asked, "Can you please explain to me how an entire baby is going to come out of that tiny opening?" We try to explain that millions upon millions of women's bodies have risen to the challenge. Nature designed us for this. Ideally, a woman's pelvis is shaped to allow the easy passage of the fetus. The vaginal skin and muscles are incredibly elastic and can stretch open more than ten centimeters wide to accommodate the baby's head. A birthing mirror can help a woman better understand when and where to push; if she's looking at her baby's head descending and watching the opening expand, it can tell her that she's pushing correctly. In other cases, like in Sandra's, a birthing mirror can add to a woman's sense of panic and fear. We always leave the decision up to our patients.

Natural Birth

We frequently are asked, "Am I going to have my baby naturally?" This question requires some investigation before we can answer it. It turns out that people have different definitions of "natural." Some women want to know if they are going to have a vaginal birth or a cesarean, while others want to know if they are going to have an unmedicated delivery.

The choice to have an unmedicated, less-interventional birth is a personal one. Some moms know that they definitely don't want to feel the pain of contractions, but others do a great deal of preparation to find other ways to cope with labor.

In the United States, 20 to 30 percent of babies are born by cesarean section. In most cases, whether your baby comes out vaginally or by cesarean is not determined until you are in labor. In a few cases, cesareans are scheduled: for breech or transverse lie babies, multiple gestations, placenta previa, active herpes outbreak, or elective repeat cesarean delivery. But especially for first-time moms, we often do not know how the labor will progress until it happens. The two most common reasons why the baby must be born by cesarean are that the baby doesn't fit through the birth canal or that the baby experiences distress during labor.

Whether the baby can navigate through the birth canal depends on the size of the baby, the size of the mom, and the position of the baby. We can get a general sense of the baby's weight and the size of the mom's pelvis, but we cannot predict how the baby will attempt to come through this area. For example, if the baby's head is cocked slightly off-center or its neck is extended, the width of the part of the head that is coming first is increased by a few millimeters, and this can make a huge difference when you are dealing with a confined space. The ability of the baby to tuck its chin and corkscrew through the pelvis is not something we can control or predict.

In the same way, we cannot predict how your baby will tolerate labor. When you have a contraction, the blood flow to the placenta decreases dramatically. Because a contraction lasts only for a minute, most babies adapt to this decrease without any problem. Some babies, however, are not able to keep up with this change for hours on end. They will begin to experience fetal distress and will need to be delivered by cesarean. We hope that all moms who want a vaginal birth get their wish, but we also recognize that the other player in this game—the baby—may have other plans.

Bowel Movements

Many of our moms-to-be fear that they might have a bowel movement while they're pushing. Yes, this is possible, and believe it or not, it's just fine if it happens. In fact, most of our patients are surprised to hear that we think it's a good thing because it tells us that they're pushing correctly. From a mom's point of view, it can be embarrassing. But from a doctor's point of view, it's reassuring.

Wrapped Umbilical Cord

myth: If you walk over electrical cords when you are pregnant, your baby will get twisted in the umbilical cord.

FACT: As many as 25 percent of babies will wrap the umbilical cord around some part of their body. However, it is not related to any activity that the mother does. So you don't need to be superstitious and worry about that electrical cord when you are vacuuming!

A *nuchal cord* is an umbilical cord that is looped around the baby's neck. We doubt that most expecting parents realize that a full 25 percent of babies are born with the cord wrapped around their necks, with no adverse outcome. If you think about it, it makes perfect sense. You are talking about a two-foot-long garden hose floating around in a confined space, next to a busy, gymnastic baby. If the baby twists in a certain way, it can soon find itself wearing an umbilical cord necklace. Remember this: In the uterus, the baby is not getting oxygen by breathing through its mouth. It gets all its oxygen through blood from the placenta. So something tight around its neck isn't going to compromise its "breathing." In addition, the consistency and firmness of the cord make it hard for the cord to be pinched.

The umbilical cord is quite thin, so it can be difficult to visualize on an ultrasound. However, if it is seen around the neck, it becomes a source of tremendous unnecessary worry for many pregnant moms. We can do nothing about a wrapped umbilical cord during pregnancy. We discourage moms from trying to find out this information because it rarely affects the baby, you can't do anything about it anyway, and the cord may unloop itself because the baby is still moving all the time.

In a worst-case scenario, a nuchal cord can lower the baby's heart rate during labor, causing stress in the baby to the point sometimes that a cesarean delivery is necessary. Whether to do this depends on many factors, including the duration of the distress, the baby's heart rate, and whether the mom is close to delivery.

Over the years we've been practicing, we've had a very, very small number of babies who have died because the cord was wrapped around the neck too tightly. Please remember that 25 percent of babies have a nuchal cord and adverse outcomes are rare.

Dealing with Unplanned Surprises

Many married couples face an accidental pregnancy. Usually it happens because the couple thinks they are too old, have sex too infrequently, forget to use protection, or have had infertility issues in the past and consequently don't think they can get pregnant. These couples are then faced with an unintended pregnancy but want to continue to term.

This event can be stressful if the family hasn't had a baby for a while and are in a different phase of their life—often way past diapers with a child going to college. Perhaps financially they had planned for two and now there is a third, and they have the need for more resources.

It may be reassuring to know that most of our patients in this situation find a way to make room for another baby, even if they are nervous and uncertain during the pregnancy. In the end, they always come back to us saying, "We couldn't imagine life without our baby!"

▶ ▶ ▶ UNEXPECTED SURPRISE

Maggie, forty, and her husband Matt, fifty, were a couple with a solid marriage who had been told five years earlier that Maggie's eggs were too old to have babies. Proving the experts wrong, she went on to have two children, a girl, now five years old, and a boy, aged three, before she first came to me.

Both Maggie and Matt were shocked when she became pregnant for a third time. This was not in their plans, and Maggie confided in me that she felt unprepared and also a little resentful about the upheavals this new life would force upon her. However, there was no question that she would keep the baby. All throughout her pregnancy, she remained worried and fearful of how her life would change with a third child to care for.

After her son arrived, however, everything changed. Her instincts kicked in and she adjusted quickly. She told me at her six-week checkup that she couldn't imagine life without little Sam.

—Yvonne ◀ ◀ ◀

Stress and Your Baby

Most likely, the stresses of everyday life are not going to hurt your baby. Most of the data on this topic comes from studies of severely stressful situations, such as war, famine, or severe illness. There does *not* seem to be an association between stress and miscarriage, pre-eclampsia, preterm labor, or fetal movement. However, some studies suggest a relationship between high levels of anxiety during pregnancy and behavioral problems in children.[7] That being said, an occasional argument with your partner or a disagreement at work is not going to harm your baby.

Kegels

myth: Doing Kegel exercises will make your labor much easier.

FACT: Studies have shown that doing Kegel exercises may help prevent urinary incontinence in the postpartum period. But in terms of Kegels making the pushing harder or easier, it probably does not make a difference either way.

Kegels are an exercise in which you strengthen the pelvic floor muscles. They may help you with stress incontinence, a condition in which you leak urine when you cough, jump, or sneeze.[8] If you have experienced these symptoms during your pregnancy, it is because the extra weight of the baby and the growing uterus puts pressure on your bladder. The extra muscle tone from Kegels can help avoid a leak and keep you dry. However, Kegels will *not* help you make your vaginal delivery easier. Do them when you're pregnant only if you are trying to combat incontinence.

To do Kegels, follow these steps:

1. Locate your PC, or pubococcygeus, muscle. The easiest way to identify this muscle is while you are urinating. While the urine is coming out, stop it midstream. The muscle that you use is your PC muscle. Be sure not to use your abdominal, buttocks, or thigh muscles.
2. Squeeze the PC muscle for five seconds as hard as you can, then release for five seconds.
3. Repeat this ten times. As your muscles become stronger, you can squeeze the muscle for ten seconds.
4. Repeat each set of ten at least three times per day.

When Kegels are performed regularly, the perineal muscles that run between the vagina and rectum become strong and tight. However, when delivering a baby, you push with your *abdominal* muscles, not the vaginal muscles. In fact, the more stretchy and relaxed the vaginal muscles, the easier delivery will be. That's why women who have had babies before don't push as long or hard as first-timers. After your baby has been delivered, you can think about doing Kegels to tighten everything back up and reduce urinary incontinence. But please, unless you are experiencing incontinence, say "no" to Kegels leading up to the birth of your baby.

Cord Blood

During the past several years, saving cord blood has become a more common practice. Blood from the umbilical cord contains stem cells and can be collected after delivery. These cells have been shown to be useful in treating some genetic disorders of the blood and immune system. According to the American Academy of Pediatrics, somewhere between one in one thousand and one in twenty thousand babies eventually use their stored cord blood.

You can find both public and private cord blood banks. Public banks store cord blood to help the general population, and most public banks use the National Marrow Donor Program to find matches for patients in need. Private cord blood banks are for-profit businesses that store cord blood for the private use of the donor's family.

We've saved cord blood for some of our own kids. We counsel our patients to think of saving and storing cord blood in the same vein as having insurance for their child—you hope you'll never have to use it, but who knows what will happen in the future? But it's also wise to consider that cord blood is expensive to store and maintain, with a low likelihood that you will one day need to use it.

Your Former Body

Some women worry that they will never get their prebaby bodies back. "Will I ever look the same again?" they ask us. We assure our moms that yes, they can return to normal but it will take, on average, nine months to return to your prepregnancy weight. The uterus will go back to its normal size by about six to eight weeks postpartum. At this point, you can return to your prepregnancy routines, including taking baths, having sex, and exercising more intensely. However, because most women have lost a lot of physical stamina during the last part of the pregnancy, we recommend that they take everything more slowly and build up gradually to where they were before their pregnancy. We've given the crucial months right after the baby is born a name of their own, "the Fourth Trimester," and we'll address it and its many unique concerns in Chapter 7.

The Birth Plan

Preparing for your baby's entry into the world involves visualizing your ideal birth but also thinking about how you will adapt if the unexpected should occur. These days, many moms and their partners often come to the hospital—and sometimes, to their very first obstetrician visit!—with some vision of what their ideal birth will be.

Unfortunately, it wasn't long ago in the history of hospital births that women would arrive to deliver their babies and discover that the staff seemed to treat them as bit players in the ensuing drama. Nurses and doctors would take over most, if not all, of the decision making and the mother would find she had little say in the process. Our profession has come a long way since those days, and it's our philosophy (and that of most of our fellow ob-gyns) that a woman should have as much choice as possible in how she delivers her baby.

One way women have taken back control of the process is by writing and sharing with their doctors a personal birth plan—a list or statement of their preferences to be used as a guide for how they would like their labor and delivery to proceed.

Preparing a birth plan has several advantages. A birth plan encourages patients to be informed, to ask questions of their doctors and hospitals, and to have a calm, logical dialogue in preparation for a day during which decisions may have to be made quickly and under pressure. Birth plans can help a mom remember and stay focused on a number of important items that she might not have given much thought to otherwise.

For us, a birth plan gives us insight into the fears and concerns of our moms-to-be. We find it interesting to observe the various ways our different patients approach the plan. Some moms hand us one sheet of paper with a few scrawled sentences, while others come in with a fully formatted, printed three-page plan. Over the years, we've come to realize that no matter what form the birth plan takes, it gives us a starting point for addressing questions and trepidations women have about their big day. There's also nothing wrong with not having a birth plan written or printed. Many of our patients communicate with us verbally whatever concerns they may have; that works just fine for us, too.

Plans May Change

A birth plan allows a woman to play a more active role in her delivery care, but at the end of the day, it can describe only an idealized version of the birth. We advise all our patients to be flexible and to be ready to make immediate adjustments to their plans—or even be prepared to throw everything out completely—if their birthing circumstances throw everyone a big curveball.

We've had moms determined to go through a drug-free, natural childbirth who end up in labor for forty-eight hours, cry for an epidural, and ultimately undergo a cesarean delivery because their baby just didn't fit. On the other hand, we've scheduled moms for cesareans due to their baby's breech position, only to find the baby flipped into the right position in the hours before their scheduled surgery. Unexpectedly, these moms were able to deliver vaginally after all.

Be aware that parts of your birth plan may be at odds with hospital policy or insurance company rules, so please share your plan with your doctor well in advance so you can make any needed modifications, including changing hospitals if need be.

Creating the Plan

In this section, we describe the general areas of our patients' birth plans. If you want to create a birth plan, ask yourself (and your partner) the following questions.

Labor: This section allows you to describe your vision for your labor process. Do you want a birth with minimal medical intervention? Do you want to minimize vaginal exams? Is it important for you to be able to walk around? Do you want an IV? Do you want to keep the room quiet? Who do you want to have in the labor room with you? Do you want to be able to get in a tub or shower?

Fetal monitoring: While in labor, your contractions and your baby's heart rate will by monitored by a machine. This can be accomplished with a handheld Doppler, with disks that are held against your abdomen by a belt, or with a device that connects to the baby internally. The information can be collected continuously or intermittently. You can specify your preference for the type of monitoring you would like.

Labor augmentation or induction: If your labor must be induced for a medical reason, how would you prefer that we do it? Would you like to have the water broken, use Pitocin, or try more natural methods such as castor oil or nipple stimulation. (Walking doesn't induce labor.)

Anesthesia or pain medication: Do you want to avoid pain medications if possible? Do you want an epidural as soon as you get to the hospital?

Cesarean delivery: If you need a cesarean, who do you want in the room with you? Do you want to have the operating drapes lowered so you can watch the baby come out?

Episiotomy: An episiotomy is the cut made between the vagina and rectum to allow more room for the baby to pass. Would you prefer to tear naturally or have the doctor use an episiotomy?

Delivery: Do you have a preference for the position in which you will deliver? Do you want to watch the birth with a mirror? Do you want the baby to be placed on your chest immediately or would you rather have the baby cleaned and dried first?

Immediately after delivery: Who should cut the cord?

Baby care after delivery: Do you want the baby to receive antibiotic eyedrops and vitamin K injections? Are you planning to breastfeed? Do you want the baby to use a pacifier? Do you want all exams with the baby performed in the delivery room? Do you want your newborn to stay with you the entire time?

Birth plans are like snowflakes—no two are alike. Table 5-2 is a sample of an actual birth plan we received from one of our patients. It's detailed, and fairly typical.

The woman who presented us with the birth plan in Table 5-2 was one of Alane's patients, and she did end up with a drug-free, natural, vaginal birth, almost exactly according to her plan.

However, whenever anyone presents us with such a detailed plan, an underlying reason is usually behind it. When Alane sat down with

Table 5-2: A Sample Birth Plan

LABOR

I would like to be allowed to labor at home for as long as possible before coming to the hospital.

I would prefer to keep the number of vaginal exams to a minimum.

I would like to wear glasses or my contacts, whichever I feel more comfortable in.

I would prefer to have the lights low for labor and delivery.

I would like to drink fluids if I can, or suck on ice chips or a wet rag soaked in water, instead of receiving an IV.

MONITORING

I do *not* want constant fetal monitoring. This includes an internal monitor. Intermittent and as little as possible will be okay.

LABOR AUGMENTATION/INDUCTION

I do *not* want my amniotic membrane ruptured artificially.

I do *not* want Pitocin to be administered; I would prefer to use natural methods.

ANESTHESIA/PAIN MEDICATION

I do *not* want a continuous IV or any kind of medication.

I am okay with a precautionary saline lock being placed in the vein in case of an emergency.

CESAREAN

Unless there is no other option, I want to avoid a cesarean delivery.

If a cesarean is necessary, I would like to be fully informed and to participate in the decision process.

If a cesarean is necessary, I would like my husband present at all times.

EPISIOTOMY

I do *not* want to be cut but be allowed to risk tearing instead.

DELIVERY

I would like to be in the sitting squat for delivery and do *not* want my feet in stirrups.

I do *not* want the use of forceps, a vacuum, or any other foreign object during the delivery of the baby.

I would like guidance in when to push and when to stop pushing so the perineum can stretch.

I would like my husband or mother to support my legs and me during the pushing stage.

I would like to hold my baby while I deliver the placenta and any tissue repairs are made.

(continues)

Table 5-2: (*continued*)

IMMEDIATELY AFTER DELIVERY

I want to hold the baby immediately after delivery, with the baby placed on my chest or stomach.

I want the cord blood to go to my baby and not be cut too soon.

I would like my husband to cut the baby's cord.

I would like to breastfeed right away.

I would like to naturally birth the placenta and do *not* want my stomach to be pushed on or the placenta to be forced out in an unnatural manner. *No* routine injection of Pitocin.

I do *not* want silver nitrate or antibiotics used in my baby's eyes.

I do *not* want the baby to be given a hepatitis immunization or any other shot.

I would prefer to hold my baby rather than have him placed under heat lamps.

If my baby must be taken from me to receive medical treatment, my husband or mother must accompany my baby at all times.

I plan to keep my baby near me following the birth and would appreciate it if the evaluation of my baby can be performed with him on my abdomen, with both of us covered by a warm blanket, unless there is an unusual situation.

I want my baby evaluated and bathed in my presence.

I would prefer not to be shown the placenta after it is birthed.

After birth, I would prefer to be given a few moments of privacy to urinate on my own before being catheterized.

BREASTFEEDING

I plan to breastfeed and do *not* want my baby given any bottles, including glucose water or formula.

CIRCUMCISION

I would like circumcision of my baby to happen before we leave the hospital and to have my husband or mother present for the procedure.

PHOTO/VIDEO

I would like a photo taken of the first moment I hold my baby right after birth.

OTHER

My support persons are my husband and mother and I would like them present during labor and delivery.

---

this woman and her husband, she learned that they had both had negative experiences with medical treatment in the past and had felt ignored and left out of the decision-making process. They were both fearful that they would feel similarly powerless with the birth of their first child, one of the most significant moments in their lives.

Ultimately, what they really wanted was just for us to keep them informed of what was happening all the time. Their birth plan was a cry for help, "Can you please just let us know what's happening?" They had been considering a home birth, but after realizing that Alane was on their side and was going to do everything in her power to make sure the delivery went the way they wanted it to, they decided to stay at the hospital. Their baby boy is now one year old and doing great.

▶ ▶ ▶ A BIRTH PLAN GOES AWRY

Our patient Gemma is one of those women who projects such a serene and positive attitude that she soothes the spirits of everyone around her. A thirty-year-old ballet teacher, Gemma is incredibly in touch with her body and did everything she could throughout her pregnancy to keep herself healthy and well prepared for the rigors of delivery. We all thought she would have no problem with a natural childbirth.

But despite all her prep work and healthy habits, nature had a different plan in mind for Gemma. Her labor lasted for almost three and a half days. She labored at home in the beginning, and by the time she came to the hospital, she had gone from calm, unflappable, and buoyant to exhausted, miserable, and desperate.

Gemma clung to her natural, drug-free birth plan for as long as humanly possible, but after more long hours of pain and struggle, she finally accepted the epidural that would allow her some much-needed rest. She slept, reenergized, and finally did end up delivering vaginally. At first, she felt disappointed. She had so much riding on her vision of what her perfect delivery day was supposed to be like, and it all fell apart. We had to reassure her that veering from her ideal path wasn't anybody's fault and couldn't be predicted—it's just the hand she was dealt.

Talking about her delivery afterward, Gemma told us, "You know what? I get it now. I could not fix any of what happened or control it or change it in any way. It was just how it was going to be, and I had to finally decide to just ride it out and let go." The end of the story is what counts, and Gemma ended up with a healthy baby boy.

Gemma's story is a reminder to all moms-to-be that on delivery day, the best preparation is to expect the unexpected, and trust that you will get through it.   ◀ ◀ ◀

What to Bring to the Hospital

It's a good idea to have a bag packed before you go into labor. We recommend bringing the following items with you to the hospital.

For mom:
- Nursing bra.
- Lanolin ointment (our favorite is the Lansinoh brand, smooth and easily applied).
- Slippers and socks.
- Personal comfortable clothes or PJs. But remember, you may get a little messy during labor and delivery. You can always use the gown the hospital will provide for you.
- Small portable fan to cool off during labor.
- Bottle of mineral oil or vitamin E oil with safflower base. We use these oils to slowly stretch your perineum (vaginal area) during pushing. Some hospitals may have this in stock.
- Toiletries (shampoo, conditioner, soap, toothpaste, hairbrush). Hospitals may provide these, but many moms prefer their regular brands.
- Personal CDs or an iPod for music.
- Camera or video recorder or both.
- Birthing ball.
- Birth plan, if you have one.
- Insurance card if you have not preregistered.
- Pillows for you and your partner. Hospital pillows are not the most comfortable.
- Lip moisturizer.

For baby:[9]
- Infant car seat. Don't buy a cheap one. We like Graco for newborn infants and Britax when they are a little older.

- Neck support pillow for the car seat. Try the Kiddopotamus brand. It's nice and soft.
- Infant mittens. Babies tend to scratch themselves with their fingernails.
- Infant nail clippers. If the nails are very long, you may need to clip their fingernails in the hospital so the baby does not repeatedly scratch his or her face.
- A cute outfit to take your newborn home in.

Hospital provides:
- Diapers.
- Wipes.
- Receiving blankets.
- A kimono-type top and a cute hat.
- Pacifiers.
- Bottles and formula.

Delivery Timetable

The truth is, despite all the incredible advances in modern obstetrics, we still can't pinpoint the exact time when you are going to have your baby, unless you've scheduled a cesarean delivery for a specific day. The mechanism by which someone goes into labor is not fully understood. A component is related to the production of hormones by the fetus, which increase hormone production in the placenta, which make the uterus more sensitive to oxytocin. However, the timing and trigger of this cascade currently remain among nature's mysteries.

Sometimes a mom will have a completely closed cervix and go into labor that night. On the other hand, a mom may be three or four centimeters dilated and walk around like that for weeks. The majority of pregnant moms will deliver at term, which is anytime three weeks before and two weeks after their due date. The following list shows you the percentage of women who go into labor at different times:

Less than thirty-seven weeks: 13 percent
Thirty-seven to thirty-nine weeks: 54 percent
Forty weeks: 19 percent
Forty-one weeks or more: 14 percent

If a woman has already had at least one baby, reviewing what happened during her first pregnancy can help us identify certain patterns. Did the mom have the baby early or late? Was it a slow, hard labor or was it a relatively quick and not terribly painful one? If you've had an early baby once, you will be more prone to having another early baby. These statements are the closest to predictions we can make.

Dropping

"When am I going to drop?" When a baby drops, it means that the baby has moved lower into the birth canal. You may feel like there's less pressure underneath your ribs or diaphragm, you may suddenly have less heartburn, or you may feel more pressure on your bladder or pubic bone.

myth: After you've dropped or if you are carrying low, you are on the verge of having the baby.

FACT: There is no clear correlation between when your baby moves into the pelvis and when it ultimately comes out.

For most first-time moms or women with tight abdominal muscles, the baby won't drop (see Figure 5-7) until they are in active labor and the uterine contractions are actually pushing the baby down. Women with lax abdominal wall muscles or those who have had babies before may carry the baby low throughout their pregnancies.

▶ ▶ ▶ PRELUDE TO LABOR

Along with the last trimester came bonus visits to the hospital for dehydration and unexplained pain. At least we were able to find what we believe is the fastest route to the hospital. After what felt like 101 tests, in the middle of the night the baby began moving like I had never felt before and suddenly the pain was gone. The doctors concluded the baby's position was affecting my breathing and suggested maybe next time I try some yoga moves.

Linda, Allison's patient ◀ ◀ ◀

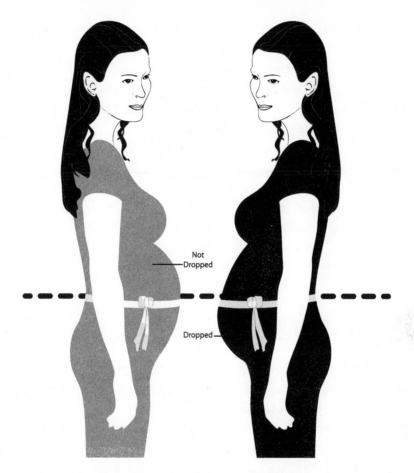

Figure 5-7: Dropped vs. Not Dropped

When to Call OB 911

As the dates of their deliveries draw nearer, our patients constantly ask us, "When should I call?" and "Is it okay if I call?"

For us, the bottom line is: *if you aren't sure, you should call.* This is even more true for first-time moms who have never experienced contractions, labor, and the other array of new sensations that occur before a baby is ready to meet the world. Don't second-guess yourself. Contact your doctor if you aren't absolutely certain about what your body is telling you. We often tell our patients: "Listen to your body. You have good instincts."

Call your OB immediately if you experience any of the following:

- Vaginal bleeding that is like a period
- Contractions that occur every ten to fifteen minutes if you are less than thirty-six weeks, or every five minutes when you are more than thirty-six weeks
- Rupture of the membranes or leaking fluid
- Severe headache not relieved with Tylenol
- Severe swelling of the face, hands, and feet
- Decreased fetal movement
- Fever higher than 100.4 Fahrenheit

▶ ▶ ▶ SPEAK UP

Lara and Diego were always a very polite couple. Throughout Lara's pregnancy, both she and her husband had seemed shy, compliant, and deferential to a fault. I sometimes even got the impression that they felt like they were intruding on my time when they came for their scheduled regular appointments. I always had to urge them to speak up and ask some of the many questions that I knew were just lingering on their lips.

Very close to Lara's due date, she called our emergency service line to report some fluid leaking and abdominal discomfort. I advised her to come in to Labor and Delivery (L&D) so we could determine if her water had broken. Lara complied and, after testing, it was determined to be a false alarm. The L&D nurses sent her home with very specific instructions, asking her to watch for symptoms such as regular contractions, decreased fetal movement, vaginal bleeding, or a fever higher than 100.4 degrees Fahrenheit. If she had any of these symptoms, she was to return to the hospital immediately. Lara nodded quietly and left, apologizing to the nurses for any inconvenience her false alarm might have caused.

Lara went home, and we didn't hear back from her. Several hours later, Diego called me, sounding very nervous. Apparently, Lara had come down with a high fever shortly after arriving home but was afraid she would be bothersome if she went back to the hospital. She decided to tough it out at home, until her husband finally intervened and called us. We advised her to come straight to the hospital, where we delivered her baby forty-five minutes after her arrival. In that short time, the baby had contracted an infection and became very sick. Lara's temperature had been a symptom of chorioamnionits (a uterine infection) that caused her baby to pass and breathe in its meconium (baby's bowel movement), resulting in pneumonia. Her new daughter had to go on a special ventilator for several months before she was allowed to leave the hospital.

Ultimately, Lara's baby thrived without any long-term consequences from her severe infection. But this case is an example of why it's important to err on the side of caution. Like Lara, many people fear that they're going to come to the hospital only to get sent home again. Always remember it's not the end of the world to be sent home, and you certainly don't have to worry that you are bothering us or wasting our time. We'd rather you come in to find out everything is okay than have you wait it out at home, not knowing if there is a serious problem. Trust your instincts and let us know if something doesn't feel right.

◀ ◀ ◀

If you call your doctor with a real question or concern, even if it's the same question and concern you've had a thousand times before, you still deserve an answer. That's why you have a doctor or midwife, someone who can help give you advice. People should understand that no question is foolish, and when you're on the verge of delivery, no trip to the hospital is unnecessary. If you are concerned about what's happening in your body, a professional needs to confirm that you and your baby are okay.

Let Us Do the Worrying

As the birth day approaches, some patients feel fearful and become obsessed with everything that could possibly go wrong. The more these moms educate themselves by surfing the net and reading every worst-case scenario that the Web can serve up, the more terrified they often grow. We agree with a phrase that originated with a nursing bra company and was then picked up and repeated on maternity blogs across the Internet: "Google doesn't have children."[10] There's such a thing as too much information, especially when it hasn't been filtered through the perspective of an experienced professional.

Worries are normal. You are about to undergo one of the most monumental and profound experiences of your life. We're here to reassure you that the things you may be worrying about will probably never come to pass. If you have been diligent about taking care of yourself, coming to your prenatal visits, and sharing your concerns with your doctor from the beginning, your well-informed and experienced ob team will be there to guide you through any glitches or emergencies that might occur on your big day.

That's what we're here for.

▶ ▶ ▶ WAITING FOR THE BIG DAY

The hardest part of the third trimester is not the swollen feet, contractions, frequent trips to the restroom, heartburn, hot flashes, or insanely huge belly. Rather, it's the insomnia and anxiety. I have been told that this is nature's way of getting you ready for what is to come. I get up at night to use the restroom and then can't go back to sleep. I look out the window and feel like I am the only person awake in the world. Everyone tells me to rest now before the baby comes, as if it were really that easy.

My mind begins to race; some nights I have anxiety about the labor and birth. I like to think I have some control over it, but the truth is I know that I don't. It can happen at any moment and no matter how I organize my packed bag or how detailed my birth plan is, anything can happen.

Other nights I am up thinking about how my entire life is going to suddenly change. Will I be a good mother? How will this affect my career and my marriage? What will my identity be? The scariest question I ask myself is, will I instantly fall in love with my baby like everyone tells me I will?

It is 3:00 a.m. I make a cup of tea, take a deep breath, and remind myself of how excited I was when I first saw those two lines appear on the pregnancy test. I remember the first ultrasound and the first time I heard the heartbeat. I turn on the lamp in the nursery and take it all in. Peace fills my mind and I know I can't wait to meet him.

—Kerry, Alane's patient ◀ ◀ ◀

chapter six

THE BIRTH DAY

▶ ▶ ▶ THE WAITING GAME

Today is my due date, and so far, all of my attempts to convince this baby to make her debut have failed! I'm not even officially a parent yet, and I've already resorted to threats ("If you don't come out today, you can never stay out past curfew!") and bribes ("If you come out today, I'll buy you a pony").

Everyone keeps telling us to relax and enjoy these last days, and even though I know it's good advice, it's impossible to be patient when we can't wait to meet our daughter. How am I supposed to think about anything else with this giant watermelon sitting on my thighs? It doesn't help that people's eyes go wide whenever my belly rounds a corner, or that I keep having visions of my water breaking all over my coworker's open-toed shoes. One minute, I'm excited about how soon I'll get to see whether our daughter really has her daddy's nose like she does in the ultrasound picture, and the next minute, I'm terrified about the impending act of childbirth, not to mention everything after. I've been avoiding squats and breathing exercises like they're geometry homework, so how will I ever be a good parent? My mom says this is something I'll never stop worrying about, so for now, I'm just trying to focus on the present.

We've cleaned the house for the "last" time, bathed the dogs for the "last" time, and cooked the "last" of the freezer meals. Maybe I'll do all of these "lasts" again this weekend. I know no one stays pregnant forever, but sometimes it feels like I might be the first. I just want to hold our baby in my arms instead of my belly. When, when, when?

—Caitlin, Alane's patient ◀ ◀ ◀

You've prepped and you've planned for nine months or more. Your nutrition has been excellent and you've never forgotten to take your vitamins. You've stretched and toned your body with prenatal yoga and puffed to perfection in birthing class. You've toured the hospital where you'll be delivering and figured out the fastest route to get there. You've discussed all your plans with your doctor. Your suitcase is packed and the baby's room is painted. You're as ready as you can possibly be.

Now, prepare yourself for the idea that *anything* could happen.

The vast majority of pregnancies are completely normal. You get pregnant, you go into labor, you deliver the baby, and you go home. On the other hand, although the chances are low, it's possible to be a fit, healthy woman and experience a complication that ends up with you in the operating room having a cesarean. In many cases, we never know exactly why an ordinary pregnancy veers from its expected path, but from our shared years of experience, we do know that it can happen to anybody. Each of the three of us experienced unforeseen issues—some of them serious—in delivering our own children, but we are all here to tell the story. And you will be, too.

Whether your goal is to deliver vaginally, have a natural childbirth without pain medication, have a scheduled cesarean, or have your child at home, chances are you won't know until the birth day arrives what your experience will be. We'll ask our married patients to think back to their wedding day, and recall all the months of preparation that went into making that event come off as perfectly as possible. Then we ask them to remember all the unexpected surprises, snags, and hurdles that occurred, despite their plans and expectations. Now, these same women are about to face the rigors of a day that can be far more unpredictable.

You could deliver your baby as early as twenty-four weeks or as late as forty-two weeks. Your due date is merely an estimate, with most babies coming in the two weeks before or after the estimated date. The labor experience is just as unpredictable. On average, deliveries take up to twenty-four hours for first-time moms, and up to twelve hours for moms who've previously given birth, but your labor could last from a few hours to a few days. We also can't foretell the time, day, length, or intensity of the delivery. This doesn't mean that something bad will happen; it just means there's a wide range of possibilities. The variety of labor experiences is remarkable considering that the distance of your baby's trip through the birth canal is only a matter of inches.

No matter what, we recommend that you try to savor the birth experience, think positive thoughts, and visualize having a great birth. It's our job to make sure you are prepared physically, mentally, and emotionally for the possible surprises that could be in store.

▶ ▶ ▶ THE BIG DAY: AN OB'S POINT OF VIEW

We deliver about thirty to forty babies a month, but the birth day never ceases to be like the opening night of a Broadway show for us. When a patient of mine arrives at the hospital, the nurse usually will send me a text message with the patient's name and information. The first thoughts that go through my mind are "Is this her first baby or has she had kids before?" "What was her exam last time I saw her in the office?" I take into account how often she's contracting, whether her water has broken. Then my mental calculator starts crunching the numbers, and I try to estimate how many hours she has until delivery. "Okay she's going to deliver in about six hours, right around three in the morning." We get pretty good at estimating after fifteen years. So then I make the judgment, "Should I drive in now and sleep on the sofa in my office or wait until she makes a little more progress?" No matter which I choose, I'm on pins and needles until that baby makes its entrance into the world.

—Allison ◀ ◀ ◀

Labor

myth: Most babies are born at night.

FACT: Today, between induced labors and the fact that roughly 30 percent of all births are by cesarean delivery, more babies are born during daylight hours in the United States.[1]

The basics of labor confuse a lot of people, but they don't have to. In this section we describe what you need to know.

Labor, or parturition, is the process of childbirth in which the uterus contracts and the cervix opens to allow the baby to pass to the outside world. The complicated chain of events—from hormonal changes to involuntary muscle contractions to the baby's transition to breathing air—are nothing short of remarkable. The most common signs that you are on the verge of having your baby are uterine contractions, back pain, vaginal bleeding, or leakage of fluid.

Cervical Changes

You body begins to prepare for labor weeks before the onset of any painful contractions. We can determine how much your body has prepared by manually examining the cervix and assigning the Bishop's score, which describes several characteristics of your cervix:

- Effacement
- Dilation
- Station of fetal head
- Consistency
- Position

Effacement refers to how thin your cervix has become. Before labor, the cervix is like a long cylinder, typically three to five centimeters in length. As the cervix effaces, it becomes shorter, so by the time you are ready to deliver, the cylinder is like a thin piece of paper with a hole in the middle, or 100 percent effaced. When the cervix is 50 percent effaced, it has shortened or thinned to 50 percent of its original size. So when it comes to delivering the baby, the more effaced the better (see Figure 6-1).

Dilation is the process by which your cervix opens. Your cervix is closed, or zero centimeters dilated, before you go into labor. Complete dilation is when the cervix is ten centimeters open.

Station describes how low the baby's head is in the birth canal. We use a landmark called the ischial spines, which are part of your pelvic bones. The baby's head is at 0 station when it is at the level of the ischial spine, -2 station means the baby's head is two centimeters above

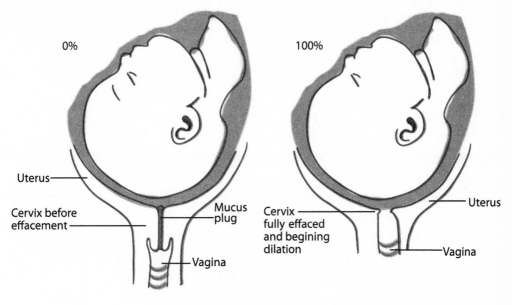

0%   100%

Uterus

Cervix before effacement

Mucus plug

Vagina

Cervix fully effaced and begining dilation

Uterus

Vagina

Figure 6-1: Effacement

the ischial spines. When the baby's head is crowning, it is at +4 station, four centimeters below the landmark.

Consistency refers to the firmness of the cervical tissue. Before labor, the tissue is firm like the tip of your nose. As the cervix prepares for labor, it softens, which allows it to dilate more effectively.

Position refers to the angle of your cervix in the vagina. As the cervix prepares for labor, its position changes from pointing toward your spine to angling forward toward your pubic bone.

We assign a score to each of the previous five characteristics, as shown in Table 6-1, and then add them. A Bishop's score of 8 or more means that your cervix is fully prepared, or ripe. However, the Bishop's score does not necessarily predict *when* you will go into labor. The score is used to predict the success of an induced labor. For example, some women will have a Bishop's score of 8 or more and be dilated three centimeters, and walk around like that for weeks. However, if you have a high Bishop's score, we generally recommend packing your bag because you may be in labor soon.

Table 6-1: The Bishop's Score

Score	Dilation (cm)	Effacement (%)	Station	Consistency	Position
0	closed	0–30	-3	firm	posterior
1	1–2	40–50	-2	medium	mid
2	3–4	60–70	-1 to 0	soft	anterior
3	5–6	80	+1 to +2	n/a	n/a

Contractions

Contractions are a tightening and relaxing of the muscles of the uterus that assist in dilating the cervix and pushing the baby through the birth canal. Some women liken the sensation of contractions to cramping, while others feel it as a growing pressure that wraps around their abdomen to their back. Contractions last about sixty seconds each and are rhythmic and painful. Oxytocin, which is made in the mother's brain, is the hormone that causes uterine contractions. It aids also in keeping the uterus firm after delivery to prevent excessive blood loss and is a critical part of breast milk letdown, or release.

False labor

In Chapter 4 we talked about Braxton Hicks contractions, also known as false labor. Braxton Hicks contractions can start as early as twenty weeks of pregnancy. We've had patients experiencing Braxton Hicks through the entire second half of their pregnancy. They feel their whole belly tighten, and then release after about a minute. A few minutes later, it repeats. Traditionally, these sensations are irregular and painless, and more importantly, they do not cause the cervix to open.

Real labor

"How will I know when I'm really in labor?" This is one of the most common questions we hear from new moms. And our answer is always the same: Unfortunately, you'll know. Labor hurts. There is no way around it. You will look back on it saying, "Oh yes. This is what everyone was talking about."

Like Braxton Hicks, true labor contractions also start as a feeling of tightness, in the front or the back. With time, they become rhythmic, happening every two to five minutes. In addition, the pain of the contraction intensifies as labor progresses, to the point where most women find it difficult to speak during the contraction. If you can easily carry on a conversation while contracting, it is probably not the real thing yet. When you are in true labor, we observe a change in your cervix as it opens (dilates) and shortens (effaces).

Confusion arises because a woman may be unsure when her contractions are regular or painful enough that she should call her doctor or go to the hospital. So let us give you some guidelines.

Timing contractions

Timing a contraction has two parts: You time the duration of the contraction itself and the length of time between contractions.

You determine the duration of the contraction by timing from the moment it begins to the moment it ends. Then you also need to time from the beginning of one contraction to the beginning of the next. If you can, have your partner assist you with timing your contractions.

The 5-1-1 Rule

We use the 5-1-1 rule to determine when you should call your doctor or go to the hospital. This rule means that you are having contractions every *five* minutes, with each contraction lasting about *one* minute, and those regular minute-long contractions repeat consistently for *one* hour. This pattern usually indicates that it's the real deal—and we encourage our patients to come to the hospital at this point. And remember, laboring and delivering a baby can be long and hard work!

Laboring at Home

What if you want to stay at home and labor there? Doing so is a personal choice. The main reason why women want to stay at home as long as possible is to avoid unnecessary medical interventions. In addition, some women are afraid they will not feel comfortable in the sterile environment of the hospital. However, although many women plan to stay at home, few do because laboring alone, especially if this is your first baby, can be frightening. A first-time mom, after the throes of contractions are underway, might ask, "How do I know how far dilated I am? Is the baby okay? Is this bleeding normal?" You decide when you want to come in. If you have spoken to your doctor beforehand about your wishes to make the hospital environment as comfortable as possible, coming to the hospital can be an easy transition that makes you feel safe.

◗ ◗ ◗ LABOR PAINS: TWO STORIES

Diligent, perfectionist Sandy was a first-time mom. She had been a model patient, coming on time to all of her OB visits, asking thoughtful questions, eating healthy, taking her vitamins, exercising regularly, and reading to educate herself about her pregnancy, labor, and delivery. Then, the big day arrived. Her labor began at home and she and her husband toughed it out through the night—laboring so hard, in fact, that neither one of them had a wink of sleep.

Sandy called us in the morning and said she thought it was time to come in. Alane performed a cervical exam, and told her she was two centimeters dilated. She still had eight more centimeters to go! Sandy's face fell with shock and disbelief. After all her hard work and a night of agony, how could she only be two centimeters dilated? We explained to her that, no matter how much homework a mom does, she can't do much on her own to control the pace of how her labor will go. Sandy decided to stay in the hospital, labored valiantly throughout the day, and finally had the vaginal delivery she had been hoping for.

Pearl is a labor and delivery nurse in our hospital. Slender and petite, she carries herself with an ease and confidence that inspires trust from both doctors and patients on the hospital floor. Pregnant with her *own* first child, however, all her training and experience went out the window. At full term, she phoned Alane one morning and said, "I think I might be in *labor*." Hearing the heaviness of her breathing, including the frequent breaks she took mid-sentence to breathe through her contractions, Alane determined she was in active labor and advised her to come in immediately. On arrival, she was already seven to eight centimeters dilated, and delivered less than two hours after arriving at the hospital.

Sandy and Pearl, Alane's patients ◗ ◗ ◗

We counsel our patients not to have any expectations about how far dilated they may be when they come in for an exam. That way, they won't be too disappointed if it turns out they aren't as far along into their labor as they had hoped.

Mucous Plug and Bloody Show

Soon after conception, thick mucous accumulates in the cervical canal to protect the baby from potential infection from vaginal bacteria. As the cervix softens and opens in preparation for labor, this mucous comes out as a thick, gooey discharge from your vagina, called the *mucous plug*. Unfortunately, the release of the mucous plug does not come with a fixed appointment time for you to go into active labor. It can happen just as you are starting labor or a week or two before.

In many cases, the release of the mucous plug is also accompanied by bleeding, or *bloody show*. As the cervix opens, some of the enlarged blood vessels within it will break and bleed. The blood may appear bright red, pink, or brown. Bloody show is not dangerous in any way. And like the mucous plug, it doesn't mean that your real labor is the next item on the program. Bloody show could be a sign that you may go into labor in the next few hours—or in the next few days or weeks. We know how frustrating not knowing your labor schedule can be. Think of the mucous plug and the bloody show as the cable repairmen of pregnancy. They'll offer you a wide window of time in which your labor is probably going to begin, but you're going to have to hang around waiting anyway, because you can never pin them down to the specific hour.

Water Break

myth: When your water breaks, that means you are in labor.

FACT: The water bag breaking doesn't necessarily mean you have to come rushing to the hospital right away. But the majority of women will go into spontaneous labor within twenty-four hours after breaking their bag of water.

For the past nine months, your baby has been surrounded and protected by fluid in the amniotic sac. As the uterus becomes more distended, or if it has more muscular contractions, the sac will be stretched to the point where it cannot stretch anymore, so it eventually pops. Most women will go into labor within twenty-four hours after their bag of water breaks, so it's a more reliable predictor of labor than the mucous plug or the bloody show.

At term, about 10 percent of moms will break the bag of water before they have any contractions, while 90 percent will have contractions that precede the water breaking. And the water breaking can happen in many ways. Sometimes, there is a distinct pop, followed by a large gush of water running down your legs to a puddle on the floor, leaving no doubt that the amniotic sac has broken. Other times, your water breaking may not be as obvious. You may have a high leak, meaning the break in the amniotic sac has occurred near the top of the uterus, and not near the cervical canal, causing an intermittent, slow leak of amniotic fluid. Because women tend to have more vaginal discharge and occasional urinary incontinence during pregnancy, this kind of break can be confusing. (Did my water just break? Or is it just vaginal discharge again?) Amniotic fluid should be clear and has an odor that is distinctly different from the ammonia scent of urine. Some say it smells like Comet. At term, your uterus holds nearly one liter of amniotic fluid.

If you want to know whether your water has broken:

- Take the cough test. If you cough and more fluid comes out, it is more likely to be amniotic fluid than mucous or urine.
- Do Kegels. See page 204. If you squeeze your pelvic floor muscles, as in Kegel exercises, you can stop the flow of fluid if it is urine. If the water continues to come out despite Kegels, it is probably amniotic fluid.
- Walk around for thirty minutes wearing a sanitary pad. If the pad is soaked, your water has probably broken.

Always remember: When in doubt, call your doctor or go to the hospital for further evaluation.

After your water has broken, the protective barrier between the bacteria-filled vagina and the baby is now lost. A longer interval between the water breaking and delivery increases the chance that the mother or baby could get an infection. If more than twenty-four hours passes, 25 percent of women will develop an infection. For this reason, we recommend calling your doctor for advice about when to go to the hospital.

In the following situations, you need to get to a hospital after your bag of water breaks. Prepare what you need and go to the hospital quickly when any of the following is true:

- You know that your baby is not in a head-down position.
- You see a loop of umbilical cord coming out of your vagina. This condition is known as cord prolapse and is an emergency. If you see this, call 911.
- You are a Group B strep carrier (refer to page 172).
- You have a fever of 100.4 degrees Fahrenheit or greater.
- The amniotic fluid appears green, which means your baby has passed stool, called meconium.
- Your baby is not moving.
- Vaginal bleeding is excessive.
- You are less than thirty-six weeks pregnant.

Ideally, after the bag of water breaks, you will go into labor in a timely manner. If you don't, you may need to receive antibiotics to prevent infection or Pitocin to induce labor. Fortunately, these interventions are not typically needed because your body will likely do what is necessary to deliver a healthy baby.

▶ ▶ ▶ WATERFALL

One of the most loyal workers in our office is Tish, who has earned the nickname "Martha Stewart" because of her tidiness and efficiency. I remember her working one day while pregnant with her first daughter. She was at term, quite near her due date, but still going strong, making sure everything was perfect in the office before she left on maternity leave. I was just finishing up my day at work when a few of our employees came running in to tell me that Tish's bag of water may have just broken. I walked over to the exam room where Tish was just finishing up cleaning. She had a cascade of amniotic fluid coming down her legs but she was standing on a towel to be sure she did not make a mess of her nice clean floor! Tish successfully delivered her first daughter, Emily, later that evening.

—Alane ◀ ◀ ◀

First-Time Moms and Childbirth Veterans

Deciding when to come to the hospital is also dependent on whether you are *nulliparous* (a first-time mom) or *multiparous* (have had children before).

Friendly warning: Most women will be in labor for a long time— sometimes twenty hours or more—if this is their first child. There's no way around it—a first delivery is almost always incredibly hard work. Although labor times vary from woman to woman and from pregnancy to pregnancy, on average, first-time moms will labor for about fourteen hours, while veteran moms will labor for about seven hours. So please reassure your partner that he or she doesn't have to speed like a NASCAR driver so that you won't deliver the baby in the backseat of your car instead of the hospital.

If you are multiparous, you will probably deliver the baby much more quickly. After the path has been carved, it is much easier the next time around. We've had moms that have progressed from a cervix dilated at five centimeters to a baby in their arms in as little as one hour. Multiparous moms should use their instincts and recall their prior labor history. If contractions are ten minutes apart but are already intense, you should come to the hospital, especially if you've had rapid labors in the past. If you're afraid of going to the hospital too early only to be sent home, tell your nurses that your instinct tells you that you may have this baby soon. Be sure to mention if you live far away and are concerned about making it back in time. Good nurses will always listen to their patients' instincts.

Precipitous Labor

Precipitous labor is defined as a labor that lasts three hours or less. A quick and easy birth like this sounds great, but it occurs in less than 2 percent of births. We do not know why some women progress so quickly through the labor process, but if you've had precipitous labor before, you are likely to have it again. Some women just seem to have a uterus that is incredibly efficient, and everything about their labor process is fast and furious.

▶ ▶ ▶ **TWO FOR THE ROAD**

I first met Deirdre, thirty-four, when she was pregnant with her second baby. She worked for a motion picture distribution company, and her husband, Larry, was an attorney. Deirdre relayed the dramatic story of the birth of her first son to me on our first visit. She had been seeing another doctor at our hospital during that pregnancy. Everything about the pregnancy was normal—until it came to the delivery day.

Deirdre went into labor while she was at home with her mother and Larry. Within an hour, her labor was off to the races. Unlike a typical first labor, the contractions came one after another without any break. With her mother in tow, she got into the backseat of the car and Larry drove them quickly to the hospital. As they pulled up to the emergency room entrance, her water broke, and before he could stop the car, the baby started coming out. Deirdre's mom helped guide the baby out while Larry called for help. Mom and baby were taken by wheelchair up to Labor and Delivery. Everyone was dazed, but happy and safe. They had to sell the car.

With her second pregnancy, Deirdre was naturally concerned that she could follow the same path. It turns out her mother also had experienced extremely rapid labors with all three of her children. As Deirdre's thirty-eighth week approached, we talked about a plan—when to come to the hospital, how to get there quickly, and what signs of early labor to watch for.

Deirdre called me on a Saturday morning to say that she was having some mild contractions. I asked her to come to the hospital right away. When she arrived, the nurse found that she was two centimeters dilated and contracting only every ten minutes. Deirdre felt that the contractions were not as strong as earlier and asked if she could go home. I told her I was afraid things could change quickly, but she insisted that she could get back just as quickly if need be.

Two hours later, I received another call from Deirdre. This time I could hear a lot of background noise and commotion. She was talking rapidly, saying that she and Larry were on their way back to the hospital and the contractions were out of control. Suddenly she cried, "My water broke!" I heard the phone drop and an intense scream. The next thing I heard was the cry of a baby. She had pulled the baby out of herself in the front seat of the car on the 110 Freeway. Larry never stopped driving, and by the time they arrived at the hospital ten minutes later, their second son was in her arms, after his dramatic entrance into the world.

—Yvonne ◀ ◀ ◀

Laboring Alone

"Quick! Boil some water!" Everybody's heard this line from childbirth scenes in old television and movies, but the truth is, the three of us still aren't sure what that water was supposed to be for. If you do find yourself going into labor away from the hospital, rest assured that you won't have to worry about finding a pot to put on the stove.

Emergency childbirth situations, however, aren't a Hollywood concoction. As Deirdre's story indicates, they really do happen from time to time. If you go into labor and no one is available to help get you to a hospital, don't panic. Call 911 and tell the emergency dispatcher about your situation. They will send EMTs or paramedics to help you and get you to the hospital.

The 911 dispatcher should stay on the line to help you until the emergency team arrives. In the meantime, you should get yourself in a comfortable location such as your bed and have some warm towels or a blanket handy. Lie on your back with your shoulders propped up by a pillow. If you need to push, remember to push as if you were having a bowel movement. After the baby's head comes through, reach through your legs and gently guide the baby out. Then place the baby on your bare skin and cover him or her with a towel for additional warmth. If the baby has not cried or is blue, gently rub the back of the baby and keep the baby warm. You don't need to worry about cutting the cord or delivering the placenta until emergency help arrives.

We truly hope that you never find yourself in a situation like this, but unless you have an incredibly quick labor like Deirdre's, emergency help should almost always be able to get to you in time.

▶ ▶ ▶ MY PARKING LOT DELIVERY

One Saturday, I was on my way to make rounds at the hospital after a long hike. On the way, I stopped at the nearby market for some groceries. As I got out of my car, I heard a man screaming "My wife is having a baby!" I looked around, thinking this must be a joke. Am I being filmed? But sure enough, I saw a man near a car with the back door of the car open, and two feet sticking out. I ran over to find a woman on her back in the back seat—half-dressed—and a baby crowning. I quickly told her I was a doctor and reached down to pull her baby out. Her husband and I wrapped the baby in her pants and drove the few blocks to the hospital. I am happy to report that mom and baby were perfect— but I have never shopped at that particular market again.

—Allison ◀ ◀ ◀

At the Hospital

After you're pretty sure that your big event is about to happen, it's time to call your doctor (and any friends or family members you want to alert!), pack the car, and set out for the hospital to begin the final phase of your pregnancy journey. Soon, that empty car seat you've installed in the backseat will hold your very own little one.

The Labor and Delivery Floor

When you first arrive on the labor and delivery unit, you might feel overwhelmed. Often, if the ward is busy, you will see a few patients walking the halls, encounter some nervous family members, and hear the unmistaken first cry of a new baby. Understanding what will happen after you arrive will help soothe your nerves.

1. Check in at the admitting desk on the labor and deliver (L&D) floor.
2. Your nurse will take you into a triage room unless it's obvious that you are in active labor, in which case you will be admitted directly into a labor and delivery room (LDR).
3. You will be given a hospital gown to change into.
4. Your nurse will ask you questions regarding what brought you in, your contraction pattern, bag of water status, vaginal bleeding, and medical history.

5. Your vital signs will be checked.
6. You will be connected to an external fetal monitor to check the baby's heartbeat and contraction pattern.
7. Your nurse will do a cervical exam.
8. Your doctor will be notified.
9. You may be admitted, discharged home, or monitored. Some moms may not be very dilated, but appear to be uncomfortable enough that they need further monitoring. In these instances, the nurse may ask you to walk around for an hour or two and then recheck your cervix. If there has been a change in your cervix, you will most likely be admitted.

The Birthing Room

You should check with the hospital regarding their policy on guests in the birthing room. Some hospitals are liberal, while others may have a maximum. Other than that, it's up to you to be the policymaker in this arena.

You'd be amazed at how many people some women want to invite to participate in their baby's birth. We've had as many as a dozen family members and friends crowding the place. Having more people crammed into the room doesn't necessarily make for a happier birth experience. Generally, we find friends and family aren't able to stay silent for very long. If you have ten people with you, sooner rather than later they'll start talking to one another. We often find that the patient can't focus when several conversations are going on in the room.

We recommend bringing your partner and perhaps one other friend or family member who can help get water, ice chips, or a towel. This person can also support you while pushing if you need extra assistance. We recommend that expectant mothers surround themselves with people who project good energy and who have a positive and calming influence on them. Negative, bossy, or excitable people are not going be of any use to a mom who is tired and in pain and trying to push her baby out.

You may have some really good reasons for *not* wanting certain people in the room with you. Other times, you may have no good reason—maybe you just don't want them there. However, some women find it impossible to tell their mother, or their father, or even their spouse, that they don't want them in the birthing room. When that happens, we're happy to step in and become the excuse. We can say, "I'm sorry, but as Ellen's doctor, I am asking that no one except Ted be with her." We don't mind playing the bad guy if it means we'll have a calmer, happier mom in the delivery room with us. So make sure to talk about your preferences with your partner ahead of time, and then let your doctor know well in advance who you've chosen to allow in the room with you on your big day.

Vaginal Delivery

When moms-to-be ask us whether they will have a vaginal delivery, the short answer is that we don't know yet. Even without understanding the details of labor's trigger, we know that the relationship between the baby, the mother's pelvis, and the force of contractions determines whether a vaginal delivery will be successful. For example, the baby must fit through the mother's pelvis properly with strong uterine contractions to be able to successfully enter the world vaginally. If one of these variables is abnormal—such as the baby is too big, the pelvis is too narrow, or the contractions are weak—a cesarean delivery may be needed.

Most women prefer to deliver their baby vaginally. The chance of a successful vaginal delivery depends on these factors:

- Size of the baby
- Position of the baby
- Shape and size of the mom's pelvis
- Mom's ability to push effectively
- Whether there is an infection
- How the baby is tolerating the contractions
- Whether the baby is descending through the birth canal properly
- Whether the amount of vaginal bleeding is unusual
- Whether the mom's blood pressure is normal

As you read through this chapter, you will see how each of these different variables comes into play.

▶ ▶ ▶ MY PLEASANT SURPRISE

Our favorite stories are the ones where we are pleasantly surprised by a pregnancy outcome. For example, twenty-six-year-old Sienna is a fun-loving young woman who enjoys traveling. She was married in Rome but lives in Los Angeles. Despite our advice to first-time moms to take childbirth classes, her busy schedule never gave her the chance. Sienna passed her due date and came in for her routine checkup one day. Her cervix was nowhere near ready—or so we thought.

The very next day, Sienna came back into the office. As I was walking down the hallway to see one of my other patients, I saw Sienna writhing in one of the chairs in a treatment room while getting her blood pressure taken. Sienna looked up and said, "I think I might be in labor." I examined her and found that she was three centimeters dilated, so I admitted her to Labor and Delivery, anticipating that she would deliver much later that evening. Remember, Sienna and her partner did not take a single class and were completely unprepared. I thought the labor process—which can often take fifteen hours or more—might overwhelm her.

Just a few hours after I sent Sienna to the hospital, I got a call to come up for a delivery. I was confused—which of our patients could possibly be delivering now? It was Sienna, ready to push her baby out. She pushed like a champ and in a relatively short period of time, she was a new mom. Despite little preparation, Sienna had an easy pregnancy and a completely unexpected easy delivery. Her case shows us that nature usually tells a new mom exactly what to do. Your DNA will kick in and you will probably find yourself instinctually knowing how to breathe, how to push, and how to take care of your baby.

—Alane ◀ ◀ ◀

Fetal Monitoring

In some way, shape, or form, your baby's heart rate and your contractions will be electronically monitored while you are in labor. Fetal monitoring can be performed continuously or intermittently.

The purpose of fetal monitoring is to alert your medical team to possible fetal distress that could lead to brain damage and cerebral palsy. When a contraction occurs, the placenta is squeezed, with a corresponding decrease in blood flow through this important organ.

Most babies can easily tolerate this decreased flow without any consequence. In some cases, however, contractions cause the fetal heart rate to drop, with the baby receiving less oxygen. If this continues for too long a period of time, *cerebral palsy* (CP), a permanent disorder affecting movement, may result. CP is caused by damage to the motor system of the brain, which can happen during pregnancy, during labor, or in early childhood.

Usefulness of fetal monitoring

There's an ongoing debate about the usefulness of continuous fetal monitoring. Does it improve the outcome of pregnancies and prevent birth injuries such as cerebral palsy? It is important to keep in mind that, in most cases, we do not know the exact cause of cerebral palsy. Only about 10 percent of cases are linked to events of labor. In fact, the incidence of cerebral palsy has slightly increased since the 1950s despite the use of fetal monitoring because we have the ability to improve the survival of very preterm infants, who are at the highest risk for this condition.

Despite the fact that continuous fetal monitoring may not improve fetal outcome, the majority of obstetricians in the United States use continuous monitoring as an added safety measure. Remember, we're here to make your labor and delivery as smooth and trouble-free as possible for you and your baby. However, because today's sensitive technology allows us to spot even the smallest signs of fetal distress, it's fair to say that the use of continuous monitoring has increased the cesarean rate; most doctors (and parents) would rather be on the safe side if they perceive what could be a serious sign of trouble.

Continuous versus intermittent monitoring

Some women balk at the idea of continuous monitoring because their ability to move around during labor is limited by a belt that is attached to the fetal monitor. An alternative to continuous monitoring, called intermittent monitoring, uses a Doppler to listen to the baby's heart rate every thirty minutes during the first stage of labor and every fifteen minutes while the mother is pushing. Intermittent monitoring allows the mother to have greater mobility. Especially in low-risk

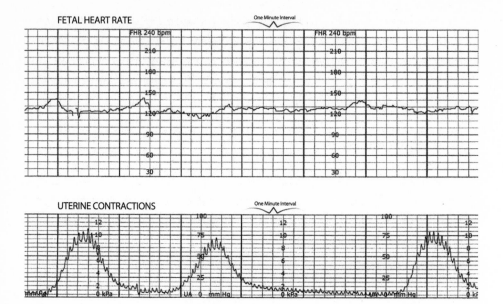

Figure 6-2: Fetal Heart Rate Strip

pregnancies, listening intermittently can be as effective as continuous monitoring in detecting fetal distress during labor.

Continuous fetal monitoring can be performed using one of two methods: external or internal.

Figure 6-2 is an example of what you will see when you are in the hospital being monitored during your labor, whether you are continuously or intermittently monitored. The top portion of the fetal monitoring strip shows the baby's heart rate, and the bottom portion shows the contractions.

External monitoring

A Doppler—in the form of a handheld device for intermittent monitoring or a disc that can be held against the mom's abdomen with a belt for continuous monitoring—monitors the baby's heart rate to ensure that the baby is tolerating the contractions well. If you are a high-risk patient, are receiving Pitocin, or have an epidural, your doctor may recommend that the baby be monitored continuously. Please check with your doctor and hospital for their rules and guidelines.

To monitor contractions externally, a second disc (called a toco-dynomometer) is held with a belt on the mom's abdomen. This monitor measures the change in the shape of the mom's abdomen as the uterus contracts. It can tell us the duration, frequency, and relative strength of the contractions.

Internal monitoring

We do not regularly use internal monitors unless we have a difficult time monitoring the baby's heartbeat, contractions, or both externally.

A *fetal scalp electrode* (FSE) is the internal monitor that monitors the baby's heartbeat. It has a small spiral metal wire that is screwed onto the baby's scalp. No, this does not sound like something you would want on the head of your soon-to-be-born child. The most it leaves is a little scab on the baby's scalp and will not leave any permanent scars on your little one.

An *intrauterine pressure catheter* (IUPC) is the internal monitor that measures the strength and frequency of your contractions. It is a sterile tube, like an IV line, that we thread into the uterus. In addition to measuring the contractions, the IUPC can be used for an amnioinfusion, where sterile water is infused into the uterus if the baby is showing signs of distress due to low amniotic fluid. By replenishing the fluid in this way, there is a larger cushion around the baby and umbilical cord and less chance that the cord can be squeezed. (A squeezed cord without the extra fluid can lead to fetal distress.)

The risks involved with internal monitors are low, but they can cause infection in the mother and the baby. In addition, after internal monitors are in place, the mother will no longer have the ability to move around and will be bed-bound. For these reasons, we try not to place internal monitors unless medically necessary.

Intravenous Line

It's important for moms to remain adequately hydrated when they're going through labor. That's why we sometimes use an IV (intravenous line) to administer fluids, such as sugar water, during the process. Because most women are not eating or drinking very much as they're laboring, and are doing a lot of heavy breathing, dehydration can happen easily. However, if you are a low-risk patient and can take in some fluids orally, you do not necessarily need an IV while you are in labor. Being attached to an IV pole can be cumbersome and limits mobility. In our practice, we recommend that you have an IV heplock placed. A heplock is a small IV tube with a cap on the end that allows us to have an easy access point in case of an emergency or the need for hydration. In cases of a true emergency, every minute counts for your baby's well-being. Again, the likelihood that an emergency may happen is quite low, so if you really do not want an IV line or a heplock in place, talk to your doctor. If you are on Pitocin, are a high-risk patient, or you want an epidural, you need an IV in place.

Eating during Labor

After our patients are in real labor, with painful contractions occurring every two to three minutes, we encourage them not to eat anything too heavy. If your stomach is full and you are contracting, you may become nauseous and may even vomit. Drinking small to moderate amounts of juice or water, sucking on ice chips, having a few crackers, or enjoying a lollipop is fine. But most laboring women aren't hungry anyway.

The Stages of Labor

Labor is a complex process involving mother and baby. As the uterus contracts and the cervix opens, the baby descends through the birth canal and rotates to find its path of least resistance into the world. Despite most moms' anxiety and fear about how all these complex processes will work in their own bodies, the good news is that nature and our bodies have it worked out so that most of us can have a vaginal delivery. Labor consists of three stages, as outlined in this section. (See Figure 6-3.)

First Stage of Labor

The first stage of labor is the period between onset of labor and full cervical dilation (ten centimeters). This stage is divided into two phases, the latent phase and the active phase.

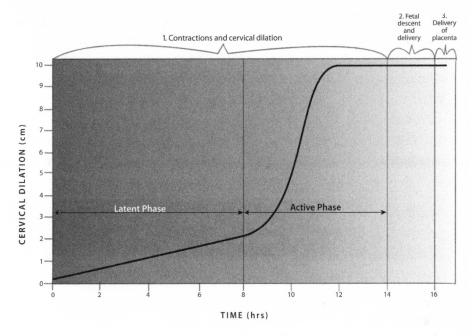

Figure 6-3: Stages of Labor

The latent phase

The latent phase, in which the cervix dilates from zero to four centimeters, is the most unpredictable part of your labor, primarily because it's hard to tell precisely when the latent phase begins. This phase generally lasts from six to twenty hours for first-time moms, and four to fourteen hours for veterans. The contractions become more regular, starting twenty to thirty minutes apart and becoming four to five minutes apart, lasting between thirty to sixty seconds.

During this time, you may be trying to figure out if this is the real thing or only Braxton Hicks contractions. You may also see bloody show or the release of the mucous plug. The amniotic sac could also break during this phase, resulting in a leak of fluid.

As true labor in the latent phase progresses, the contractions become stronger and more frequent. Lying down, resting, or drinking fluids will not slow down or alleviate the pain. If you are not ready to come into the hospital and would like to remain home for as long as possible as you go through the initial phase, several techniques can help you tolerate the labor pains: walking, taking a warm shower, sitting on a birthing ball, getting your lower back massaged, or doing breathing exercises with assistance from your partner or a doula.

Over the years, we've seen moms undergo hypnosis, have acupuncture, or practice chanting with their partners and doulas to make labor pains more bearable. If you desire a natural birth without pain medications, we will support you in whatever works for you as long as we feel that you and the baby are safe and healthy. If your natural techniques aren't working and you are in significant discomfort, you may want to consider getting an epidural or using IV pain medications.

myth: Because my mom had a very difficult labor, I will surely face a difficult one, too.

FACT: Don't worry unnecessarily. What your mom or sister went through is not necessarily a prediction of how your labor will go. However, we believe genetics does play some role. For instance, if you come from a family of people who are quite tall, you may have a large baby, and possibly a more difficult labor.

The active phase

Active labor is characterized by increased regularity and intensity of contractions. The now thunderous contractions cause the rate of dilation to increase significantly. Some refer to this phase as the transition. Women may find themselves nauseous, huffing and puffing, sweating, and overwhelmed by the idea that they cannot take it anymore. You may ask for an epidural or IV pain medication during this phase. However, this is also the time that support from your doctor, nurse, doula, and partner is the most useful—to encourage you to stay calm and focused, keeping in mind that the end is in sight. Although this is the time when some women become desperate for pain relief, it's also the time when we've witnessed our patients who choose an unmedicated birth demonstrate an enormous amount of focus, determination, and strength.

During the active phase, first-time moms generally dilate at least 1 to 1.2 centimeters per hour, while second- and third-time moms could dilate at least 1.5 centimeters per hour, and sometimes more.

Clearly, not every baby has read the book on exactly how its labor is supposed to progress. In days past, doctors were quite strict with their evaluation of how a woman was progressing through these different stages. If you hadn't pushed the baby out during a certain time period, you were likely to be whisked down the hall to surgery for a cesarean. Today, if you're continuing to make progress and the baby is not in any distress, the progress of your labor does not need to follow such rigid guidelines and you'll have more flexibility in your options. Talk to your doctor about his or her philosophy on labor and ask what that doctor might recommend if your labor stalls out.

▶ ▶ ▶ A LABOR AND DELIVERY NURSE'S PERSPECTIVE

I can't begin to explain my passion for nursing without recounting my own labor and delivery experience. When I had my first child, Isabella, I had been a labor and delivery nurse for two years. I had requested to be induced on my due date because I could not bear being pregnant for one more day. My journey began with twelve hours of Cervidil to ripen my cervix, followed by intense contractions, and an epidural at one centimeter. After about twelve more hours of Pitocin, I started feeling the contractions and the urge to push just as my night shift colleagues arrived fresh for their shift. What I didn't expect was all my fellow nurses would invite themselves to join my pushing extravaganza!

Because I had seen the labor and delivery process so many times, I had confidence in knowing what do. Little did I know that I would be doing it for almost three hours! Shortly after I started pushing, I began to feel every excruciating contraction in my abdomen and the intense pressure in my bottom. Everyone kept yelling, "Here she comes!" "You got it!" "You're almost there!" But after the first hour, it was hard for me to believe anymore. Soon, more of my coworkers entered the room and started joining in on the encouragements. Finally, with the aid of a vacuum and an episiotomy, I delivered my six-pound, eight-ounce giant. The feelings of triumph, exhaustion, and wonderment of finally having my baby in my arms were overwhelming. I will never be able to forget the empowerment and the comfort that my fellow nurses gave me on that day. Never once did they tell me to give up. They might have been thinking about it, but their words and encouragement never faltered.

My personal labor and delivery experience made a huge effect on my work as a labor and delivery nurse. I know how exciting and scary it is to come to the hospital to have your baby. I know about the anguish, the pain, and the tears in enduring the labor process. I know what it feels like when someone is telling you, "You're almost there" and you're thinking "No, I'm not!" I feel that my role as a nurse is to be a woman's guide, someone whom she can trust and count on. What can I say to make my patient more at ease? If I change my patient's position will it affect the outcome? Will my patient dilate more quickly if I do certain interventions? Because of my friends' and colleagues' dedication to me, I feel this same responsibility to my patients.

—Jinnie Noh Shim, Labor and Delivery Nurse ◀ ◀ ◀

myth: Walking makes you go through labor faster.

FACT: Studies have shown that walking does not make a difference in the duration of labor. In our practice, however, we do encourage moms to walk if they desire a natural experience without pain medications because walking may help with pain control.

Second Stage of Labor

The second stage of labor is the period between full cervical dilation (ten centimeters) and delivery of the infant. This is where the pushing comes in. Pushing is harder work than most people anticipate, especially for first-time moms. You may be lucky and push for only fifteen minutes, while others may be at it for three hours! On average, first-time moms push for about fifty minutes, and multip moms push for twenty minutes.

You will know when it is time to push because you will have a sensation similar to the one that occurs when you have a bowel movement. Even with an epidural in place, most women will be able to feel when the baby has moved out of the uterus and into the vaginal canal. They experience a distinct pressure sensation and have a natural urge to push with each contraction.

The motion of pushing is similar to the action of having a bowel movement. The direction of your forceful push, using all the strength of your abdominal muscles, is toward the rectum so that the baby can slip under the pubic bone. A long, sustained push lasting for about ten seconds is the most effective means of moving the baby through the birth canal.

Following are some tips when pushing:

1. Find a position that is comfortable for you with your pelvis opened and relaxed. This may be on your back, on your side, squatting, or on your hands and knees. (See Figures 6-6 through 6-10 on pages 268–270.)
2. Curl over the baby, with your chin down to your chest. This allows the angle of the push to be most effective. Do not arch your back.
3. As each contraction begins, take in a deep breath. Hold your breath as you push for about ten seconds. Let the air out and quickly take another breath and repeat the push. Do this three to four times with each contraction.
4. Do not let your air out until you finish the push; otherwise, you will lose your force.
5. As you are waiting for the next contraction to start, let all your muscles and your mind relax. Have a sip of water or have your partner put a moist cloth on your forehead.
6. Push with your abdominal muscles, not with your legs or into your face. The motion of the push is toward the rectum, as if you are having a bowel movement.

Over the years, we've noticed that most moms have focused all their energy on the first stage of labor—the breathing and relaxing techniques—and have done little to prepare for the pushing phase. It may be helpful to watch birthing videos or do some reading about how the baby comes out so you can better visualize what you are trying to do. Please, do not forget about this important facet of your labor. We'd hate for you to work so hard to get to ten centimeters only to find out that you are now too tired to push through all the way. The key is in pacing yourself. During the latent and active phases, allow yourself to relax completely between contractions. You need to save your energy for the physical act of pushing.

Some women who have an extremely long first stage, especially one that goes on for a few days, may not have enough strength left to push. In these cases, an epidural and a greatly needed nap may revitalize and rejuvenate a mom so she can get through the important second stage. Only you know how much energy and stamina you have left, and you need to let your partner, doctor, nurse, and doula know where you are on the energy spectrum.

Television and movies haven't helped at all on the pushing front. Even our show is guilty of it, but what movie or TV series is going to feature two hours of a woman trying to push her baby out? So in most TV shows and movies, the mom pushes three times and then the baby comes out, misleading many new parents into thinking that is how the delivery will be. Frequently, the amount of force needed to push the baby out completely takes women by surprise.

▶ ▶ ▶ THE LONG PUSH

Claudine and Jean, with their charming, elegant French accents, had recently moved to the United States from Paris and were overjoyed about having their first baby together. Claudine's pregnancy had been textbook perfect. Her due date came and went, but just five days later, her labor started at around 6:00 a.m. By 11:00 a.m., Claudine's water broke and she was really in the heat of it. When the couple arrived at the hospital, she was already six centimeters dilated. The baby looked great. Because we allow moms to labor in water at our hospital, to help relax them and lessen their labor pains, Claudine was able to get in the warm Jacuzzi for a little while, and within a few hours, she was ten centimeters dilated.

By this time, Claudine was feeling a lot of pressure and had the urge to push. She got herself into a comfortable position and began the process. She pushed well, with little coaching. It all came naturally to her.

But after three strong pushes, Jean looked at me strangely and asked with concern, "Where is the baby? Why isn't she out yet?'

I reassured him that this was all normal and that sometimes moms will push for a few hours with their first baby. He furrowed his brow with some doubt and said, "You mean to tell me you, me, her, and the nurse are going to be in this room, with her pushing like this, for hours? There is no way that she can do that!"

"Birth takes time," I explained to them. "We are trying to squeeze a round peg through a square hole. It's not like in the movies where the mom pushes a few times and the baby flies out. The hard work has been edited out—even out of our own show, which is documentary-style! It's just not that interesting to watch a woman pushing for more than a few minutes."

Claudine, of course, *was* able to do it. After an hour and twenty minutes of sweating and pushing her heart out, she gave birth to a beautiful girl named Sabine, who weighed eight pounds, thirteen ounces. My French couple couldn't have been happier, and the struggle of the journey—including the long push—faded quickly into memory for them.

—Allison ◀ ◀ ◀

Episiotomy

An *episiotomy* is an incision the doctor makes in the vaginal opening to allow for delivery of the baby's head. The incision is usually made from the bottom of the vaginal opening toward the anus. There are no official guidelines on how big an episiotomy should be. Women with an epidural usually will not feel an episiotomy. For women without an epidural, a local injection of numbing medicine can be given before the incision.

Years ago, episiotomy was a routine part of a vaginal delivery. In fact, old obstetrical text books list "cut a generous episiotomy" as step one in the delivery of a baby. As time has marched on, the medical community has come to agree that an episiotomy is rarely necessary. In a few situations, however, an episiotomy is appropriate. For example, if the baby has fetal distress and needs to be delivered immediately, the episiotomy can give the necessary room for the baby to come out quickly. In addition, if we see too much tension on the skin as the head is crowning and we are concerned that tearing may occur in all directions, we may suggest an episiotomy. As you can see, the decision to make an episiotomy does not happen until the last few minutes of the labor process.

Many women, especially first-time moms, will tear, or lacerate, the vaginal tissue during delivery. Unfortunately, you do not have complete control over this tearing. It is affected by many factors, including:

- The size of your baby in relation to your birth canal
- The consistency of your vaginal tissue (stretchy or tight)

- Whether your baby is coming through the vaginal opening slowly, to allow time for the tissue to stretch
- The need for a vacuum or forceps

There are four levels of potential tearing during delivery:

- First-degree laceration: tear of the skin only
- Second-degree laceration: tear of the skin and underlying muscle
- Third-degree laceration: tear of the skin, muscle, and the anal sphincter muscle
- Fourth-degree laceration: tear extends all the way from the vagina into the rectum

Your doctor or midwife will use dissolving stitches to repair any lacerations, so you won't need to worry about having them removed. You may receive local anesthesia for pain relief during the repair. After the repair is completed, we use ice packs and numbing sprays to keep the swelling down. The vaginal tissue heals within a few weeks of delivery. You do not need to clean the area in any special way other than rinsing it with warm water and using a gentle soap when you shower.

▶ ▶ ▶ MY BIRTH EXPERIENCE

I was quite lucky with my first pregnancy. I had a terrific pregnancy overall. Then the big day arrived: my bag of water broke in the middle of my sleep, and I went into the hospital.

One of my concerns about the delivery had always been "How badly would I tear?" I told my obstetrician that if he thought I was going to have a third or a fourth degree tear, he should do a cesarean delivery. I feared the potential pain and problems that might result. But being an obstetrician myself, I knew no one could predict how badly I would tear. So even though I pushed Matthew out with relative ease, I ended up with a third-degree tear.

I won't lie: It was uncomfortable for the first two weeks or so. And that first bowel movement was a little scary—you wonder, "Can things open up again?" But being an obstetrician, I also knew that the blood supply in your perineal area is pretty terrific and that women are designed to heal well there. That's exactly what happened for me.

If you have discomfort during the first two weeks after a vaginal birth, my advice is to use the anesthetic spray or foam that the hospital gives you, apply ice packs to help with the swelling, take ibuprofen for pain, try raisin bran cereal for the constipation, and do warm sitz baths with witch hazel several times a day until your perineum starts to feel better. I promise, it will.

—Alane ◀ ◀ ◀

Third Stage of Labor

The third stage of labor is the period between delivery of the infant and delivery of the placenta. Most placentas come out within a few minutes of delivery. The placenta naturally detaches from the uterus and will by expelled by the force of continued uterine contractions. Thankfully, the placenta is smaller and softer than the baby, so there is little discomfort with its delivery. Your doctor will examine the placenta to be certain that it has been delivered in its entirety without any small parts being left behind.

Inducing Labor

myth: Eating spicy foods or a special balsamic dressing can help induce labor.

FACT: We've seen no evidence to prove a connection between what you put in your stomach and when your body goes into labor.

Despite modern medicine's miraculous strides, years of research, and innovation, we have yet to understand the sequence of events that cause labor to begin. The general thought is that a hormone released by the fetal adrenal gland somehow initiates the chain of events that become labor. But we don't know how to turn on the system. And we also haven't discovered an off switch to stop labor if it happens prematurely.

Spontaneous labor is always preferable because it allows the baby to settle down properly into the birth canal, while the natural uterine contractions help to efface and dilate the cervix most efficiently. However, inducing labor may be indicated if any of the following is true:

- You have developed high blood pressure (preeclampsia or eclampsia).
- You are past your due date (post-term).
- Your baby isn't growing normally (fetal growth restriction).
- You have certain medical conditions, such as diabetes, blood clotting disorders, lung and heart conditions, lupus, or cholestasis.
- You have low amniotic fluid (oligohydramnios) because your placenta isn't working well and the baby isn't producing amniotic fluid.
- You have a history of stillbirth.
- You have a history of very rapid births.
- You live far away from your hospital.
- You have had six prior vaginal deliveries (grand multips).

The reasons for labor induction include situations where staying pregnant would be harmful to the mom or to the baby. We try to balance the risks to the mother or baby if she stays pregnant against the risks associated with induction or prematurity. This is often a fine line. For example, if a woman develops severe preeclampsia at thirty weeks, she has an increased risk of stroke or seizures if she stays pregnant. At the same time, there are risks to the baby if it is born at only thirty weeks. When the risk to the mother outweighs the risk to the baby, we recommend induction.

Some cases have little to do with medical issues and everything to do with equally important psychosocial factors. For instance, some patients live significantly far from the hospital. They may have other children at home or a history of very rapid births. These patients will often ask for an induction for fear of leaving their other children alone if their labor begins in the middle of the night or of potentially delivering en route to the hospital.

Finally, some women simply want their baby to be born on a certain day for cultural reasons, superstitions, availability of family members, or just because they can't take it anymore. Inducing for these "social" reasons is controversial and must be discussed with your doctor.

Ways to Induce

myth: Having a foot massage will make you go into labor.

FACT: Oh, how we wish labor induction was this simple! Although an acupuncture site on the foot is associated with the uterus, we have yet to see a patient go into labor because her feet were rubbed.

Several basic methods can accelerate the process of cervical ripening and initiation of labor. In nonmedical terms, the following methods can help get your labor rolling when it's not happening on its own:

- Prostaglandin agents
- Oxytocin
- Mechanical cervical dilators
- Membrane stripping
- Amniotomy
- Nipple stimulation
- Nonmedical methods

Prostaglandins, natural chemicals that your body produces, play a critical role in the preparation of your cervix for labor, causing effacement, softening, and dilation in the weeks leading up to delivery. So how do we ripen a cervix if you have to be induced? We use prostaglandins manufactured as a gel (Prepidil) or as a vaginal insert (Cervidil).

Prostaglandins are administered in the hospital while you are observed with a fetal monitor. For example, if your doctor has decided to use Cervidil, it is placed in your vagina next to the cervix. You will not be able to feel it. Cervidil stays in place for twelve hours, and can be replaced by a second insert if the cervix hasn't changed. Do not be disappointed if you are told that your cervix has not changed significantly after the Cervidil is removed. Remember, the goal of this process is to ripen your cervix, not to put you into active labor. On occasion, Cervidil can cause active labor, but this is not common.

Oxytocin is a small but powerful hormone made in your brain that causes uterine contractions. During induction, we can mimic the effects of this hormone by using an identical synthetic agent called *Pitocin*. Because Pitocin has the same chemical structure as oxytocin, the medicine itself is not harmful to the baby. However, if Pitocin causes overly frequent or strong contractions, it can lead to distress in the baby. These strong contractions can happen with natural oxytocin as well. The key here is monitoring and supervision.

We administer Pitocin through a continuous IV pump. The protocols vary from hospital to hospital, but generally we start Pitocin at a low level and increase it slowly over time. After you are contracting every two to three minutes, we maintain the dosage at that level. Pitocin is great at causing your uterus to contract but not that great at ripening your cervix.

Beyond medications to induce labor, several physical methods are also available.

Mechanical cervical dilators are tools we can place into the cervical canal to physically open the cervix. These dilators include the laminaria, the Foley balloon, and the double balloon device.

Membrane stripping is a procedure by which your obstetrician or midwife manually separates the amniotic sac from the cervix during a cervical exam. In this process, natural chemicals (prostaglandins) are released that could help initiate labor. The procedure has no risks but can cause some discomfort and bleeding. Scientific studies show that women who have undergone membrane stripping went into labor earlier compared to women who did not undergo this procedure.[2]

Amniotomy is another physical means of induction. In this procedure, a device called an *amniohook* (essentially a long handle with a small hook at the end) is used to break your bag of water during a cervical exam. Again, this may release the chemicals involved in initiating and augmenting labor. In addition, after the water has been released from the bag, the baby's head can more strongly push down against the cervix. The firm head is a more effective dilator of the cervix than the soft bag of water. Often, combining Pitocin with amniotomy will shorten the interval between the start of induction and the delivery of the baby. The amniotomy itself is not painful; it feels like a regular cervical exam.

Nipple stimulation causes your natural oxytocin to be released from the brain to stimulate labor. Your baby's heart rate should be monitored in case you contract vigorously with this method.

Nonmedical methods of labor induction have been tried by some people. Acupuncture, intercourse, evening primrose oil, and castor oil have been tried to induce labor. Be aware that no scientific findings prove that any of these methods are successful in helping labor to commence.[3]

▶ ▶ ▶ PATIENCE PAYS OFF

Svetlana and Benjamin were a happily married couple already in their late thirties when they decided to have their first baby. When Svetlana was thirty-four weeks pregnant, she confided in me during an office visit that something didn't feel right. She knew that Benjamin was thrilled about the little boy she was carrying. But Svetlana confessed that she just didn't feel these emotions that strongly yet. I told her that many other patients have admitted these fears to me, but it was never anything to worry about—as soon as the baby comes out, something just clicks and moms instantly fall in love. Our maternal instincts kick in too, thank goodness!

Unfortunately, Svetlana's baby was in no hurry to make his entrance and assuage his mother's fears. Svetlana passed her due date and was monitored every three days to check her amniotic fluid levels and undergo a nonstress test. Her testing was always perfect and she had abundant amniotic fluid. Her uterus even showed us that it was contracting regularly but her cervix wasn't yet ready to budge. Each time they would come in, Benjamin was hoping I would find some reason to induce Svetlana, but I just couldn't. Everything was perfect with the baby.

Finally Svetlana got to forty-two weeks, with still no signs of change in her cervix. I told her we were at a stage when I usually recommend induction because, at this late date, the risk of stillbirth begins to increase slightly.

Svetlana prepared herself for a long induction. First, I gave her Cervidil—a prostaglandin to soften her cervix—for twelve hours. Then I started her on Pitocin. I told the nervous couple that they may have to wait a day and a half longer before meeting their newborn son in person. Because they did not want a cesarean, they patiently went through the process.

After Svetlana got an epidural, her water broke. She then progressed nicely with the aid of Pitocin to full dilation (ten centimeters). She pushed like a veteran, and after only an hour of hard work, she delivered a perfect, healthy eight-pound, eleven-ounce boy named Alexei. It was such a triumphant moment for all of us. Svetlana proved my prophecy true—she immediately felt the magic and instantly fell in love with Alexei. I was so proud of the new parents and impressed with their patience. They never gave up or wavered and they got the vaginal delivery—and the "love at first sight" experience—that they were hoping for.

—Yvonne ◀ ◀ ◀

Pain and Induction

When a patient learns that we have to induce her labor, one of her first questions is always, "Will this hurt more than natural labor?"

The first part of the answer to this question is that unfortunately, labor hurts, period. Whether your labor happens naturally or you're in a hospital bed being induced with Pitocin, the uterus must generate a certain amount of force for your cervix to open. And that force is painful. You might be cringing at the thought of the pain you will be enduring, but it has to hurt or the cervix won't open.

That being said, induced labor *does* differ from natural labor in a few key areas. When you go into spontaneous labor, your body prepares the cervix by softening it over time, as the baby moves into the optimal position to maneuver through the birth canal. In induced labor, we are forcing the cervix to open before it is really ready, so the baby may not be in the ideal position.

When we measure the strength of an effective induced contraction, we find that it is essentially the same as the contractions that occur spontaneously. However, in natural labor, oxytocin is released in small bursts, whereas in induced labor, we give Pitocin continuously. In addition, spontaneous labor is coupled with the release of natural endorphins, which nature designed to help women adjust to the pain. These endorphins are not released in the same way during induced labor, making it more difficult for the woman to cope. Although we try to mimic the body's natural processes as much as possible, we can't get it exactly the same way as nature intended it.

In our combined years of practice, we have never seen a baby come out without the mom experiencing some degree of pain with an un-medicated vaginal birth. However, we have observed that, while in-duced labor is not necessarily "stronger," the woman's perception of the pain and the ability to cope with it are different. For this reason, inductions should be proposed for clear medical reasons only. And, of course, whether your labor is spontaneous or induced, a variety of pain management options are available.

▶ ▶ ▶ IN THE ZONE

I have known Bonnie for a number of years. She's a beautiful, caring, smart woman who happens to be a patient of mine, but she also is a labor and deliv-ery nurse at our hospital. Bonnie's pregnancy progressed without much diffi-culty. She had voiced to me that she would like to have as natural a delivery as possible. And because she's a labor and delivery nurse, she knew what to ex-pect. I very much hoped she would go into spontaneous, natural labor. Yet as her due date approached, I was beginning to get concerned about the size of her baby and that her cervix was not ripening.

Her due date approached and then passed. Bonnie was well aware of the risks associated with being post-term (see Chapter 9 for details), so after ten days, we finally gave up and decided on an induction date. Luckily, by this time, her cervix had finally effaced and dilated to one centimeter.

Bonnie was admitted to the hospital in the evening and began her induc-tion with Pitocin. In the morning, I came by to break her bag of water. She seemed disheartened that she was not in much pain, despite being on Pitocin all night. She was afraid the induction would not work. I reassured her that it is common for women not to be in significant pain until the bag of water has broken.

About fifty minutes after her bag of water was broken, Bonnie started feeling much more uncomfortable and knew she was now in active labor. By her side were two L&D nurses, Jessica and Karole—both friends from the hospital—acting as her labor support. Thanks to Jessica and Karole, the room had great positive energy for Bonnie and for me as well. I had also delivered Jessica's son and daughter and Karole's little girl. They all did phenomenal jobs pushing their babies out vaginally, but they had epidurals during their births, as I did.

Throughout the first hours of her labor, with Pitocin going strong, Bonnie remained in the zone. She was in tune with her body, breathing through the contractions and relaxing when they would subside. As it became harder for her to endure the pain, she asked me to examine her, hoping that she had made some progress. I happily reported that she'd dilated from three to six centimeters in about four hours. Bonnie could see the light at the end of that tunnel. She then progressed to ten centimeters, without any IV pain meds, without an epidural, and with Pitocin on board. I watched her face as we pushed together, noticing that she looked tired but completed focused. And after about thirty minutes of pushing, she birthed a beautiful baby girl, nearly eight pounds.

Bonnie performed like a champ that day, and I told her so. She had a Pitocin-induced labor and delivery without an epidural, without any pain medications. I've seen induced and pain medication–free labors more than once. I am certain that if you asked her, she'd tell you she was in a world of pain. She has participated in hundreds of births herself. So to see her deliver her beautiful daughter the way she envisioned it, even with the Pitocin . . . Wow! is all I can say. I get to see the strength that women are capable of, every day.

—Alane ◀ ◀ ◀

Induced labors are responsible for higher cesarean rates. When your body is not yet prepared for labor, with a Bishop's score of 5 or less (see page 224), the chance that an induction will lead to a cesarean is 30 to 40 percent. In addition, if the induction is performed for a medical condition such as fetal growth restriction, the baby may not be able to tolerate the labor process anyway, leading to a cesarean. In this case, the very medical issue that caused us to induce in the first place—slow fetal growth due to a poorly functioning placenta—increases the chance that the baby wouldn't tolerate labor.

The most important point about induction is to be clear about why your doctor is recommending it. Don't hesitate to ask questions, find out about any alternatives, and have a discussion about the risks and benefits of the method your doctor will be using.

Pain Management

myth: A drug-free, natural childbirth is always best.

FACT: Although natural childbirth is a laudable goal, pain medications may be used during childbirth for many legitimate emotional and medical reasons. Patients with high-risk conditions may require labor induction or cesareans. In addition, many women simply do not want to feel the pain associated with labor. The bottom line is, there is no right or wrong way to deliver your baby. Your mission—and ours—comes down to this: a healthy baby and a healthy mom.

Some mothers are determined to have the most natural deliveries possible and choose to forego pain medications. Millions of mothers have been having babies without medications for thousands of years, but in some places in the world, childbirth is a risky proposition for both mother and baby. Modern hospital births have changed that.

Our first-time moms hear a lot of labor stories by the time they're ready to deliver. Some people try to make them feel guilty if they don't choose to tough it out and go all natural. Others regale them with stories of indescribable pain more suitable for the plot of a slasher horror movie. When our patients ask us how painful labor is, we reply that labor hurts but people perceive labor pain differently. Some women have almost no pain up to ten centimeters, but others are straining at only one centimeter. Labor pain can be controlled and doesn't have to be associated with all those nightmarish stories.

Alane's son Matthew's preschool teacher has a saying that "There are no 'bad' feelings." By this she means that *all* our feelings—from happiness to sadness to pain—are valid and natural states of our emotional being. Labor and delivery is a finite experience. You will not feel the pain forever.

You know your temperament and tolerance for pain. Don't let the pressure of family or friends persuade you. Do what *you* want to do.

The experience of a drug-free birth is vitally important for some women but it's not for everybody. Remember that no matter what you decide, your birth experience will be unforgettable.

It's not uncommon for a mom-to-be to tell us, "I wouldn't go to the dentist and have them work on my teeth without numbing medicine just because I can. Why should I go through labor without some pain relief?" We've also had patients who have gone through a fairly easy, drug-free natural childbirth with every one of their pregnancies. These days, more than 50 percent of women in America give birth with an epidural or a spinal block. But nonpharmacologic pain management alternatives do exist: relaxation, hypnosis, breathing, massage, acupuncture, labor coach, doula participation, walking, showering, bathtubs, and birthing balls. You do have other choices.

▶ ▶ ▶ SO THIS IS WHAT IT FEELS LIKE?

I remember asking my doctor early on how I would know when the contractions are real. She told me I would know, and she was right.

During the drive to the hospital, I yelled and screamed while my husband told me to breathe. Just breathe, as if it were that easy. Everything I had learned in the birthing classes was long forgotten. After we arrived at the hospital, I continued yelling and even started cursing. The pain was scary. At 4 p.m. the nurse checked to see how dilated I was, and I learned I was six centimeters! Only six centimeters? Then, like a gift from the heavens, the anesthesiologist appeared. He was here to save me from the pain.

By 5 p.m. the pain had disappeared. I began to look around and suddenly felt embarrassed. I realized that I had looked and acted like a complete lunatic. I apologized to all the nurses and anyone else who was nearby. I felt like myself again and wanted them to know that the crazy woman was gone.

I would like to applaud all those women who can manage to have a baby without the aid of medication. They are my heroes.

—*Linda, Allison's patient* ◀ ◀ ◀

Pain medications are optional, but if you don't want a painful labor, you don't have to have one. Following are several methods of pain management that you may have access to in your hospital.

- Regional anesthesia (epidural or spinal)
- IV narcotics
- General anesthesia
- Local anesthesia
- Doula support

We describe each of these methods in the following sections.

Regional Anesthesia

The two types of regional anesthesia are epidurals and spinals. Epidurals are normally used to control labor pain for the duration of the labor. Spinals are primarily used for cesareans, take effect more quickly than epidurals, but wear off in a few hours. In an *epidural,* a small catheter or tubing is placed in the epidural space (in front of the spinal nerves, as shown in Figure 6-4). In a *spinal,* the anesthetic is placed directly into the compartment containing spinal fluid.

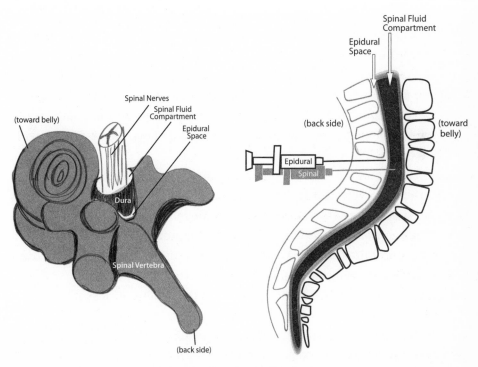

Figure 6-4: Spinal vs. Epidural

Epidural procedure

From the time you first make the request for an epidural to the time you're pain free takes about thirty to forty-five minutes. So don't wait to ask for an epidural until the pain is so severe that you're at your wit's end. Some doctors recommend waiting to get an epidural after you are at least four centimeters dilated; others allow epidural placement when you are having regular painful contractions, regardless of the dilation. You should talk to your doctor about his or her preferences.

The first step in getting regional pain management is to request it from your labor nurse, who will contact your doctor or midwife and then your anesthesiologist. Some advice: If you know you want an epidural from the beginning, make sure you ask your nurse to check out the activity on the L&D floor. If cesareans are scheduled and many laboring moms are requesting epidurals, your L&D nurse can find out how many women are ahead of you, waiting for an overbooked anesthesiologist to get to them.

Next, your nurse will start IV fluids to make sure you are well hydrated, to help prevent a drop in your blood pressure. When the anesthesiologist arrives, he or she will usually ask you to sit on the edge of the bed with your legs hanging off or lie on your side on the bed. You will curl over the baby in the shape of a *C*, like someone with really bad posture, to try to open up the space between each vertebrae. The anesthesiologist then injects numbing medicine into the skin where the spinal needle will be inserted (see Figure 6-5). This injection feels like a pinch or it may burn.

The spinal needle is inserted into the epidural space, and a catheter (a very thin, long tube) is threaded through the needle into the space. The catheter is then taped to your back and connected to a pump containing the anesthetic medication. The catheter stays in place until the delivery. When the catheter is removed, it doesn't hurt.

In some hospitals, you may have an epidural pump that you can control by pushing a button to give yourself more or less medication. Some women prefer to be completely pain free; others want to feel some of the contractions.

Many women fall asleep right after they've had an epidural because they've been in a lot of discomfort and are simply worn out

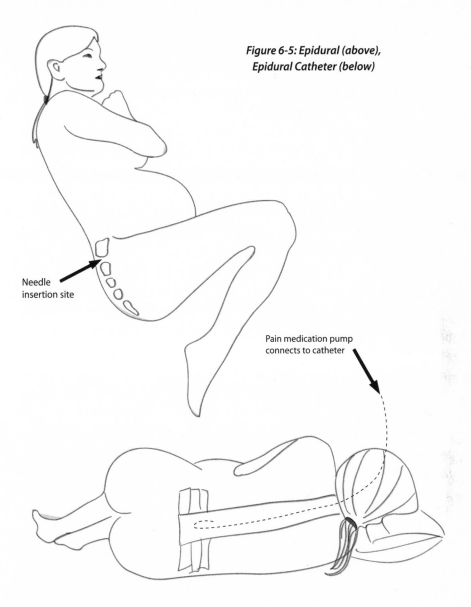

Figure 6-5: Epidural (above),
Epidural Catheter (below)

Needle
insertion site

Pain medication pump
connects to catheter

myth: Epidurals cause back pain.

FACT: Epidurals virtually never create back problems. Sometimes doctors will
give an epidural specifically *because* a patient is experiencing back pain.

from the labor process. After a mother gets an epidural, it allows her a welcome break from the struggle and some precious moments to rest.

Pros and cons of epidurals

The most obvious advantage to having an epidural is pain relief. An epidural can be helpful precisely because it allows a tense patient to relax. It can be exactly what a mother needs to get her through her labor. Sometimes, just letting go of that pain-created tension allows the cervix to open up quickly. As we've mentioned before, pushing is a lot of work, so pacing yourself is a smart idea.

On the other hand, epidurals have some potential disadvantages, as outlined in the following paragraphs.

Pushing can be more difficult if you have had an epidural because you do not have physical feedback telling you where and how hard to push. Moms, especially first-time moms, can find it difficult to coordinate their movements when they can't feel their muscles. In these situations, we may lower the epidural dosage. Sensation returns in about thirty to sixty minutes. At that time, the patient will know where to push. Sometimes, we use a mirror to help the mom coordinate her pushing effort so she can see what happens when she pushes. The visual feedback can help a great deal when physical sensation is diminished. Reaching down and touching your baby's head in the vaginal canal may help motivate you to push harder, because you can sense that the finish line is right in front of you.

Hypotension, or a drop in blood pressure, is another potential side effect of an epidural. The medications used for the epidural relax the blood vessels, which can cause blood pressure to drop. In turn, this can lead to a decrease in the baby's heart rate. To keep your blood pressure from falling too low, you will often be given a large amount of IV fluids just before the epidural placement. At other times, the anesthesiologist may give you a medication to increase your blood pressure.

Spinal headaches occur because some of your spinal fluid leaks out during the anesthesia placement. Spinal headaches hurt when you are sitting or standing but disappear when lying down. If you have a headache like this, notify your doctor. If the headache is mild, you will be asked to try some caffeine (coffee) and Tylenol or Motrin. If the headache is not relieved with these measures, you may need a blood patch. In this procedure, your anesthesiologist uses a small amount of your blood to patch the small hole where the spinal fluid is leaking. Think of it as a Band-Aid over the leak. This procedure has minimal complications, and you will notice an immediate improvement in your headache.

Labor duration may be affected by the use of epidurals. In some studies, epidurals have been associated with an increase in the duration of the first stage of labor by thirty to ninety minutes and the second stage of labor by fifteen to twenty minutes.[4] However, most moms will gladly labor an extra hour if they can do it comfortably. Epidurals also increase the need for Pitocin and the use of the vacuum.

Fever may result if you have an epidural. The exact cause is uncertain: It may be due to infection or your body's inability to control your temperature from the medications used in the epidural space. Whatever the reason, if you do develop a fever, your doctor will most likely recommend IV antibiotics.

Finally, some moms are terrified of an epidural—just the thought that someone is going to put a needle near their spine is more than they can handle.

▶ ▶ ▶ DADDY GOES DOWN

My patient Erin, a petite gymnastics teacher, had brought her tall, masculine pro-football player husband, Lance, with her to every prenatal appointment. Both first-time parents-to-be, they went through every stage of Erin's pregnancy with flying colors. Lance seemed fascinated with the details of what would happen at the birth, where he could stand, and what he could see. His excitement was palpable.

One week before the due date, Erin's water broke and her contractions came hard and furious. By the time the couple arrived at the hospital, she was five centimeters dilated and in serious pain. Lance did his best to comfort her, but she soon needed more than soothing words. Finally, an agonized Erin called out for an epidural.

She sat on the edge of the bed with her legs hanging off the side as Lance was engaged in conversation with the anesthesiologist. What was the medicine he was using? Where would the catheter go? How does he know he's in the right spot? Lance was full of curiosity about the procedure.

As the doctor pulled the spinal needle out of its box, Lance glanced over Erin's shoulder to look at it. He had no idea it would be so long! The next thing we knew, Lance felt nauseous, sweaty, and wobbly. He started to lose his balance as he began to faint, and he reached for Erin in one desperate effort to stay on his feet. However, it was too late. He hit the floor and pulled Erin off the bed with him. She tumbled over him, landing chin-first on the hardwood floor.

Lance was taken to the emergency room, and Erin, through one contraction after another, was helped back into bed, with a bleeding gash on her chin. She finally received her epidural and got some pain relief, but her chin continued to bleed. A plastic surgeon was called, and she received ten stitches.

A few hours later, I went to the room to deliver the baby. I found Lance lying on the sofa with an IV in his arm and Erin sitting in her bed with a giant ice pack and bandage taped to her chin. Needless to say, the delivery was a walk in the park compared to what they had been through before that. And everyone agreed—in a few years it would make for a great birth story.

—Allison ◀ ◀ ◀

What epidurals won't do

A common misconception is that epidurals put a halt to the labor process—that they somehow stop everything—so that a person with an epidural will inevitably end up with a cesarean. Scientific studies have proven that this is not true. When adjusting for other variables, epidurals do not increase the cesarean rate. For women who end up with a cesarean after a long labor, likely something was dysfunctional about the labor from the start. Perhaps the baby was just too big or wasn't coming through the birth canal in the proper position. The epidural did not cause the problem.

In addition, studies have not shown *early* epidural placement to be associated with increased cesarean rates. However, as mentioned, early epidurals have been associated with longer labors and pushing time.

Another misconception about epidurals is that they affect the baby. Unlike IV medications that can make the baby sleepy, epidurals do not have a significant effect on the baby because the amount of medication absorbed into the bloodstream is minimal. Babies born to moms with epidurals are alert and active immediately after delivery.

Pregnant women are also concerned that somehow the epidural or spinal may cause chronic backaches. This, too, is a myth. Remember that the process of being pregnant and delivering a child puts a lot of strain on a woman's back. Patients often come in postpartum and complain that their back is hurting, and attribute it to their epidural. We remind them they've been carrying around extra weight the last few months of their pregnancy. Now they are carrying around a newborn, and a car seat, and a stroller, and a diaper bag, and they may be hunched over trying their best to breastfeed. This is what is most likely causing their sore back, *not* the epidural. It's true that after an epidural, a patient can experience a little soreness or bruising at the insertion site for a few days to a few weeks, but this soreness does not cause long-term chronic back pain.

In a few situations, an epidural is not advised or isn't possible. Women who are on blood thinners, have a low platelet count, have difficulty with blood clotting, or have abnormalities of the spine such as severe scoliosis may not be candidates for an epidural. In addition, if you have had spinal surgery, any accident or injury affecting your back, or disc problems, you should discuss the safety of an epidural with your anesthesiologist.

IV Drugs

We can also deliver pain medications through an intravenous line directly into the bloodstream. These drugs are narcotics, from the morphine family. The medications take effect within a few minutes after they have been administered by the nurse. Although the feeling of pain is lessened, it does not totally disappear, allowing the mom to have the ability to push. However, IV medications affect mental clarity, causing the woman to feel drowsy. In addition, they cross the placenta to the baby, also leading to drowsiness in the newborn. If they are given too close to delivery of the baby, the newborn may be drowsy and have difficulty breathing. The pediatrician can give the baby a medication to reverse this effect. The pain medications do not have any long-term consequences for the baby.

General Anesthesia

As a rule, we try not to use general anesthesia during delivery because the medication crosses the placenta to the baby, making the baby very drowsy. In general anesthesia, a woman is completely asleep, on a breathing machine, and receiving anesthesia in the form of a gas. It is used only in emergency situations where the baby needs to be delivered quickly, and there is no time for the placement of an epidural or a spinal or the mother's medical condition does not allow an epidural.

Local Anesthesia

Local anesthesia is medication that is injected directly into the vaginal tissue. It is most commonly used before an episiotomy or during repairs of any tears you may have developed during the birth. It is similar to medicine used for dental procedures.

Doula Support

A *doula* is a woman who is trained and experienced in childbirth and provides continuous physical, emotional, and informational support to a woman during labor, birth, and the immediate postpartum period.[5] Thirty or forty years ago, a doula may simply have been an experienced mother coaching a new mom through a difficult birth, but today, doulas undergo a short training course and assist with labor support and postpartum care. A doula is not a midwife and does not deliver babies, but she is well versed in relaxation, breathing, and other natural pain control techniques. Over the past few decades, doulas have become a well-accepted staple of the modern childbirth process.

Most medical schools and OB-GYN residencies don't formally teach doctors about doulas and their many skills and benefits. We think that's a shame. Experienced doulas can be a significant addition to any mom's labor and delivery process. Studies have shown that having a doula during your labor and delivery decreased the need for pain medication, Pitocin, and vacuum or forceps-assisted deliveries, and shortened the time for labor and delivery.

The excellent doulas with whom we have had the privilege of working are seasoned pros who have undergone training and have been mentored by other veteran doulas. They work hard at helping to give mom the birth experience she's wished for. Most importantly, expert doulas make sure that the most important goal to keep in sight is to have a healthy mom and baby, whether through a drug-free vaginal birth or a cesarean delivery.

Keep in mind, your unofficial doula may not be a credentialed, hired support person, but your partner, sister, or friend. We think of labor and delivery as a team effort. This team consists of the soon-to-be mom, her partner, her obstetrician (or midwife), her anesthesiologist, her L&D nurse, any

BEING A DOULA

We are all fans of doulas and have met several who've especially impressed us. Carmen Bornn is one of them, and she kindly agreed to write a description of her important work for our book:

"As a birth doula, I am blessed with the honor and privilege of helping families during one of the most special and intense times of their lives, the birth of their children. Whether I am giving suggestions to a husband on how he can help massage and stretch his wife's leg to relieve her discomfort during pregnancy, or showing him how to support her body during labor without hurting his own back, my job is all about the little things.

Many nights I have found myself with a family in the wee hours, helping a mother find her labor pattern. I've discovered that my soft touch on her forehand, a smile shared from my positive attitude, a little guidance toward a new labor position, or the repetition of her chosen hypnotic phrase—or maybe a combination of all these things—keeps her steadfast, calm, and poised on her safe birth plan. Again, all the little things help.

Being a doula is about the purity of my attention to these many little things, which all come together to help empower a family into its creation. By the same token, these little things make for such a wonder-filled, big job."

other support person she desires, whether a sister, best friend, or licensed doula. Work with your obstetrician, family, and doula ahead of time to make sure everyone is on the same team for your delivery day.

Your Delivery Position

In the traditional birthing position, shown in Figure 6-6, a woman lies on her back with her legs open and pulled back slightly toward her head. For many women, this is the most effective position for delivering the baby. It allows the baby to maneuver through the narrowest part of the pelvis. Gravity will help to pull the baby's head toward the mother's back so it can slip under the pubic bone in the front. Especially if a mom has an epidural, this position may be the most comfortable and efficient. The angle of the pelvis is straightest in this position, so it may be helpful for women who have larger babies. When you have a bigger-than-average baby, every millimeter counts.

myth: Lying on your back is not the most effective delivery position.

FACT: Doctors suggest using the traditional birthing position, with the mom on her back with her hips opened and her legs pulled back against herself, for good reasons. In that position, gravity pulls the baby back toward the spine so it can pass under the pubic bone, which is the path of least resistance in many births.

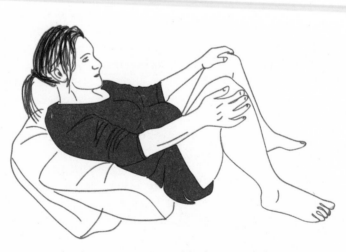

Figure 6-6: Traditional Birthing Position

However, you might want to try other positions, such as squatting with a squat bar (see Figure 6-7), on your side (see Figure 6-8), or on your hands and knees (see Figure 6-9). If your baby and pelvis are both of normal size, almost any of these positions are effective. In all cases, the same principles hold true: Bear down with your pelvis

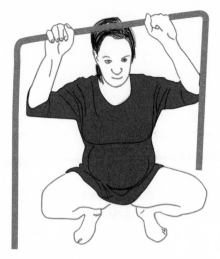

Figure 6-7:
Squatting Birthing Position

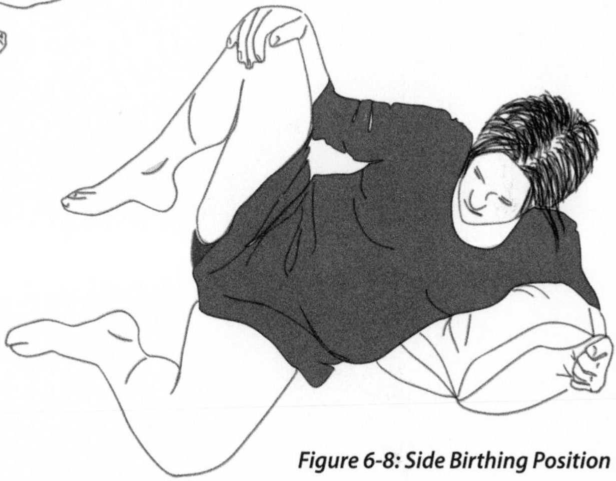

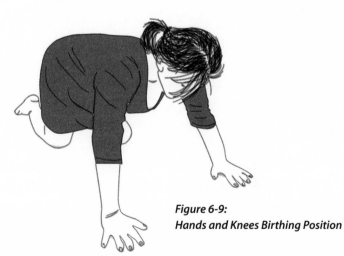

Figure 6-8: Side Birthing Position

Figure 6-9:
Hands and Knees Birthing Position

open, curling over the baby. You should start pushing in whatever position feels the most natural to you. If you are pushing strongly but not making progress in moving the baby, your doctor may suggest that you try a different position.

As we described in Chapter 5, babies in the OP (occiput posterior or sunny-side-up) position are harder to push out, particularly if your baby is large and this is your first birth. Alane pushed out her second son, Max, in the OP position. If your obstetrician or L&D nurse suspects that your baby is in the OP position, he or she may place you in an exaggerated Sim's position (see Figure 6-10), which may help your baby rotate into the easier OA (occiput anterior) position.

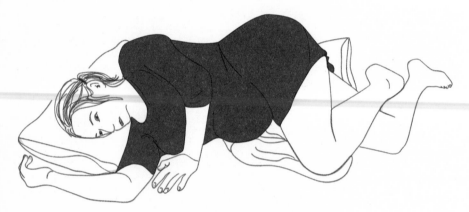

Figure 6-10: Exaggerated Sim's Birthing Position

Forceps and Vacuum Extractions

Forceps and vacuums are devices used to pull the baby out vaginally. We use vacuums and forceps when the mom is exhausted. Sometimes a mom's been pushing for quite some time but can't get to the finish line because she has no more energy. The other indication for forceps or vacuums is when the baby shows signs of distress and we must speed up the delivery.

Forceps are metal instruments that resemble large salad servers. The doctor places the forceps on each side of the baby's head and applies traction to pull the head out. Although not used as frequently these days, forceps are considered a safe route of delivery in the hands of a well-trained obstetrician and can be lifesaving. Complications from forceps can include lacerations to the baby's face, injuries to the skull, and lacerations to the mother's vagina.

The *vacuum extractor* is a handheld plastic cup that is placed on the baby's head. The doctor applies suction and then, as the mom pushes, gently pulls on the device to allow for the delivery of the head. Like forceps, vacuums can cause trauma to the vagina as well as bleeding and bruising of the baby's scalp.

Cesarean Delivery

In the United States, approximately 30 percent of all babies are delivered by cesarean. Most women prefer a vaginal delivery because it feels natural to them, the recovery is easier, and there are no surgical risks. However, we can't forget that "natural," in the days before modern medicine, meant that childbirth was one of the riskiest and potentially deadliest times in a woman's life. Even today, women in third-world countries routinely lose a baby or their own lives during delivery. In developing countries, the mortality rate (deaths associated with childbirth) can be as high as 1,400 per 100,000 births; in the United States, the maternal mortality rate is 24 per 100,000 births.[6] Doctors, midwives, and medical technology can intervene when, for whatever reason, nature isn't coming through.

Common Cesarean Myths

myth: Doctors perform cesareans so they can go home earlier.

FACT: Some doctors may have performed a cesarean for this reason, but we can assure you that this behavior is not the norm.

When our patients ask us why we perform a cesarean, we always answer that we do so for medical indications only. The majority of cesareans are decided about five minutes before they happen. Sometimes we can speculate on the need for a cesarean based on the size of the baby and the size of the mom, but we never know for sure until we see how the labor progresses. Near their due date, moms often ask us whether we think they will end up with a cesarean. On rare occasions, we may have a feeling one way or the other, but we always counsel our patients that we won't really know until they try giving birth vaginally.

---

myth: Doctors want to do a cesarean because they get paid more.

FACT: Not true. The insurance company pays your doctor the same whether the delivery is vaginal or by cesarean. Doctors have no financial incentive to do a cesarean.

Medical Indications for Cesarean Deliveries

You may need a cesarean delivery for many reasons. In this section, we describe the most common ones.

History of previous cesarean: After being counseled by your obstetrician about the risks and benefits of a trial VBAC (vaginal birth after cesarean) versus an elective repeat cesarean, you may decide that you want an elective repeat cesarean. (We describe VBAC later in this chapter.)

Failed VBAC: In this situation, you tried to deliver vaginally after a previous cesarean, but the baby shows signs of distress, you haven't dilated enough, or your baby hasn't descended through the vagina.

Arrest of dilation: In this circumstance, your cervix fails to dilate to the full ten centimeters, which is often a sign that your baby and your pelvis are not a good fit or that the baby is not coming down straight. A few millimeters makes a huge difference when you are fitting a larger infant through a small opening.

Arrest of descent: In this situation, you've dilated to ten centimeters but your little one just won't descend through the birth canal despite your best pushing efforts. Again, this is a sign that your baby and your pelvis are not a good fit.

Fetal distress: When your baby is intermittently or continuously monitored, we can detect whether the baby is getting enough oxygen. Fetal distress can occur for a variety of reasons. Perhaps the umbilical cord is wrapped around the neck of the baby a little too tightly or the baby is grabbing on to the cord. Maybe the cord is positioned such that it is getting squeezed during contractions. Or the placenta might not be providing adequate oxygen to the baby during labor.

Multiples: If you have twins or other multiples, your doctor may suggest that a cesarean is the safest route of delivery.

Breech, oblique, or transverse baby: If your baby is positioned breech, oblique, or transverse and the ECV (in which we try to turn the baby to a head-down position) fails or you have decided not to attempt an ECV, you might need a cesarean.

Chorioamnionitis: When an infection develops in the uterus—called chorioamnionitis—the mother and baby can be affected. If you are close to delivery, you may still be able to have a vaginal birth. However, if the delivery is many hours away, the risk of the infection spreading to the baby is higher, and your doctor may recommend a cesarean delivery. Remember that a newborn does not have the immune system that we adults have. An intrauterine infection is a risk factor for cerebral palsy.

Placenta previa: For information on this high-risk condition, see Chapter 9, page 388.

Active outbreak or prodromal symptoms of genital herpes: If you have an outbreak of genital herpes when you go into labor, you must have a cesarean to prevent transmission of the virus to the newborn. Neonatal herpes is a serious disease that can cause permanent neurologic damage or death.

Placental abruption: In this condition, the placenta detaches from the uterus prematurely and the baby does not receive enough oxygen. Placental abruption is characterized by excessive vaginal bleeding and fetal distress.

Maternal medical problems: If the mother has a medical condition, such as certain heart, lung, or musculoskeletal conditions, the act of pushing could be dangerous to the mother.

We always try to correct the problem before we resort to cesarean delivery. For example, we can alter the mother's position to untangle an umbilical cord, give her extra oxygen to deliver more oxygen to the baby, increase the intensity and frequency of contractions if they are not strong enough to dilate the cervix, and help her relax with pain medication if she's overly tense. Nonetheless, in some cases, nothing helps and a cesarean is the only option.

Requesting a Cesarean Delivery

Some women are terrified of labor in general and simply don't want to feel pain or have no desire to go through the process. Others are afraid of the consequences of vaginal injuries, such as urinary or fecal incontinence or changes in sexual function. Still others may have had a bad vaginal delivery experience. In our opinion, no matter what the reason, choosing to have a cesarean is the right of every mother. Before we will proceed with one, however, we have a thorough discussion about her reasons for wanting the elective cesarean and we describe the risks and benefits of cesarean versus a vaginal birth. After we are confident that our patient is well informed, we feel it's our job to support whatever choice she makes.

Risks of a Cesarean Delivery

So what are the risks associated with cesarean births? As with any surgical procedure, a cesarean has a risk of infection, either in the uterus or skin. You may need a blood transfusion if the bleeding during the procedure is excessive. You risk forming a deep venous thrombosis (blood clot) in your legs or damage to the organs surrounding the uterus, including the bowel and bladder. All of these except the last are complications that can occur with vaginal births as well but are more common after cesarean births.

The ultimate goal of any delivery, whether vaginal or by a cesarean, is a healthy mom and a healthy baby. If your doctor recommends a cesarean, make sure you thoroughly understand the reasons why. Ask lots of questions, and make sure that all your alternatives have been exhausted. In the end, we hope that you trust our recommendations from years of training and experience.

▶ ▶ ▶ LAST RESORT, HAPPY ENDING

Energetic, active, and outdoorsy, Julia and Al were having their first baby, a son they hoped to take hiking in Yosemite one day. All throughout her pregnancy, Julia took excellent care of herself, following our directions about diet and exercise to the letter. Because of her high level of fitness, and also taking into account her tall build, we all felt confident that she would be a strong pusher, successfully capable of pushing out a large baby.

What we did not anticipate was Julia going two weeks past her due date, with no sign that her cervix was ripening. Starting around her due date, Julia did everything under the sun to get her cervix ready for the work ahead, including walking, hiking, taking evening primrose oil, and undergoing acupuncture. She had intercourse with her husband often; so frequently, in fact, that Al said, "I'm not sure I can keep this up." The couple even went to a pizza place in Studio City to eat "the" salad, at Alane's suggestion. (Local rumor says something in the salad dressing can trigger labor.)

Alane started seeing Julia twice weekly after her due date passed to check that her amniotic fluid was still plentiful, and to check the baby's heartbeat with a fetal heart monitor using a nonstress test (NST). This test reassured us that the baby was happy in mom's uterus and getting plenty of oxygen. Alane considered membrane stripping, but because Julia's cervix remained tightly closed, the procedure could not be performed.

We finally set a date for induction. Julia was aware that she was going in with an unripe cervix and that she would need Cervidil to help ripen it. Alane suggested that we use Cervidil for an extra twelve hours—a total of twenty-four hours—to maximize Julia's chances of successful cervical ripening. Unfortunately, Julia's nurse called after twenty-four hours to tell Dr. Park that the patient's cervix was still the same, disappointing news for both Julia and Alane.

Alane delivered Julia the next day by cesarean, birthing a beautiful baby boy weighing nine pounds. Tears of joy and smiles were all around the OR, as Al looked lovingly at the son who'd finally arrived. "You're late," he said, clutching his new baby in his arms, "and you're grounded."

The Process of a Cesarean Delivery

While a cesarean may not be your first choice of delivery routes, the miracle of birth is still just that: a miracle. You finally get to meet your baby for the first time and welcome him into the world.

When a woman agrees to have a cesarean, she signs the consent forms and is then taken to the operating room. The first thing she'll notice is that the room is quite cold to prevent the spread of infection. She receives her anesthesia, either a spinal or an increase in medication through an already-placed epidural. After she is completely numb from the chest down, a Foley catheter is placed into the bladder to drain the urine. The nurse will clean her belly with a sterile solution and cover her in a blue operating drape. At this point, we ask her

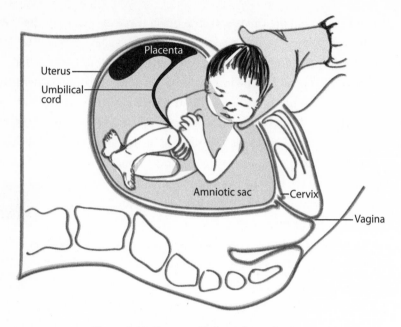

Figure 6-11: Cesarean Delivery Procedure

husband, partner, family member, or doula to come into the OR to be with their loved one.

The skin incision needs to be roughly the size of the baby's head, usually about twelve centimeters (about five inches). Normally this is a bikini cut, a low horizontal incision made at the top of the pubic hairline. Next, we open the many layers between the skin and the uterus. However, we do not cut the abdominal muscles because the midline has a natural separation that we simply stretch apart.

After we are inside the abdominal cavity, we make an opening in the uterus. One doctor guides the head and body, as seen in Figure 6-11, while a second doctor applies pressure on top of the uterus to push the baby through the incision. You may feel pressure, like someone is sitting on your chest. The umbilical cord is cut, and your baby has officially entered the world! At this point, you may hear the voice of your baby for the first time. The baby is then handed to a pediatric team awaiting the delivery in the OR.

Next, we remove the placenta and repair the uterine opening with stitches. Often we pull the uterus outside the abdomen to do this. When finished, we place the uterus back inside, and then sew closed each layer from inside out. The surgery usually lasts approximately thirty minutes, but may take longer if you have scar tissue from a previous surgery.

The hardest part of recovery from a cesarean is the pain at the incision site, but you can take medication to ease the pain. We also recommend not lifting anything heavier than your baby and no strenuous exercise for four to six weeks.

▶ ▶ ▶ CESAREAN DELIVERY VERSUS VAGINAL DELIVERY

I had a normal vaginal delivery with my son and a cesarean delivery with my daughter. I needed the cesarean because I had placenta previa. If I had gone into labor with the placenta covering the cervix, I would have hemorrhaged. Would I rather have had a vaginal delivery with my daughter? Ideally, yes, but that wasn't in the cards for me. After my cesarean delivery, the first few days were painful, but the pain went away quickly. I went back to work when my daughter was four weeks old.

I quickly got over my disappointment over not having a vaginal delivery. In the end, it didn't matter which way she was delivered. What I really cared about was that she was happy, healthy, and all smiles.

—Yvonne ◀ ◀ ◀

The VBAC Controversy

myth: After you have a cesarean, you must have cesarean deliveries for any future pregnancies.

FACT: Not necessarily. Read on about VBACs.

Some moms who've had a cesarean in the past prefer to try a vaginal birth the next time around, called a vaginal birth after cesarean, or VBAC. These days, some physicians and hospitals do not offer this option, so check with your provider early in your pregnancy.

Preference for VBAC

In general, the recovery from a vaginal birth is easier than the recovery from surgery. Recovery time is especially important when you already have a toddler at home who needs your attention. Also, for women who want large families, having multiple cesareans places them at higher risk for bleeding complications. Multiple cesareans also increase the likelihood of having *placenta accreta,* where the placenta grows into the uterine scar, which may ultimately require a hysterectomy. (For more on placenta accreta, refer to Chapter 9.)

Safety of VBAC

The chances of a complication from a VBAC after only one cesarean delivery are slim. The main risk is uterine rupture. Even though the incision made on your uterus during your cesarean was sewn together during the original surgery, the strength of the uterine muscle is never the same as before it was cut open. With one previous low transverse incision on your uterus, there's less than a 1 percent chance (0.7 percent) that the uterus will open at the weak point of the previous scar. If uterine rupture occurs, the chances are one in one thousand that the baby could die or become brain damaged. Ultimately, only you can decide if this small risk is worth taking.

The following characteristics make you a good potential candidate for VBAC:

- You have had only one prior cesarean delivery.
- You have an average-sized pelvis and average-sized baby.
- You have an obstetrician, an anesthesiologist, and a nursing/surgical team to handle emergency cesarean at all times.
- The incision on your uterus was made from side-to-side (low transverse).

And these characteristics make you *not* a good candidate for VBAC:

- The incision on your uterus was made up and down (classical). This type of cesarean is usually performed with very premature babies, small babies, or during an emergency cesarean delivery, where the baby has to be delivered more rapidly.
- You do not have access to an obstetrician, an anesthesiologist, and a nursing/surgical team at all times.

- Your baby is expected to be large and you had a previous cesarean delivery because your baby would not fit (you didn't dilate all the way or the baby didn't descend).
- You have had more than one cesarean.

Women who are undergoing a VBAC have to be monitored continuously with a fetal monitor so we can watch for changes in the fetal heart rate or in the contraction pattern that might suggest an early rupture. Therefore, having a VBAC limits your mobility.

▶ ▶ ▶ MY THOUGHTS ON VBACS

My patients who are considering VBACs sometimes ask me, "Would you have one yourself?" My answer is "No," because for me, having the vaginal birth experience wasn't my highest priority. My highest priority was just having my baby as safe and healthy as possible. But I'm supportive of a mom who wants to attempt a VBAC as long as she understands the risks. I also need to be sure that she knows that I'm going to be conservative when it comes to what I see during labor. If anything is out of the ordinary, I will recommend a cesarean. In this situation, when something goes wrong, it can *really* go wrong and go wrong fast. A VBAC is ultimately a woman's choice, but I want to be sure my patients are informed and understand why we're so cautious about doing this procedure.

—Allison ◀ ◀ ◀

The Baby Arrives

▶ ▶ ▶ LOVE AT FIRST SIGHT

Nothing compares to the moment when you were first placed in my arms and I kissed your sweet baby breath. Complete love and indescribable joy filled my heart from that instant on, and as your cries quieted with the soothing sound of my voice, I knew I was forever changed. I drank you in, memorizing every detail of your beautiful face, perfect lips, rosy red cheeks, and big blue round eyes. I knew that my life had begun the moment you were born.

—Tiffany, Yvonne's patient ◀ ◀ ◀

Whether you deliver vaginally or by cesarean, whether labor was fast and furious or slow and prolonged, whether the process was exactly as you hoped or nothing like you had imagined, those precious first few hours with your new baby are a time you will never forget. You will probably want to record it with photos or video and send out your first text message: "He—or she—is here!"

The first two priorities for the newborn are breathing air and staying warm. The baby is immediately dried with a towel or blanket and placed against his mother's chest, preferably skin-to-skin. The mouth and nose of the baby are suctioned to remove excess fluid. The baby will cry to expand his or her lungs and move the extra amniotic fluid and mucous up and out of the airways. We want the baby to cry vigorously. In days past, doctors would actually spank a baby to incite a cry. Thankfully, we don't do that anymore. Instead, a flick to the bottom of the feet or a vigorous rub on the back will get most babies to speak their first words.

Within the first thirty minutes in the life of a healthy baby, the infant will show signs that he or she is interested in feeding. The baby will turn his head toward any object that strokes his cheek and search for it with an open mouth, called rooting. Ideally, before a new mom and baby leave the delivery room, the baby will have latched on and nursed from both breasts.

Your Baby's First Breath

While the baby is floating in the womb, the placenta acts as the baby's lungs. The placenta is where all food, nutrition, and oxygen are transferred to the baby. At the baby's first breath, all that changes. As the lungs expand with that first inhalation, the blood vessels in the lungs open. Blood now freely flows from the right side of the heart into the lungs and then to the left side of the heart. The increase in blood in the left side of the heart causes the instant closure of a connection between the right and left sides of the heart, which is seen only in the fetal circulation. (See Figure 6-12.)

Meanwhile, the newborn's blood contains more oxygen from breathing air. This immediately causes a shunt, or passage, between the aorta and lungs to close forever. Now the circulation through the

Baby's Heart Before Birth

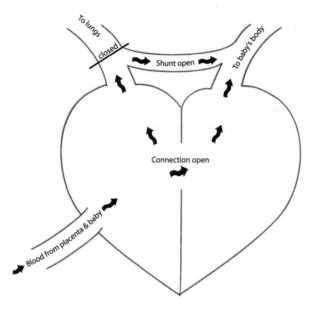

Baby's Heart After Birth

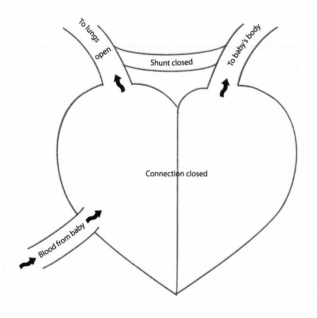

Figure 6-12: Baby's Heart Change at First Breath

lungs is separate from the rest of the body. It never ceases to amaze us how seamlessly nature has designed a newborn to transition from the womb to the outside world.

Cutting the Cord

Cutting the umbilical cord separates the baby from its mother for the first time, and culturally has become a moment of ceremony, usually carried out by the father as others in attendance take pictures. Traditionally, the cord is cut within the first minute after delivery. However, some studies suggest that delaying this procedure for a few minutes may be beneficial to the baby. Blood through the cord will naturally stop pulsating after approximately three minutes. During those first minutes, blood from the placenta continues to flow to the baby, increasing the amount of red blood cells and possibly preventing anemia. Other studies suggest that delaying the cord cutting may increase the risk of jaundice. Whether or not to delay is a personal decision you should discuss with your doctor.

Warmers

Baby warmers are in every delivery and operating room. When babies first come out, they are wet and cold. Imagine how you would feel if you had been lounged in a soothing, warm bath for forty weeks, but then suddenly found yourself stark naked in a cold institutional setting? If for some reason we can't place the baby on mom's chest to warm up, we will put the baby under the warmer.

First Impressions

When your baby comes out, chances are he or she will not look like the photo on the cover of *Parenting* magazine right away. Often, you will see a white cottage cheese–like substance called *vernix* all over his or her body. The role of *vernix* has been to waterproof your baby for the last forty weeks. After all, your baby has been floating in water, and you know what your fingers look like after an hour or so in the pool. Vernix can be creamy or sticky. Sometimes there's not much; other times, babies seem coated with it. Some moms want to have the baby bathed right away to wash off the vernix. Other moms want to rub it into the baby's skin like a cream.

The most common aesthetic problems we see right after vaginal birth are caput succedaneum and molding. *Caput succedaneum* is the swelling of the part of the scalp that is just over the cervix as the cervix dilates and the baby comes down the birth canal. *Molding* is the change in shape of the baby's head and skull as it fits through the birth canal. Especially with a first-time birth, the baby often has significant caput and molding, giving the baby the familiar conehead appearance. We've seen many moms and dads aghast at the first sight of their baby. Don't worry: The conehead usually goes away within the first few days.

Often, babies enter the world with small bruises on their head or on their faces, which can be a little scary for parents. These marks are just temporary reminders of the baby's epic journey through the birth canal, maneuvering him- or herself either against the cervix or going through the vagina. Sometimes, a mom's hormones can make a baby boy's scrotum swell temporarily. Lastly, if the baby has any birthmarks, they'll appear right away.

Birth Day Tests and Treatments

While still in the delivery room, your baby will undergo his first set of exams. In most situations, the baby will remain with you during these tests and treatments.

Apgar

When the baby comes out, we immediately check the vital signs to make sure your little one is transitioning well to the outside world. The primary tests performed on your baby's birth day are tallied up in the *Apgar score,* which evaluates five characteristics of the newborn. The Apgar score can be assigned while the baby is on your chest after a vaginal delivery or in the warmer if you had a cesarean. The characteristics are:

Appearance (color)
Pulse (heart rate)
Grimace (reflexes)
Activity (muscle tone)
Respirations (breathing effort)

A score of 0, 1, or 2 is assigned for each of these characteristics after one minute and five minutes of life. The maximum score is 10. A score greater than 7 means the baby has made the transition well.

Antibiotic eye ointment and vitamin K injection

The American Academy of Pediatrics and American College of Obstetrics and Gynecology recommend that two medications be given to babies in the delivery room. One is erythromycin or tetracycline eye ointment, which prevent eye infections from bacteria in the vagina. The second is a vitamin K injection to prevent vitamin K–dependent bleeding disorder in the newborn. Although this disorder is rare, occurring in only one out of ten thousand babies, it can cause serious bleeding problems such as brain hemorrhages. Unfortunately, oral vitamin K is not as effective.

Some moms decline the administration of these medications because the chance of eye infections and bleeding disorders are low. We recommend that your baby receive these, but it is a personal choice that you should talk to your doctor about.

▶ ▶ ▶ THE PERFECT ENDING

My eyes fill up with tears just thinking about how perfect the setting was. The lights were dim, and my husband and a nurse held my legs as I pushed. I could hear nothing except the voices of my doctor and husband guiding me and reassuring me. It was so comforting. I'd had my epidural, but by the time I had to push, it was turned down just enough so I could feel the contractions. I found it so strange that when I pushed with the contractions I felt zero pain. In fact, I felt nothing. My doctor kept saying, "Good job, he is coming down." I actually thought she was lying because I didn't feel a thing. However, I did feel the baby's head crowning. Doctors call it "the ring of fire." It was a short pain, and then my doctor said, "Okay, one more big push." Everything went silent. I locked eyes with my husband. Nine months had come down to this moment. From the home pregnancy test to the doctor visits, ultrasounds, back pain, swollen feet, uncomfortable sleep, all of it—it was all over. My doctor told me to look down, and there he was. My husband placed him on my chest and everything just melted away. As he lay on my chest crying I felt an instant connection. I looked in his eyes and said, "I know you. I love you." At 8:36 p.m. on September 29, 2010, I met my son for the first time, a moment I will never forget.

—Linda, Allison's patient ◀ ◀ ◀

After You Deliver

If your delivery went off without a hitch, whether vaginal or cesarean, you and your baby will stay in a delivery/recovery room for the first few hours. During this time, your newborn will make the adjustment to the outside world and your body will begin its journey back to prepregnancy form.

The Shakes

About 20 percent of women will experience the "shakes" during the last part of labor or immediately after delivery. This uncontrolled shivering often leaves them wondering if something is wrong. We do not know what causes the shaking. Most women have a normal temperature and do not feel cold. The shaking does not appear to be related to epidural placement or an infection. The shaking could be caused by hormonal changes, adrenaline, or fatigue. If the shakes are debilitating or upsetting to the mother, we assure her that they will pass, but sometimes an injection of intravenous pain medicine will make them stop. The good news is that the shakes usually last for only about an hour after delivery.

Your Shrinking Uterus

After delivery, you may look down at your belly and notice that you look deflated. The large squirmy baby is now replaced by a hard ball that can be felt below the belly button. You may wonder whether something was left behind. Actually, this is your uterus.

Whether you deliver vaginally or by cesarean, the uterus goes from the size of a large watermelon to a cantaloupe in a matter of minutes. In this process, called involution, the uterine muscle contracts, constricting the large blood vessels in the uterus to minimize blood loss.

We can help the uterine muscle remain firm and contracted after delivery by performing a fundal massage. Your nurse will firmly rub the uterus below the belly button. Because the uterus has just gone through the most intense workout of its life, a fundal massage can often be quite uncomfortable. However, this simple procedure can greatly decrease the amount of bleeding after delivery.

With the delivery of the baby and the placenta and the loss of amniotic fluid and blood, you can expect to lose ten to twelve pounds in the delivery room. And by about four weeks after giving birth, your uterus should return to its original prepregnancy size.

▶ ▶ ▶ I'M MISSING YOUR KICKS

I remember waking up the first day after my daughter Kate was born. She had slept most of the night, stirring only every few hours to eat. I was happy to see that we had both made it through night number one without a hitch, but what I noticed right away was that I didn't feel her moving inside me. And surprisingly, I missed it! Every morning for the past twenty weeks, I had enjoyed lying in my bed on still, quiet mornings and reveling in all her kicks, rolls, and subtle tickles. Those feelings were gone. And although I could now see her and touch her, something about the absence of her movements struck me with a pang of sadness. I knew Kate would most likely be my last baby, and the reality quickly set in that I would never feel that unique sensation again.

—Allison ◀ ◀ ◀

Before You Bring Your Baby Home

Before your baby is discharged from the hospital, he or she will undergo a physical exam. Normally, this takes place on the birth day or the following day. At this point, we, your faithful ob-gyns, revert back to our "gyn" role in your care, and the total care and medical treatment of your baby is passed on to your experienced pediatrician. During your baby's first checkup, your pediatrician will be checking for the normal newborn reflexes: rooting, sucking, grasping, and the startle reflex. After the exam, the doctor will answer any questions you may have.

A baby will not be able to leave the hospital until he has urinated and passed meconium, the first bowel movement. Both events usually take place within the first twenty-four to forty-eight hours and ensure that the baby is well hydrated and the intestinal tract is working. Meconium appears dark green or black, but with time, the stools will turn mustard colored and may occur after every feeding.

Hepatitis B Vaccine

Another medication routinely offered to your baby in the hospital is the hepatitis B vaccine. All moms are screened for hepatitis B during their pregnancy. If a woman is a carrier of hepatitis B, her baby will get the vaccine and a second injection called hepatitis B immunoglobulin to prevent the baby from contracting the virus from the mother. However, if the mom is not a carrier, the baby will be offered only the vaccine.

Newborns are offered the vaccine in the hospital because the baby might be exposed to other household contacts who do not know that they are hepatitis B carriers. Some parents decline this vaccine. We recommend discussing this decision with your pediatrician.

Universal Newborn Screening

Your baby will be screened for a panel of diseases before you leave the hospital. The diseases in the panel vary from state to state. The panel of tests is performed by taking a drop of blood from your baby's heel. The results of these tests will be sent to your pediatrician within a month.

Hearing Test

Your little one may also be hooked up to a machine to check his or her hearing. Don't worry, this will not cause your baby any pain.

Jaundice Screening

Jaundice, a yellow discoloration of the skin and whites of the eyes, occurs when bilirubin builds up in a baby's body. Bilirubin is a yellowish by-product of the breakdown of red blood cells. The body normally gets rid of bilirubin through stool and urine. In some cases, the baby's liver is not mature enough to process the bilirubin or it cannot come out in the urine because the baby is dehydrated. Premature babies are more prone to jaundice, primarily because their livers are more immature. Because jaundice can be hard to detect in a newborn, all babies are screened in the hospital before discharge.

Jaundice is more commonly found in Asian babies, boys, exclusively breastfed babies, and when mom and baby don't have the same blood type (ABO incompatibility or Rh disease). For example, in ABO incompatibility, if a mom's blood type is O and her baby's blood type is A or B, that baby is more likely to develop jaundice. Jaundice is also more common when the baby's Rh blood type is positive, but the mom's Rh is negative. If the mom and the baby have the same blood type, jaundice is less likely.

If left untreated, jaundice can cause serious complications, such as deafness, cerebral palsy, or brain damage. Mild cases usually will resolve on their own, as the liver catches up with the metabolism of bilirubin. The simplest treatment of jaundice is hydration, to flush the bilirubin out through the urine and stool. In some cases, a baby will need to be supplemented with formula for a few days, especially if the mother's milk volume is inadequate. Another treatment is phototherapy, where the baby is placed in filtered sunlight by a window at home (if jaundice is only mild and this is what your pediatrician recommends) or placed under bili-lights in the hospital (usually recommended if jaundice is more severe). The light waves help break down bilirubin into its by-products through the skin. In severe cases, the baby may need a blood transfusion to replace its bilirubin-filled blood with fresh blood.

Switched at Birth?

Who hasn't heard the stories of babies getting mixed up in the hospital and parents taking home some other family's offspring? Although these stories aren't a myth, a baby from the time it is born is tracked with so many checks and balances that it is next to impossible for this to happen. Every hospital has a system for identifying which baby belongs with which family. The baby and the parents are tagged with bracelets immediately after delivery. Some hospitals even use electronic tags that set off an alarm if a baby is taken from the maternity ward.

Bringing Baby Home

Hospitals often have a video of "child care 101" that they ask all new parents to watch. They'll also give out flyers with tips about breast-feeding and breast milk storage, danger signs to look for in the newborn, and when to call your obstetrician or pediatrician.

All infants discharged from the hospital must go home in a rear-facing infant car seat. Some hospitals will give a car seat to all new parents, but most people purchase them beforehand and have them properly installed in their cars before going home. You can find more information and federal guidelines for infant and car seat safety at http://www.nhtsa.gov/Safety/CPS.

▶ ▶ ▶ MY "HAPPY BIRTHDAY!"

I get the honor of speaking these words far more often than the average person; sometimes, more than once a day. Back when our practice was first beginning, I started saying "Happy Birthday" every time I held a groggy newborn in my hands. I know the babies don't understand anything I am saying, but I like saying something personal to the lives I help bring into the world. Something about uttering that joyful phrase makes me feel happy, involved, and connected.

I got to "catch" my first baby in my third year of medical school, with a resident watching over me to ensure that everything would go smoothly. I remember how my heart raced as I prayed I wouldn't make any mistakes. Sixteen years and many, many babies later, that anxiety has been replaced by the joy and the sense of calm I get when I am at a birth. As I coach my patient to push harder and finally see the head crowning, I can only imagine what their partner and family members are feeling. I've always wished I could have a heart monitor on the partner to see how fast his or her heart is beating. Then the joy and tears you see on everyone's faces after the baby is delivered is like no other experience in the world.

—Alane ◀ ◀ ◀

chapter seven

THE FOURTH
TRIMESTER

▶ ▶ ▶ **A NEW DAD'S DIARY: DAYS ONE TO THREE**

Cesarean day. The delivery was exciting; our obstetrician did an awesome job. I was surprised that I didn't cry like I thought I would, but I think the sheer excitement of finally seeing my baby's face overwhelmed me. Every parent thinks his child is beautiful, but I really did believe that with all my heart. He looked gorgeous.

Jacob slept a lot the first day. Audry breastfed and we could see colostrum was easily coming out. It's so amazing how a woman's body works during pregnancy. Little did we know most of my wife's difficulties with early motherhood would soon be related to breastfeeding.

At home, we were on our own. Those days were hard! No nursing help. No lactation consultants. No daily visits from Dr. Park or our pediatrician, Dr. Asnani. We had to figure things out on our own. Probably because I didn't know what else to do, I walked with Jacob in my arms, bouncing him for an hour at a time. It kept him quiet and sleeping peacefully. I was exhausted walking him in the middle of the night, but seeing his face, with his rhythmic breathing and little chirps and squeaks, was so rewarding. I could look at him like that for hours.

—*Dominic, Alane's patient* ◀ ◀ ◀

Welcome to the Fourth Trimester!

In some ways, we believe that this chapter is one of the most important. One of our patients said it best: "Nobody ever warns you about the fourth trimester."

Pregnancy lasts for forty weeks. The birth day is a mere twenty-four hours. But becoming a mother takes a lifetime. After you have your baby, you must give yourself permission to take the time for the parent in you to develop. You don't have to get everything right the first time, and in many cases, there is more than one right way to do things. The fourth trimester, and the years that follow, will be life changing, overwhelming, frustrating, incredible, and probably the most meaningful time of your life.

So often, we're led to believe that pregnancy is the hardest part of the process. After all, you, your family, and your doctors have prepared for months for the big day. Having brought thousands of babies into the world, and having gone through the process more than once ourselves, we can tell you that the pregnancy is only the beginning. Even the physical ordeal of delivering the baby isn't the most challenging part.

We believe there's a real need to shift some of the focus of our attention from the birth itself to the myriad events that follow it. The segment of the childbirth journey that everybody seems to forget to think about is the succession of stresses and experiences that unfurl immediately afterward.

Having a baby is like winning the Super Bowl. You train for months, labor, and give birth to your baby. The big pregnancy game is over, the champagne flows . . . but what happens the morning after? You still have a lifetime ahead of you to take care of this child. Caring for your child includes figuring out who is going to help you, when you are going to sleep, and how you are going to manage the details of everyday life. These challenges are the real tests that every mother will face. However, sometimes we find that the couples who overprepare for the birth are often the ones who don't look any further down the road and get hit hardest by the part that comes next—"the Fourth Trimester."

In our practice, we define the fourth trimester as the time frame from the birth of your baby to three months of life. You will likely spend many sleepless nights trying to figure out why your baby is crying, followed by long days attempting to keep up with the mundane details of life, such as shopping, cooking, and the always multiplying laundry. Finding quiet time for yourself and your partner can be nearly impossible during these early weeks.

By three months, however, the baby's digestive system has become more regular. Infants are not as fussy, and are not pooping after every feeding. They're sleeping for longer stretches at a time, and although your life will not return to normal by then, some basic and comforting routines will start to set in. These crucial three months will ease you, the new parents, into a lifetime of a new kind of normal, one that is not all about you. You're carrying the weight of responsibility for a new life as well as your own, but that weight doesn't have to feel like a burden as long as you and your partner prepare yourselves and make the right plans.

Your First Days Home

After you leave the hospital and are back in your own home, it's important to know that your body will continue to go through some significant physical changes. Your uterus will continue to shrink rapidly, the blood flow through your body will shift, and your hormones will do cartwheels. Here are some basic recommendations during this time:

1. No sex. Yes, we know it is probably the last thing on your mind, but medically, sex may be dangerous. While your uterus is healing and the cervix is still open, you have a heightened chance of developing an infection from intercourse. It's safer to resume sexual activity at the six-week point.

2. Wear sanitary pads, not tampons, for the same reason just listed.

3. Start your Kegels (see Chapter 5, page 204). You can begin these on the day after delivery to strengthen your vaginal and pelvic floor muscles to prevent long-term urinary incontinence.

4. Take care of your perineum and any vaginal tears. Because of the excellent blood flow to this part of your body, injuries in this area heal quite rapidly. You should rinse your perineum with warm water from a plastic squeeze bottle, especially after urination or a bowel movement. Use sitz baths, cold packs, anesthetic sprays or foam, or witch hazel to decrease pain and swelling. Avoid sitting on hard surfaces. If your hospital provides a sitz bath bowl (a plastic bowl that fits over your toilet), take it home and use it several times a day until you heal. No matter how big or small your tear, you will feel much better about two weeks after your delivery. Your doctor will use dissolvable sutures to repair any tears, and the stitches will have disappeared by the time you go to your postpartum visit.

5. Avoid constipation by using stool softeners and drinking lots of water. Prunes, prune juice, and high-fiber cereals also work well. Hemorrhoids can occur even a few months after delivery. Many women are terrified of having their first bowel movement because they are scared that they are going to pull apart their stitches. Be reassured that the vaginal repairs are quite strong and heal quickly.

6. Use an abdominal binder or girdle. This is an undergarment made of pliant material that wraps around the lower belly and braces the abdomen and back. Although it does not help your belly shrink any faster, it can give some much-needed extra support when you feel like everything is overstretched.

7. Do not sit in a bath or Jacuzzi for the first four weeks. If you are completely submerged, water can be forced into the healing uterus through the vagina and cause an infection.

8. You can drive a car within a few days of a vaginal delivery and within one or two weeks after a cesarean. If you can sit in the driver's seat comfortably and turn from side to side without pain, you can drive.

Recovering from a Cesarean

If you delivered by cesarean, your bandage will be removed before you are discharged from the hospital. If you have skin staples, they will be removed three to seven days after surgery. As early as the next day after surgery, you can take a shower and get the incision wet with water and mild soap. After your shower, dry the incision with a towel. You do not need to clean the incision with anything other than warm water. Rubbing alcohol, betadine, and antibiotic creams are not necessary unless your doctor specifically recommends them. You should keep the incision exposed to the air to keep it dry. If your incision lies directly in the crease of your skin, you can help keep it dry by placing gauze or a sanitary pad in the crease to absorb the extra moisture.

Your incision will probably be the major source of pain during your recovery time. You will feel 90 percent better and nearly back to normal in the first six weeks after delivery, but it may take six months for the surgical wound to heal completely. The skin around the incision may be numb, or it may tingle, burn, or itch as the nerves regrow. Sometimes, one side of the incision hurts more than the other side due to internal scar tissue formation .

For the first four weeks, try not to lift anything heavier than the baby. Getting in and out of bed is difficult because you need to use your sore abdominal muscles, so try to push yourself up with your arms. You can go up and down the stairs—slowly.

Finally, don't skimp on the pain medications. You will not become addicted to them if you use them according to your doctor's instructions. Many women benefit from a combination of an anti-inflammatory, such as ibuprofen, and a narcotic, which are perfectly safe when nursing. The more relaxed and comfortable you are, the faster you will heal.

▶ ▶ ▶ A NEW DAD'S DIARY: SUPPORTING MOM

Audry had a cesarean section for Jacob's delivery. This was another thing I hadn't thought about before Jacob's birthday. You realize pretty fast that you not only have a baby who needs taking care of but also a wife who's recuperating from what is essentially major abdominal surgery. Her spinal anesthesia kept her relatively pain-free the first twenty-four hours, but after that it hurt her to get up, lay down, walk, cough, and more. Her medication (Motrin) helped, but there's only so much a new mom can do when she can't even stand up straight without significant pain.

Her discomfort meant that a lot of the things that needed to be taken care of at home fell on my shoulders: cleaning, laundry, cooking, grocery shopping, all of which I needed to do continuously. To be honest, I didn't care for the cooking (which really involved reheating my mother-in-law's delivered food), I enjoyed the cleaning and laundry. It was constant and repetitive and boring, but it satisfied my nesting instinct.

I had a hard time with the hours after midnight. I was exhausted after spending the entire day taking care of the baby. I just wanted to go to sleep in my bed. That's when Jacob would be wide awake and fussy. Essentially, Jacob's daytime started at our nighttime.

—Dominic, Alane's patient ◀ ◀ ◀

Postpartum Swelling

"Help! My legs look like tree trunks," is one of the most common calls we get from our newly discharged moms. Even if you didn't have any swelling during pregnancy, swollen feet, ankles, and lower legs are normal after having a baby. When you are pregnant, your blood volume is 50 percent higher. This extra blood goes to the enlarged uterus and placenta. However, when the baby and placenta are gone, the blood has no place to go, so the extra fluid leaks into the tissues. With walking, the fluid will be reabsorbed and eliminated through the urine during the next few weeks. Depending on its severity, however, swelling can last up to a month.

If one leg is significantly more swollen or red than the other or if you have severe pain in the calf, you could have a deep vein thrombosis (a clot in the deep veins of the leg). *Anyone with these symptoms needs to be evaluated immediately by a physician.*

Postpartum Bleeding

After the placenta delivers, the uterus contracts so that the amount of bleeding slows down considerably. However, for the first several days, a woman will continue to have intermittent episodes of heavy bleeding and will occasionally pass small clots. The heaviest bleeding will subside after three or four days. Then there will be a red-brown discharge, called *lochia serosa*, which may have a foul odor. This lasts for the next three to four weeks. Some women experience a return to bright red bleeding from days seven to fourteen, as the "scab" of the placenta sloughs off. The bleeding may go away completely for a day or two and then return again, bright red and heavy. At four to six weeks postpartum, the discharge becomes yellow or white, called the *lochia alba*. This pattern will be seen whether you deliver vaginally or by cesarean.

The first thing in the morning, a woman may notice that a larger clot comes out. When you are lying down to sleep, the blood pools inside the vagina, so when you first stand up in the morning, gravity will force the accumulated blood out as a clot. This is normal and is not cause for alarm.

So how much bleeding is too much? As a general rule, if you are completely soaking a sanitary pad within one hour, you should contact your doctor, especially if you are also feeling dizzy.

> ### WHEN TO CALL YOUR DOCTOR
>
> Especially if you have had your first baby, you may find it hard to distinguish between what is normal and what may signal a true emergency. If you have recently given birth and are experiencing any of the following conditions, notify your doctor:
>
> - Fever of 100.4 degrees Fahrenheit or higher
> - Blurred vision or a headache that is not relieved by ibuprofen or acetaminophen
> - Pain in your chest
> - Swelling or pain in one leg
> - Excessive crying or anger, especially if you are unable to care for the baby
> - Red streaks or patches on the skin of the breast
> - Pain with urination
> - Changing more than one sanitary pad per hour

Hot Flushes and Sweats

After the placenta is removed, the hormone factory starts to close down. The high levels of progesterone and estrogen that were coursing through your body for forty weeks plummet to very low levels and stay that way for quite some time, especially if you are breastfeeding. Because of this, you may have episodes of severe sweats or hot flushes. These symptoms typically last a few days and then subside. Don't worry and think you have just gone from pregnant to menopausal overnight. Your body is adjusting to lower hormone levels.

Ovulation and Menses

If you are breastfeeding more than eight times per day, you will probably not have regular menstrual cycles. The elevated prolactin levels of nursing suppress ovulation during this time. Some breastfeeding moms have irregular spotting, others occasional heavy flow, and still others have no bleeding. Essentially, anything goes. After you begin to wean your baby or introduce solids—usually around six months— your menstrual cycles will resume. However, some women will not have a period until they have completely stopped nursing.

If you are not breastfeeding, your periods will start about six to ten weeks after delivery. However, keep in mind that *you might resume ovulation as early as three weeks after delivery* whether or not you are breastfeeding and even if you haven't yet had a period. So if you are not ready to have another child, you must use contraception.

A Baby's Life: Sleeping, Eating, Peeing, and Pooping

During the first hours in the world outside your womb, your baby probably won't be the life of the party. In fact, most babies sleep for much of the first twenty-four hours, and mothers often worry that their babies are sleeping too much. The baby may not want to eat, or even cry much. Don't worry—usually, this is normal newborn behavior. Your nurses and pediatricians are there to monitor the baby's activity and will alert you if anything seems unusual.

After the baby goes home on the second or third day, it may suddenly seem as though he or she has come to life and is a completely different baby than the one that was in the hospital. We see it all the time—in the hospital, everybody's making comments like, "This baby is so good!" "My baby is an angel." "The baby just sleeps all the time!" Or "What an easy baby! She never cries!" Then, a few days later, the new parents are exclaiming, "Did we bring home the right baby? This one is screaming constantly!"

That said, your baby will do a lot of sleeping during his or her first two weeks of life. In fact, the baby spends most of his or her hours sleeping—up to sixteen to eighteen hours a day. In addition, much of the baby's energy is used for growing. The average baby will double in weight by the time he or she is six months old—some babies double in weight in three months. When your mom was trying to put you to bed as a kid, did she ever tell you that you had to sleep to grow? Well, she was right.

As the weeks pass, the baby spends less time sleeping and more time awake. By the time the baby is three months old, you have a very different baby than the one you brought home from the hospital.

Generally, newborns eat every two to three hours for the first six weeks of their lives. Feeding intervals depend on many factors, including whether or not the baby is going through a growth spurt, requiring more frequent feedings. Formula-fed babies eat less often because formula is digested more slowly.

To get an idea of how challenging life with a newborn can be, Table 7-1 presents a real-life diary from one of our patients, Lorelei, a working mom who took off the first eight weeks postpartum to attend to her newborn's needs full time. To prepare for her eventual return to work, Lorelei both breastfed and bottle fed pumped breast milk to her daughter during that interval. The diary outlines a typical day in Lorelei's life, when her daughter was about three weeks old.

For Lorelei's three-week-old, each three-hour cycle of feeding, diaper changing, burping, and keeping her baby upright after feeding (to prevent the baby from spitting up) took about forty minutes. Then pumping and washing the pumping pieces took twenty minutes. So the parent sleep time/other activity time was between one and a half and two hours each three-hour cycle.

Yikes! Don't you get out of breath just reading the schedule in Table 7-1? This schedule isn't an anomaly or an exaggeration. It's absolutely typical of what most new mothers go through in the early weeks.

With multiple feedings come multiple dirty diapers. In the first few weeks, your baby will generally have a bowel movement after each meal, or eight to twelve bowel movements a day. Yes, babies pee and poop a lot, which means you'll be changing their diapers quite a bit.

Feeding Time

You would think that feeding your baby would be easy and come naturally. After all, the media image of breastfeeding moms is usually a well-groomed woman with an angelic smile on her face, looking down peacefully at her beautiful newborn breastfeeding. With practice and time, you will get there, but don't expect the Madonna and Child tableau right away because the first month or so can be challenging.

Table 7-1: Twenty-Four Hours with a Newborn

Time	Parent's activities with the infant	Parent's other activities
6:00 a.m.	Wake up.	
6:45 a.m.	Pump breast milk for 15 minutes.	
7:00 a.m.	Feed pumped breast milk and change diaper. Total time is one hour.	
8:00 a.m.	Put baby to breast for 15 minutes.	
9:00 a.m.	Put baby to breast for 30 minutes, change wet diaper .	Take shower.
9:45 a.m.	Feed baby pumped breast milk. Baby sleeps for 2 hours.	Eat breakfast.
11:45 a.m.	Pump breast milk for 15 minutes.	
12:15 p.m.	Feed baby pumped breast milk, change diaper, burp baby. Put baby to sleep for 1½ hours.	
1:00 p.m.		Sleep for 1 hour, then eat lunch.
2:40 p.m.	Pump breast milk for 15 minutes.	
3:15 p.m.	Feed baby pumped breast milk, change wet and dirty diaper. Baby sleeps for 2 hours.	Sleep.
6:15 p.m.	Feed baby pumped breast milk, change wet and dirty diaper. Baby sleeps 1 hour.	Eat dinner.
7:40 p.m.	Pump breast milk for 15 minutes.	
9:00 p.m.	Give baby a sponge bath.	
9:50 p.m.	Feed baby pumped breast milk, change wet and dirty diaper. Baby sleeps.	Pump breast milk for 15 minutes. Sleep.
12:36 a.m.	Feed baby pumped breast milk, change wet and dirty diaper. Baby sleeps.	Sleep.
1:15 a.m.	Pump breast milk for 15 minutes.	
4:00 a.m.	Feed baby pumped breast milk, change wet and dirty diaper. Baby sleeps.	Sleep.
4:55 a.m.	Pump breast milk for 15 minutes.	
6:50 a.m.	Feed baby pumped breast milk, change wet and dirty diaper. Baby sleeps.	

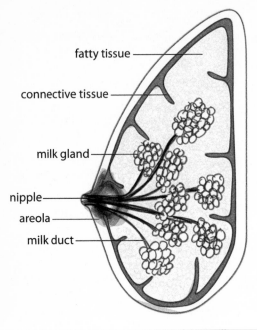

Figure 7-1: How the Breast Produces Milk

The American Academy of Pediatrics and the American College of OB/GYN recommends exclusive breastfeeding for the first six months, and breastfeeding in combination with solid foods until twelve months. Nearly all women can produce enough breast milk to sustain their newborns.

The breast begins to prepare for milk production during the first trimester, under the influence of pregnancy hormones. During the forty weeks, the breast glands and ducts grow and mature (see Figure 7-1). Colostrum is the first milk, arriving before or at delivery and continuing for four to five days after birth. It contains more minerals, protein, and antibodies but less fat and sugar than regular milk. At delivery, the level of the hormone progesterone drops and prolactin rises, triggering the regular milk to come in. This event occurs on the third or fourth postpartum day. *No matter what you do, you cannot make your milk come in any faster.* Many women are frustrated that they have little milk production during the first few days. We assure them that this is normal, and the colostrum is sufficient to satisfy most babies' needs.

Oxytocin is the hormone that causes the milk letdown, when the milk actually flows out of the breast. When the baby sucks, oxytocin levels rise. In addition, oxytocin increases when the mother is relaxed and the nursing cues are positive, such as the smell or cry of her baby. Pain, insecurity, and anxiety cause oxytocin levels to fall. Therefore, women should try to relax and nurse in a comfortable position.

During the first postpartum week, nursing will trigger painful uterine contractions. The milk-releasing oxytocin is the same hormone that causes the uterus to contract. In this way, nursing helps the uterus stay firm and decreases postpartum bleeding.

◗ ◗ ◗ OUR MILK TRIGGERS

External cues trigger milk letdown for every woman. You've heard stories of how a mother's breasts start to leak when she hears her baby cry. I pumped so much that milk would let down when I unzipped the backpack that held my pumping equipment. The sound of that zipper was my cue. After a while, my milk would let down with any zipper noise—someone in my office opening their purse or putting on a boot! Needless to say, it was annoying, but I was amazed at how much my body adapted to unusual situations.

—Allison ◖ ◖ ◖

I went to our postpartum floor to make my rounds and saw a really cute picture of one of our moms with her baby. I was thinking to myself, "Oh, what a sweet baby," and I started leaking breast milk through my shirt. Sometimes, all someone would have to do is ask me about my baby and the milk would rush in. It's an amazingly strong reflex.

—Yvonne ◖ ◖ ◖

At peak production, you make nearly one liter of milk daily. To produce this much breast milk, your body uses 800 calories per day, almost three times the caloric needs of pregnancy. Because vitamin, mineral, and caloric needs increase so much, we recommend the following in addition to your normal diet:

- Continue prenatal vitamins containing folic acid
- An extra liter of fluid
- Two cups of milk
- One slice of whole grain bread
- Half cup of dark green vegetables
- Two ounces of protein (nuts, meat, or protein bar)
- One citrus fruit
- Fish oil or DHA supplement

Breastfeeding Basics

Breast milk production follows the principle of supply and demand. The more you nurse, the more you'll make. It's that simple. For that reason, if you want to breastfeed exclusively, do not supplement with formula. When you supplement, the baby is not as hungry, so naturally you will nurse less. In addition, you may become anxious that you are not making enough milk, and the stress will also lead to decreased production.

Milk production is the same whether you have a vaginal birth or a cesarean. The route your baby takes to get into the world is not relevant; the delivery of the placenta, and subsequent hormonal changes, trigger milk production to start.

Latching On

To facilitate nursing, you must first find a comfortable position. Remember that you will potentially be breastfeeding for a year, sometimes longer, so finding a position that works for you is important. We find that many first-time moms attempt to adapt their breastfeeding style to the baby, but it's better in the long run to have the baby learn to adjust to you. Try using a pillow designed for nursing to help you maintain a relaxed physical position to breastfeed. Doing this will save you from having sore shoulders and arms.

While breastfeeding, you can hold your baby in a cradle hold (Figure 7-2), a football hold (Figure 7-3), a side-lying hold (Figure 7-4), or a crossover hold (Figure 7-5).

The baby should nurse for about fifteen minutes on each breast, six to eight times per day. With a slight touch to the cheek, a baby will turn its head and open its mouth—also known as rooting. The nipple and entire areola (the brown part) should fit into the mouth as the baby latches on (see Figure 7-6). The milk comes out because of the undulating action of the tongue. The baby will swallow 80 percent of the milk volume in the first five minutes, with the last ten minutes dedicated to ingesting the hindmilk, which contains more calories and fat.

Some women have different anatomical shapes to their nipples that can make it harder for the baby to latch on.

IS BABY EATING ENOUGH?

Your baby is getting enough nutrition if the baby:

- Appears alert
- Is nursing eight times per day or more
- Has three to four stools per day
- Produces six wet diapers per day
- Gains weight (many babies lose 10 percent of their birth weight in the first week but should regain it by day fourteen)

For example, women with inverted or flat nipples may be challenged initially. But even in these cases, special breast shields or syringes can be used to correct the condition.

▶ ▶ ▶ MY LATCHING TIP

When your baby is crying, he'll have a wide open mouth and it may seem easier to get more of the nipple in his mouth this way, but I've found that you should be careful if the baby is hysterical. In the beginning, the baby may not even know the food is there. Instead of sucking, he or she may begin thrashing or screaming even more. The baby will get frustrated and the mom will too— and any baby can sense when his or her mother is frustrated.

In my case, I had a nurse who was trying to help me to latch on while Kylie was screaming. Kylie just wouldn't do it, so I told the nurse, "Please, give us some time. I know she can do it, I'll figure this out." I had already gotten her to latch on myself earlier. I rocked her and rubbed her back and when she was calmer, I was much better at getting her to latch on. After the baby has figured out where the milk is and understands that the nipple is her route to food, she will latch on easily when she is screaming, and then calm down quickly as the sweet milk begins to flow.

—Yvonne ◀ ◀ ◀

Supplementing with Formula

A breastfed baby needs formula in only a few circumstances. In cases of severe jaundice, as mentioned, the baby may benefit from the extra fluid volume provided by formula. In addition, very large babies— those over eight and a half pounds—and babies born to diabetic mothers may have a harder time controlling their blood sugar, necessitating the use of formula.

In the hospital and during the first few weeks of life, your baby's weight will be closely monitored. Newborns commonly lose 10 percent of their birth weight within the first week but gain it back by the second week. After your milk comes in, the baby should gain about one ounce per day. If he does not follow this pattern, the milk supply may be inadequate or the baby might not be latching on well. In some of these cases of failure to thrive, formula is used as a supplement.

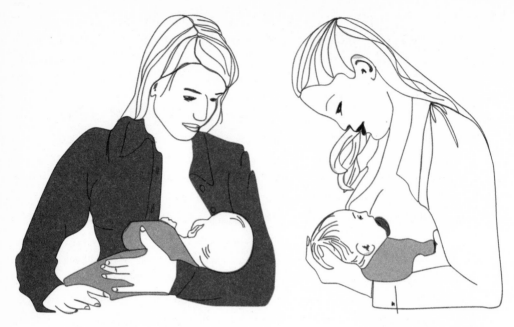

Figure 7-2: Cradle Hold

Figure 7-3: Football Hold

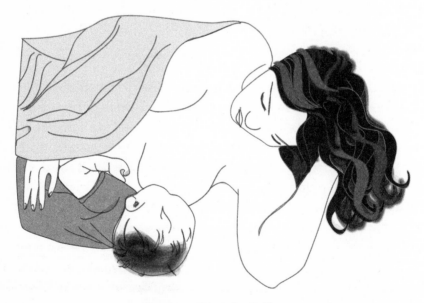

Figure 7-4: Side-Lying Hold

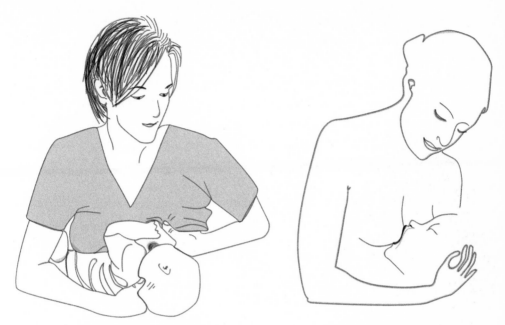

Figure 7-5: Crossover Hold   *Figure 7-6: How to Latch On*

Increasing Your Breast Milk Supply

Breastfeeding is a simple matter of supply and demand, so it follows that the simplest way to increase breast milk production is to have more demand. The amount of milk you produce is related to how much your body thinks the baby needs. If the body thinks the baby is still hungry, it will produce more milk. If you are nursing and the breast is completely empty, the baby may stop sucking. To stimulate more milk, you can then pump your breasts for an additional ten minutes after each feeding, even though no milk is coming out. The continued sucking action will trick your body into thinking the baby wants more, and within a week, you will have an increased volume. Similarly, if you are only pumping, leave the pump on for an additional ten minutes after no more milk is coming out.

What else can you do to increase milk production? There are anecdotal reports that some herbs and natural supplements may help, including Mother's Milk Tea, fenugreek, and Blessed Thistle. However, no solid scientific reports verify that these supplements are effective or explain the mechanisms by which they work.

In the United States, metoclopramide (Reglan) is the only medication currently prescribed to increase milk production. This drug increases prolactin levels in the mother, and it can reportedly increase milk production by about 60 to 70 percent. After three weeks of good milk production, and as long as the mother keeps up the frequency of feeding, her supply should be sustained. Side effects of metoclopramide are cramping, diarrhea, and depression, so it should not be used for more than four weeks.

Another anecdotal recommendation—one that is popular in the UK—is that drinking six ounces of a strong, dark beer such as Guinness increases milk production. The hops in the beer are purported to increase prolactin production. Whether or not this old wives' tale is factual, it does at least allow the mom to relax and potentially produce more milk. However, you should always be cautious about consuming alcohol while breastfeeding because alcohol is excreted into the breast milk. And according to studies, drinking excessive amounts of alcohol temporarily reduces both milk production and baby feeding.[1] Alcohol is cleared out of breast milk within two to three hours of consumption.

Unsuccessful Breastfeeding

Breastfeeding requires commitment and support from family, friends, and physicians. It is a 24/7 job that is often frustrating and exhausting. The sleep deprivation associated with feeding the baby every two to three hours can be overwhelming. A new mother may skip middle-of-the-night feedings, opting for another family member to supplement with formula. The result of this, of course, is that with less feeding, those same moms make less milk and create a cycle of breastfeeding failure.

In addition, many women quit nursing because of breast or nipple pain. Pain occurs in 70 percent of breastfeeding moms in the first month. Normally, the pain resolves after the nipple has healed and breastfeeding is well established. The pain occurs from direct nipple trauma as well as engorgement and the letdown reflex. Prevention is always the first step—provide a relaxed environment for milk letdown and a comfortable position for you and your baby. Then manually express some of your milk if your breast is too engorged or your nipple is too flat before having the baby latch on.

▶ ▶ ▶ A NEW DAD'S DIARY: BREASTFEEDING

On days two and three, Audry's breastfeeding became very painful. Her nipples were actually bleeding a little. I felt completely helpless because I could do nothing for her. Nothing. Eventually it got better. It took at least a week before the pain of breastfeeding started to subside, and that felt like a very long time. Using the breast pump we rented from the hospital helped Audry tremendously because using it didn't hurt and it allowed her nipples to heal.

—Dominic, Alane's patient ◀ ◀ ◀

Stress, worrying, and fatigue really do decrease the supply of breast milk. However, if a mom can manage to make her only focus the care of her baby, she can almost certainly make an adequate amount of milk. As the baby grows, the number of feedings decrease and the feedings are faster. You won't experience as much commotion during the night and will gradually and gratefully return to normal levels of sleep. If you really want to succeed in breastfeeding, make sure your support system allows you to make breastfeeding your primary focus for a while, until you get into a routine.

Many new moms believe breastfeeding is something that should come naturally and that they should be pros at it right away. When challenges arise, they become frustrated. We remind them that you don't go into anything in your life thinking, "I can do this perfectly the first time." Remember, you have a new baby and are trying something new, so you have to allow yourself to practice breastfeeding over and over until it truly does feel natural.

On the other hand, if you did everything in your power to breastfeed and you haven't found a rhythm with your baby, it's not the end of the world if you switch to formula. Breast milk is always preferred, but sometimes the stress of nursing can add to feelings of inadequacy, failure, and even postpartum depression. We'd rather have a formula-fed infant than a mom who has an emotional breakdown.

Bottle-Feeding Breast Milk

In some situations, a mother may choose to provide breast milk in a bottle instead of nursing. Some women love breastfeeding and get a great sense of satisfaction from the bonding that occurs during the nursing process. But for others, their priority is simply that the baby gets breast milk, not the act of nursing. For them, using a breast pump to collect the milk is an alternative. This option may be the only one for working mothers. In addition, if you've had a premature infant who was in the NICU for a long time, the baby may be accustomed to taking milk from a bottle.

The mechanics of sucking on a bottle are different than nursing from the breast. The artificial nipple is firmer, so the baby cannot use the tongue motion to draw milk out. Instead, he must generate negative pressure and will then regulate the flow of milk with the tongue. Going back and forth between bottle and breast can be difficult. Babies who have been using the bottle will use their tongue to slow down the flow. Then, when they are switched to the breast, this motion will force the nipple out of their mouth.

However, sometimes a mother must use both, especially if she is going back to work. Often with time, the baby can overcome this "nipple confusion."

Pumping breast milk

To be successful with pumping breast milk, you need to pump every three hours. You can produce as much milk with a pump as you can with nursing. The disadvantage, of course, is that it takes a lot of additional equipment to pump milk. You always have to carry the pump with you along with all the supplies, and you have to clean everything regularly. The advantage is that if you need to go back to work, someone else can feed your baby with your own breast milk.

◗ ◗ ◗ OUR BREASTFEEDING EXPERIENCES

Because both of my children were preemies and because of my breakneck schedule at the hospital, I never really nursed either of them. I chose to use the breast pump exclusively. The advantage is that you can allow somebody else to help you in a much more active way. When you have frozen breast milk, you're not as tied to the schedule of feeding. But I learned that pumping has its own pressurized schedule attached. I would set my alarm clock and get up every three hours to pump. For example, when my son was in the NICU for five weeks, I could have slept through the night. But instead, I got up every three hours—just as if my baby was there—to pump.

Once my son was home, I developed a zany system by which I would be pumping and feeding the baby from a bottle of breast milk at the same time, so that I'd have to get up only every three hours at night. It was pretty crazy. I would sit on the floor with the baby on a pillow; then holding one hand with the bottle for the baby, I'd feed him while simultaneously pumping, with my pump hooked onto me with a hands-free bra. I had a factory going on in my bathroom. But for me, it worked.

My strangest time was definitely my commuting regimen. I used the hands-free bra and a cigarette adaptor to power the pump. I would hook myself up and drive through the LA freeway system with that pump strapped on. By the time I was home, I was finished and had three full hours to enjoy my son before the next pumping session. Thank goodness I was never pulled over for anything. That would have been a hard one to explain!

—Allison ◀ ◀ ◀

I went back to work when my daughter, Kylie, was four weeks old, so I started pumping just a week after she was born. I would nurse her, and then after I nursed her I would pump because I needed to stockpile extra milk for when I went back to work. I introduced Kylie to the bottle when she was two weeks old, and she still breastfed as well. She never had an issue of not taking the breast because she preferred the bottle. I think that situation can sometimes happen when the bottle is introduced too early and the baby really doesn't get a good breastfeeding routine established.

I went back to work at four weeks and I never gave my child an ounce of formula. But I worked very hard, pumping all the time in the beginning. I had to pump driving in the car with a hands-free device, at lunch, and driving home. Breastfeeding was a commitment.

Some women don't pump because it's so much work. Washing the bottles and freezing the milk can be a chore. Others can't pump because they don't have a suitable work environment. However, the majority of people stop pumping because it's just an overwhelming amount of work.

—Yvonne ◀ ◀ ◀

Guiding my patients through their breastfeeding challenges was a part of my job that I struggled with, until I breastfed my own baby. You don't realize how hard breastfeeding is until it's your turn. I didn't understand all the details of the difficulties involved in the beginning. But I absolutely loved breastfeeding my boys, after I mastered it, which took a good month, both times. Breastfeeding is a special bonding time that only you, the mom, can provide. Your baby smells so sweet that I've always wished I could bottle that smell to save forever. It's an amazing experience to see your baby feed. You see the motion of his mouth, you hear his gulp, followed by a satisfying burp, and then he'll get that "milk drunk" look on his face . . . it's priceless. But before I was able to get to that point, I struggled.

Many times I wondered if I was going to be able to do it. I felt exhausted, sleep deprived, and insecure. I was also in some pain when Matthew was not latched on properly. He and I had to practice together, over and over again until we got it right. It took just as long to get used to breastfeeding with my second, Max. The difference was that I didn't have that insecurity. The second time around, I trusted that Max and I would eventually be able to do it.

Because I went back to work full time fairly soon after delivering my sons (five weeks after Matthew's birth, and four weeks after Max's), I had to resort to breastfeeding, pumping, and formula. Did I want to exclusively breastfeed? Absolutely. But with my work schedule, I had a hard time keeping up with the demand. And even though I had special slots carved into my workday schedule as pumping times, I eventually had to supplement with formula. It was not my ideal choice, but I had to adapt to the situation. Fortunately, both boys transitioned well from breastfeeding to pumped milk to formula. It all worked out in the end.

—Alane ◀ ◀ ◀

Many of the preemie babies in the NICU may not be able to nurse, so they will be fed pumped breast milk through a feeding tube or bottle. Of course, not all babies in the NICU have to bottle-feed long term. Many can eventually learn to nurse. Most NICUs will help the mother breastfeed her baby after the baby is able to take feedings.

We counsel our patients to think honestly about what works for their lifestyles. If a woman knows she's going back to work, she has to be realistic about her options. A woman who stays at home might have more flexibility.

Motorized pumps

Breast pumps are either manual—you have to physically pump the device like a piston—or motorized—an electric or battery-driven motor does the work. The motorized pumps are easier to use but more expensive. The motorized pumps also generate a stronger suction, so the milk is expressed faster and more efficiently. If you think you may need to pump only occasionally, the manual pump may be enough.

Following is a list of breastfeeding and breast pumping supplies:

- Electric pump such as the Medela's Pump in Style or a manual pump
- Breast pads to protect your bra from leakage
- Two or three nursing bras
- Hands-free bra
- Nipple ointment (we like Lansinoh)
- Milk storage bags
- Rubber bands or bread twist-ties if your storage bags don't zip closed
- Bottle drying rack
- Bottle brush
- Small cooler with ice pack to transport milk

You can make a hands-free bra by cutting two holes in the front of a sports bra. Then insert the plastic nipple covers of the pump into the holes and use the bra to hold the covers in place. Now you are free to do other tasks while pumping.

Complications of Breastfeeding

Beyond the challenges of latching on and finding a workable schedule and a rhythm that allows you to feed your baby every two to three hours, other breastfeeding complications involve unpleasant changes to the breast itself. Most of these problems can be overcome by following the simple steps we describe next:

Breast engorgement

Breast engorgement, the swelling of the breast caused by the pressure of new milk, first occurs three to five days after delivery. Not only does the milk come in, but the breasts retain water and enlarge tremendously. As a result, you may have significant pain. Because a hard, engorged breast may make latching on difficult, some people pump a small amount or take a warm shower to help soften the breasts before nursing. In addition, wearing a support bra and using pain medications such as ibuprofen or acetaminophen can help with the pain. This postdelivery engorgement passes after a few days.

If you are a stomach-sleeper, you may have been counting the days until delivery when you can finally lie on your belly again. However, the disappointment sets in early when you realize that your breasts are now so swollen and tender that you can't possibly lie on them. You also find that you must wear a bra at all times, even at night, or you will leak breast milk all over your bed.

Mastitis

Engorgement also occurs if you allow too much time to pass between feedings or when you're not emptying the breasts completely. Bacteria from the baby's mouth or mother's skin can easily get into the breast ducts. If the breasts are engorged and the bacteria is not flushed out with a feeding, it can cause an infection of the breast called *mastitis,* which occurs in one-third of nursing moms.

The signs of mastitis are a red patch on the breast, usually in the shape of a pie piece, fever, body aches, and pain. Mastitis needs to be treated aggressively because 3 to 4 percent of women will develop a breast abscess (a large pus collection), which may require IV antibiotics and surgical drainage.

You can treat mastitis with the following remedies:

- Use warm compresses or hot showers on the breast and massage the affected area.
- Empty the infected side every two to three hours, either by nursing or pumping.
- Increase your fluid intake.
- Evaluate your nursing technique and possibly modify the position if nipple trauma is occurring.
- Take acetaminophen or ibuprofen for fevers and pain.

If the preceding measures don't work after twenty-four hours, you may need antibiotics.

The biggest mistake that moms with mastitis make is to stop using the breast because the breast hurts or because they are worried that they will pass their infection to the baby through the milk. Don't worry, the milk is not infected, just the skin and tissue around the breast. You make the problem worse by not feeding your baby or emptying the breast. The good news about mastitis is that most cases resolve in a few days with the preceding measures. If your symptoms do not resolve in a few days, please call your doctor.

Unfortunately, about 50 percent of women who develop mastitis will stop breastfeeding because the pain and discomfort are too much to handle. Therefore, the infection needs to be addressed immediately and emotional support given to these moms.

Cracked nipples

A cracked nipple is sometimes a sign that the baby is not latched properly, but it can also occur if you use a pump regularly. The initial treatment for cracking is to place an ointment with lanolin on the nipple. Our favorite nipple ointment is made by Lansinoh. It's smooth, light, and easy to apply. Keep the nipple dry between feedings. Some women will blow dry their nipples before replacing their bra to help with this. You can also wear nipple shields or breast pads in the bra between feedings to help keep the nipple dry without any fabric touching it.

If the nipple has a serious crack that will not heal with just an ointment and is constantly reinjured, you may need to take a break from breastfeeding and pumping for a day or two to allow the nipple to heal. Thankfully, most cracks will heal within twenty-four hours if left untouched.

▶ ▶ ▶ MY STRAWBERRY MILK

I returned to work a few weeks after Kate was born, so I used a breast pump almost exclusively. I pumped everywhere—at work, in the car, at home, probably eight to ten times a day. I had a copious milk supply, but eventually my breasts paid the price. After two months, I developed cracks in both nipples. Putting the pump to the breast would literally bring tears to my eyes for the first few minutes. Then the cracks started to bleed, and there would be blood in the milk, causing it to turn pink. My freezer was full of small bags of liquid resembling strawberry milk.

Some women are afraid that blood-tinged milk is unsafe for the baby, but it's not. You can continue to feed your baby even if the milk is pink. My cracks took months to heal, because just as they would start to close, it would be time to pump again. Eventually, they did heal after I took a break from pumping for a day. The cracks resolved and the pain went away. I had made it!

—Allison ◀ ◀ ◀

Fungal infections

In addition to bacteria that can cause mastitis, the breast can also be infected with yeast. Yeast is everywhere. It's on our skin, in our intestines, in our vaginas, and can even be in our baby's mouths. The baby can transfer yeast from his mouth to the mom's breast during nursing. The nipple will feel sore and appear red, chafed, or peeling. This condition can be treated with a topical antifungal cream. Thrush, the visible fungal infection in a baby's mouth, is treated with antifungal drops.

Sometimes, a yeast infection will penetrate beyond the skin and get into the breast tissue itself. Patients describe this as a shooting electrical pain that begins in the nipple and radiates outward through the breast. Unlike mastitis, a yeast infection does not result in fever, hardness, or redness. Instead, you feel an intense discomfort that starts and continues while the baby is nursing. In severe cases, a rash of small red spots develops on the skin of the entire breast. This type of yeast infection must be treated with an oral antifungal medicine (fluconazole).

Plugged ducts

The ducts of the breast are like branches of a tree, draining to the nipple, or trunk (see Figure 7-1). When a duct gets plugged, the milk from that area cannot come out, causing the area to swell, harden, and become painful. Plugged ducts can occur if the milk is thicker or contains more mucous or if, anatomically, the ducts have sharp angles that form pockets where the milk can get stuck. After breastfeeding or pumping, the affected area will feel hard and tender, while the rest of the breast feels soft. Unlike a case of mastitis, redness and fevers do not occur. You cannot prevent ducts from getting plugged, other than emptying the breast regularly. Unfortunately, if you have an anatomic irregularity, the same ducts will become clogged over and over again.

To unplug a clogged duct, you can manually massage the area from the outer edge toward the nipple. In addition, hot compresses or standing in a hot shower can loosen the plug. Finally, nursing or using a breast pump will ultimately open up the duct and allow the milk to flow again. Your instinct may be to stop breastfeeding because of the pain, but stopping will often make the situation worse. A plugged duct that remains plugged may lead to mastitis or an abscess.

One last-ditch effort for plugged ducts is to have your partner suck from the breast to unplug it. We know this sounds crazy, but desperate times call for desperate measures. A plugged duct can be one of the most painful experiences for a new mom. Sometimes the negative pressure from a pump or the baby is just not strong enough to move the plug. We've had moms who have finally resorted to asking their partner to unplug the blockage—with almost certain success.

▶ ▶ ▶ MY PLUGGED DUCTS

I had two episodes of plugged ducts while breastfeeding Matthew. And boy, did they hurt! The sensation was sharp. I knew it was a plugged duct because after I would finish breastfeeding, my breast would feel soft and deflated except for a small area on the breast where it was still full of milk and extremely painful. You can tell which duct is plugged by using a breast pump. As you pump, you can see your nipples through the clear shield. I could see the stream of milk coming out of my opened ducts, but the plugged one would form only a small white drop of milk.

I tried vigorous massage, heat, Tylenol, and Motrin, and continued to pump and breastfeed. After doing all these steps over and over, I was able to successfully unplug my duct. How do you know your duct is unplugged? You'll know right away from the immediate relief. I got lucky with Max—no plugged ducts!

—Alane ◀ ◀ ◀

Alcohol and Breastfeeding

The American Academy of Pediatrics considers small amounts of alcohol safe while breastfeeding. Sixty minutes after consumption, alcohol is found in breast milk. One serving of beer or wine (five ounces of wine or twelve ounces of beer) is eliminated from the mother's system within a few hours. Therefore, the AAP recommends waiting two to three hours after consumption before nursing. Because the absolute amount of alcohol transferred into the milk is low, it is safe in reasonable amounts. Excessive use has been linked to drowsiness, weakness, and abnormal weight gain in infants.

Weaning

For a variety of reasons, some women need to stop nursing. The basics of weaning are the same as milk production: supply and demand. If you stop stimulating the breast, the milk supply will quickly dwindle, with cessation of milk production in one to two weeks. You can also wear a tight-fitting bra and use ice packs. Pain medications can be used to help with engorgement. Currently, no FDA-approved medications suppress lactation.

Unfortunately, you cannot prevent the breasts from changing appearance after pregnancy. Because the skin and ligaments are stretched to sometimes twice the normal size, the breasts will often appear deflated. These breast changes happen whether or not you nurse because they are just related to being pregnant. Cigarette smoking and aging make the sagging worse.

Lactation Consultants

If you've never breastfed before, it can be difficult to do it successfully without support. Reading and learning about breastfeeding before delivery is important, but there's no substitute for a consultant who can watch what you are doing with the baby in your hands and offer suggestions. Many hospitals provide this service, but often the problems aren't known until after you are discharged because the milk has not come in before you go home. Some communities offer support groups, classes, and referrals for lactation consultants.

Never hesitate to ask for help with breastfeeding, whether it's advice from your obstetrician or midwife, or from friends or family members who have breastfed. The La Leche League is dedicated to helping new mothers around the globe with breastfeeding. Their Web site, at www.llli.org, offers the best source of information for moms learning to breastfeed.

Formula Feeding

▶ ▶ ▶ A NEW DAD'S DIARY: THE TRANSITION TO FORMULA

Audry continued to struggle with breastfeeding. Jacob was latching on properly now with a deep latch, but she was still in a lot of pain. Again, I could do nothing to help, which was hard.

We started supplementing with formula, very little at first and then more and more. We wanted Jacob to be breastfed as long as possible, but it was the single hardest thing to deal with for my wife. Not only did it hurt Audry, but Jacob would suck for only a short time and then fall into a deep sleep, which meant he wasn't feeding much and wasn't getting the more nutritious hindmilk. And as a result, he would wake frequently, crying and screaming, wanting to be fed again. The frequency of this made it more painful for Audry and tiring and frustrating for the both of us.

Formula was easy for Jacob. He didn't have to work for his food, so he would easily take in an ounce or two. Then like a miracle, he would sleep deeply for two to three hours. That meant we all could finally get some sleep. It was amazing how good even an hour of restful sleep felt.

—Dominic, Alane's patient ◀ ◀ ◀

In Dominic's diary, he describes Audry's struggle in the beginning, which resulted in her needing to supplement with formula intermittently. Eventually, with continued practice, she was able to breastfeed the majority of the time. Her story illustrates the advice we give our patients: Your goal should be to try your best to exclusively breastfeed, while knowing that you always have the fallback option of formula in times of necessity.

Although manufactured infant formulas have improved significantly over the years, they never have the same quality of breast milk.

The composition of milk from the breast is different from that of soy formulas or cow's milk, especially regarding its anti-infection properties. For that reason, formula-fed infants have a higher incidence of diarrhea, ear infections, colds, and bladder infections. In addition, they have greater weight gain due to fat deposition, while breastfed babies have faster head growth.

Nonetheless, breastfeeding is impossible under some conditions, including maternal HIV, active tuberculosis, and herpes infection of the breast. If a mother is a carrier of hepatitis B or C, breastfeeding should be discussed with her pediatrician. In addition, breastfeeding women cannot use some medications, mostly chemotherapeutic agents and radioactive medications. If an alternative is not available, the woman must cease nursing. In rare cases, malformations of the breast result in breast glands that do not develop. Finally, breast augmentation or reduction can compromise the drainage of milk through the ducts, making breastfeeding more difficult.

When Your Baby Cries

During the first three months, any crying baby should be attended to. Your baby has pretty simple needs and will cry if they are not being met. The most common reasons why a baby will cry are because the baby

- is hungry
- has a wet or dirty diaper
- has gas

After you've fed your baby, burped him, and changed his diaper, you have taken care of all the basic needs. Continued crying may just mean that your baby needs to be soothed, rocked, or cuddled.

A note on overfeeding: Many families use food as the first method to soothe a crying baby, even when the baby may not be hungry. Perhaps that infant just needs to be rocked, or to hear your voice—whatever method connects you with your baby. Parents who always associate crying with hunger can overfeed their child in the first year of life. And children who are very overweight early in life can be predisposed to adult obesity.

At night, from about midnight to six in the morning, don't overly stimulate the baby when he wakes up. For example, when the baby wakes up, you don't start cooing, "Oh goo-goo gaga!" or "Oh, you're so cute!" Simply stay quiet, feed and change the baby, and then let him fall back asleep. The diaper change should occur quickly and quietly. Keep the lights dim and don't engage the baby, so that he or she comes to understand that nighttime is not a time for playing and socializing; nighttime is a time for sleeping.

The bewitching hour is not an hour, but the time from six at night to midnight, when some babies will cry inconsolably. A baby that wails for several hours straight can be an exasperating and even scary situation. Usually, this crying is just a transitional period that passes after three months, but it can be exhausting. Make sure that you have met all of the baby's basic needs, and if he's still crying, just wait it out. With gentle consoling or rocking, he will eventually be soothed.

Remember that babies make noises all the time, even while they're asleep. Often, they're not crying; they may just be grunting. Some babies make these little grunting noises nonstop. It doesn't mean they need something; the sounds may be involuntary. We don't know why some babies do this and others don't.

Pacifiers

myth: If a baby takes a pacifier, it will be hard for him or her to nurse.

FACT: After breastfeeding has been well established, most babies are able to nurse and use a pacifier without any problems.

Sucking is one of a baby's first reflexes. It is not only a means to satisfy hunger but can also be soothing and relaxing due to the repetitive motion. Infants instinctively suck on anything you put in their mouth—a nipple, a pacifier, a finger or thumb, and later, toes.

Using a pacifier is a personal decision. Some babies like pacifiers more than others. At some point, generally around a year, you will need to take the pacifiers away and go through the sometimes painful transition to a pacifier-free world. However, the later you take away the pacifier, the harder the transition.

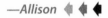 DITCHING THE PACIFIER

My pediatrician told me: "Your baby can use pacifiers, but you should get rid of them by the time he is twelve months old." Truthfully, I still used a pacifier with my son Luke after twelve months, and I even lied to my pediatrician about it. In my practice, I don't want people to feel that it's bad if they use a pacifier longer than a year because every baby is different.

—Allison

Habits become harder to break the longer we indulge in them. If you take away a pacifier when a baby is twelve months old, he will probably move on to other things within a day or so. Taking a pacifier away from a two-year-old is a completely different matter. You have to ask yourself how much you want the baby to have its pacifier right now versus how hard will it be for the baby to stop later? One of our patients put it perfectly: "Either they cry now or you cry later."

Baby's Sleep Cycle

In the womb, babies will sleep for an hour and then be awake for an hour. You may have noticed this pattern in the baby's movements while you were pregnant. In the outside world, sleep intervals increase to two to three hours with wakeful periods of one to two hours. Even as adults, it is common for us to have periods of lighter sleeping or even waking up. The difference, however, is that adults have learned how to fall back to sleep. We turn over, readjust our position or bedclothes, and soothe ourselves right back to sleep, without even knowing we did so.

Babies don't yet know the trick of how to put themselves back into the sleep state. For a little while, anyway, it is your job to rock them back to sleep. Ultimately, the baby will need to learn how to self-soothe in order to fall back to sleep independently, but this self-soothing doesn't occur immediately, especially during the newborn stage.

Some other good ways to soothe include driving the baby in a car, pushing your newborn in a stroller, or sitting him in a vibrating chair or in a motorized swing designed for newborns.

▶ ▶ ▶ MY SIX-MONTH-LONG NIGHT

Until your baby weighs at least twelve pounds, he can't physically go all night without eating because he doesn't have enough fat on his body to sustain him for more than a few hours. Twelve pounds was an important benchmark for me because both my kids were preemies. Around three months of age, a lot of babies weigh twelve pounds and start to be able to sleep much longer. My children, though, were almost six months old before they or I were able to sleep through the night. Particularly if your baby was small at birth, know that it may take longer for her to make it through an entire night without a feeding because it may be months before she reaches the twelve-pound mark.

—Allison ◀ ◀ ◀

Sleeping with Your Baby

Your baby should not sleep in your bed with you, although plenty of controversy surrounds the subject. Theoretically, you could roll over in your sleep and inadvertently suffocate the baby. The American Academy of Pediatrics instead recommends that the baby sleep in your room in a bassinet, crib, or cosleeper for the first three months. A cosleeper is a bassinet that attaches to the parents' bed so that the baby is within arm's reach and yet safely in his own protected area.

Having the baby in your room allows you to attend to his needs easily and conveniently. With cosleeping, the baby also has the comfort of having his mom right next to him, being able to smell and sense her at all times.

The following guidelines reduce the risk of suffocation and SIDS (sudden infant death syndrome):

- Lay the baby on his back.
- Do not use pillows or bumpers.
- Use a fitted bottom sheet only and keep the baby warm in sleeper pajamas.

- Use a mattress that fits tightly within the crib.
- Check the crib for any loose screws or hardware.
- Crib slats should be less than 2³/₈ inches.

Swaddling

Babies often wake themselves up and don't know how to go back to sleep. Remember, they're not used to being out in the physical world beyond the womb. They might swing an arm or a leg, get startled and awakened by their own jerky, awkward movements, and then panic because they can't get back to sleep.

For this reason, a lot of babies love being swaddled. We call it the "baby burrito." Swaddling prevents babies from making sudden movements in their sleep and gives them the feeling of being held and comforted. The technique can be a little hard to master at first, but it's worth learning. Figure 7-7 is a step-by-step illustration of how to swaddle, courtesy of our expert nurses at Good Samaritan Hospital.

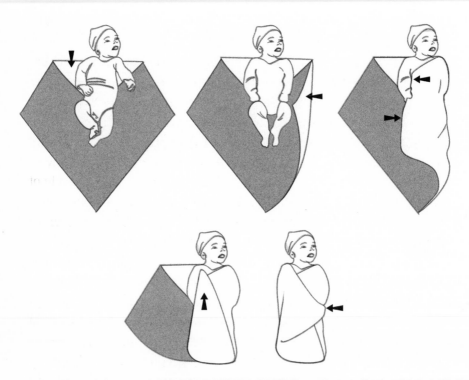

Figure 7-7: How to Swaddle

Your Sleep Cycle

Most people go to bed at night, then wake up when their alarm clock goes off in the morning. They don't usually take phone calls or get up to complete tasks at 3:00 a.m. That schedule goes out the window with a new baby in the house. A chronically disrupted sleep cycle can take its toll on everybody in the family, moms and dads alike. For some, the busiest time of day is in the middle of the night.

▶ ▶ ▶ **A NEW DAD'S DIARY: A HARD DAY'S NIGHT**

> Taking care of Jacob requires constant attention—it's so repetitive, day and night. Jacob wakes up hungry and screams until one of us satisfies his needs with breast milk or formula or both. He doesn't care if it's the middle of the night or if he's waking us up the second or third time. Jacob knows only that he is hungry, and he demands that we do something about it. No "thank you." No "sorry to have to wake you up." Not even a smile to signify appreciation. Just a sense of "take care of me now!"
>
> *—Dominic, Alane's patient* ◀ ◀ ◀

Some women feel like they are losing their minds when their babies awaken them night after night. They find it hard to remember things and complete simple tasks, and they become anxious and irritable. This phenomenon has a chemical explanation. We have a natural, circadian rhythm of sleep and wake cycles based on alternating light and dark periods. Cortisol, the stress hormone, reaches its lowest point about three hours after dark, and your body goes into a cycle of rest, physical repair, and recovery. Especially important are the cycles of light and deep dream states that occur from 2 a.m. to 6 a.m. During this time, our minds recover from the emotional stresses of the day. After six to eight hours of sleep, as the sun begins to rise, cortisol begins to peak so you have the energy to take on a new day. When this cycle is interrupted, cortisol is released in an irregular fashion at inappropriate times. Chronic sleep deprivation can be serious business and is a major factor in the development of postpartum depression.

Here's one piece of advice that new moms hate hearing: "Just sleep when your baby sleeps." First, it is difficult to fall asleep on demand

and not natural for an adult to sleep in two- to three-hour increments. In addition, the two-hour intervals leave no time for the myriad other things in life that don't involve full-time care of a baby—such as eating, showering, or laundry.

Coping with sleep deprivation is easier with good support. If you have the luxury of a family member or spouse who will be there to help you, ask that person to take over the household tasks—at least temporarily—so you can catch a quick nap after your shower. These extra bits of sleep may be just what you need to keep insanity at bay.

▶ ▶ ▶ TWO PLUS TWO

A great couple–Jill and Daniel–recently delivered twin daughters. They already had two boys at home so finding that their third pregnancy was twins was a shock. They weren't sure how they would manage, but they took it in stride and Jill made it all the way to thirty-six weeks.

Daniel decided to take a two-month paternity leave from his job at a manufacturing plant to stay home with the girls. Jill's mom came to stay with them to lend an extra hand for the first two weeks, but both of their extended families lived out of state.

Jill and Daniel came to their first postpartum visit when the girls were two weeks old. And for the first time, they had left the babies home with Jill's mom. I was running behind on my office schedule because I had to deliver a baby. So Jill and Daniel found themselves with a twenty-minute wait. By the time I walked in the room, I found both of them sound asleep in the exam room chairs. Snoring.

They stirred as I came in, and confessed that they hadn't had a quiet moment since they had been home, between the girls' new schedule and the two boys, who had become more needy than ever. They were hoping my delivery would take even longer so that they could finally catch up on some sleep!

—Allison ◀ ◀ ◀

Many women feel alone in their struggle with the stress and depression that can result from the lack of sleep. Understanding that there is a chemical reason for these feelings can help them feel normal. Even though feeling overwhelmed is common in the fourth trimester, many women never talk about it. As a result, they feel as if they're the only one who have gone through a difficult time or that somehow they're not up to the challenges of motherhood like everyone else.

▶ ▶ ▶ TAKE CARE OF YOURSELF

One of our medical colleagues, Taryn, delivered her baby with us and then went home to live a postpartum nightmare. Unable to cope well with the two- to three-hour interruptions to her sleep every night, she quickly became severely depressed and anxious. For most people, sleep deprivation is very rough.

Taryn knew that the lack of sleep was exacerbating her symptoms because she had previously suffered a period of depression that was triggered by lack of sleep. Because postpartum depression is more common in women who have had depression in the past, I recommended that she see a psychiatrist, who started her on an antidepressant. I also suggested that she hire a night nurse so she could at least catch up on her sleep. She did this for two weeks and got many nights of uninterrupted sleep, which allowed her to recover and get a better handle on things.

If you are having serious trouble handling sleep deprivation, don't hesitate to reach out for help. Ask family or friends for help, or if you have the means, hire someone even for a short time, like Taryn did.

—Yvonne ◀ ◀ ◀

A Night Nurse

A night nurse is one solution to the challenging newborn schedule that is certainly not available to all women. However, a few of our moms have successfully employed a night nurse for a few crucial weeks of their baby's infancy, so that they could have somebody to care for the baby while they grabbed a few nights of precious, uninterrupted sleep.

A night nurse can perform a variety of tasks. The nurse may sit beside the baby, and when she determines that the baby is really hungry, bring the baby to the mother. This way, the mother can breastfeed while she's in bed, and then the nurse can take the baby away when it's finished, allowing mommy to go right back to sleep. The night nurse can also change the diaper and soothe the baby back to sleep after the baby has been fed.

Some night nurses take the baby for the entire sleep period—from 11 p.m. to 6 a.m.—and feed, change, and swaddle the baby, while the mom sleeps through the night. Obviously, this scenario is more difficult to pull off if you're breastfeeding exclusively.

You don't necessarily need a registered nurse for this job; you might have a nanny, a grandmother, a sister, or a wonderful friend who volunteers to help out.

Emotional Changes

A friend without children may ask, "So, what is it that you do all day?" If you are a first-time mom, it can be difficult to understand what is so hard about taking care of a baby. Now, you are about to find out.

You may think you have prepared for this moment by listening to advice or reading books, but in truth, nothing ever compares to going through it the first time. Even though we've delivered thousands of babies and dished out a lot of sound medical advice, each one of us was amazed when we brought our first child home—overwhelmed by the stress, the sleep deprivation, and the fact that so many of our carefully laid plans and detailed preparations had to be discarded when we were faced with the day-to-day reality of new motherhood.

Women who are type A often turn to organization as a method of coping. They fuss about getting their baby on a schedule and buy all the latest gadgets. Other moms don't prepare much. Instead, they just go with the flow and figure it out as they go along. There is no right or wrong way to make the transition to motherhood.

Sleep deprivation throws nearly everyone off their game. You need to keep a close eye on your feelings during this time because it's easy to get confused, overwhelmed, anxious, or even seriously depressed, simply because you haven't had enough sleep.

Some new moms struggle immediately when they get home from the hospital. The physical and emotional stress of the pregnancy and birth opens the floodgates for all sorts of pent-up emotions. Fears that have been kept inside for so long suddenly come out in an over-whelming cascade. With other women, the pressures don't mount un-til they've been home for a few weeks. If we don't see any signs of emotional trauma in the hospital, we may not find out about their struggles until they come back to see us for their six-week postpar-tum visit. We always encourage our patients to call us before they hit an emotional wall. We can often suggest additional help either from a night nurse, lactation consultant, or family member. Sometimes, if a patient's stress reaches a critical mass, we may suggest counseling or even medication, depending on the severity of her symptoms.

▶ ▶ ▶ ROADSIDE ADVICE

My daughter's kindergarten teacher unexpectedly struggled right after she had her baby. On the job, she knew how to get a roomful of five-year-olds to fall in line, but having her newborn daughter home for one week was almost more than she could handle.

Angela is a petite, energetic woman who never skips a beat. Although she looked as wide as she was tall during the last part of her pregnancy, she worked right up until the end, giving her beloved kindergarteners all sorts of reasons to giggle about her growing belly. She delivered an eight-and-a-half-pound baby girl vaginally without any trouble.

I was out running in our neighborhood one morning when a sobbing An-gela—who was not a patient of mine—pulled her car over to the side of the street to stop me. It was about a week after her daughter's birth and she was so desperate for advice that she felt she had to flag me down to ask for help.

Among Angela's complaints—and something that we hear a lot—was that her husband was doing his best to be helpful, but when push came to shove, the responsibility for the baby and the household chores was all hers. She was feeling so much pressure to be the perfect mom, to breastfeed, to console her daughter when she cried, and to keep up the housework. It left her exhausted and scared that there was no end in sight.

I explained to her that we all try to be the perfect mom, the perfect wife, the perfect employee. Sometimes we need to give ourselves a break, to ask for help, and to take care of ourselves too.

—Allison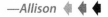

Like everything else about the birth process, remember that millions of women have made it through this transitional phase and come out triumphant on the other side. We did, and we weathered some significant bumps along our respective roads. We're confident that you can overcome these obstacles, too.

▶ ▶ ▶ SOME BABIES ARE JUST EASIER

Not every new mom has a hard time adjusting to her newborn's schedule. Some babies truly are easier than others, waking at night only to feed for fifteen minutes and then instantly falling back to sleep. These are the dream babies some of our luckier patients tell us about: They seem preprogrammed not to fuss, whine, or scream.

I remember talking with one of my patients, Colleen, right before she delivered her third daughter. I asked her if she was nervous. After all, she had two toddlers at home and now would have yet another newborn. As a veteran mom, she was well aware of the hard work that would be coming her way. But Colleen's answer surprised me. Instead of dreading the impending chaos, she was actually looking forward to the unique bonding that develops between mother and newborn during the silent hours of the night. She said that her favorite time with her first two girls was when the rest of the house was asleep. Those were the precious moments when she could hold them, rock them, and tend to them without distraction. She loved their closeness to her when they nursed, their sweet baby smells, and the peaceful expressions on their faces as they drifted off to sleep.

Colleen's answer reminded me that sometimes the most challenging times are the ones that bring us closest to our children. These simple moments allow us to experience the profound beauty of motherhood.

—Allison ◀ ◀ ◀

Baby Blues

The hormonal changes that occur after childbirth, in combination with sleep deprivation and the stresses of a newborn, can lead to postpartum blues and, more seriously, postpartum depression.

Nearly all new mothers suffer some form of postdelivery letdown. During the long months of pregnancy, the focus of everyone and everything was on you, the pregnant mom. In the delivery room, everything changes. After the baby enters the world, everyone's attention turns to the new life in the room. Parents, partners, friends, and doctors suddenly shift their focus from you—whom they've often placed on a kind of pedestal for nine months—to the baby. Many mothers describe it as feeling like they've just become invisible. Then you have to cope with the fact that right after you have a baby, your stomach is stretched out, you have hemorrhoids, your vagina hurts, and you're not exactly beauty contest–ready. You're tired, you don't have time to wash your hair, and you're wearing sweatpants because your body is sore and you can't fit into anything else. No wonder many of our patients report that their self-esteem is fragile during this time.

A baby, for everything wonderful and magical that he or she brings, is also a life-changer. Naturally, a new mom may feel sad or blue at times. You've just been handed a 24/7 commitment, so a lot of the freedom you used to take for granted in your old life seems to be gone. Remember, though, that baby blues are experienced by 50 to 80 percent of new moms, so you are not alone.

▶ ▶ ▶ THE CLOUDS ROLL IN

I learned the hard way that being an ob-gyn did not make me immune to the fourth trimester issues that so many of my patients experience. During the first two weeks after I delivered Matthew, I struggled with everything: sleep deprivation, insecurity, and difficulty in getting the hang of breastfeeding for the first time. People tell you that babies feed every two to three hours, but they don't tell you that you could struggle with breastfeeding for a full hour and then it's time to feed again, shortly after you've changed and burped your child.

During those first few weeks, I felt a shift in my body and brain that was almost unbearable during my milk letdown. The feeling, which may have been the hormone changes after delivery or related to the breastfeeding itself, was overwhelming, as if a field of massive, suffocating black clouds were rolling in and consuming me. I felt a sense of depression that I'd never experienced. After the milk letdown, the worst of it would lift and I would feel normal.

The "black clouds" were such a physical sensation—not just mood related—that I was certain the sensation had to have chemical causes. When I mentioned the feeling to my own obstetrician, he said that another patient was experiencing the same thing. With that patient, the only thing that helped was for her to stop breastfeeding. I considered doing the same, but fortunately for me, the sensation started to dissipate about two to three weeks in and eventually went away on its own.

Recently, one of our own patients admitted that during her milk letdown, she was feeling the very same way I'd felt. Before she confided in me, she had scoured the Internet hoping to find answers, but couldn't find anything. So when I shared my story with her, even though it may not have made her symptoms go away, she felt better knowing that she was not alone.

—Alane ◀ ◀ ◀

Having a baby causes most new moms to experience some sort of emotional upset, especially when the baby's requirements are much greater than anticipated or more than they have ever dealt with before. Sleep deprivation, irritability, and feeling overwhelmed and inadequate—all these emotions are normal. If you have the blues or don't feel the constant sense of joy from motherhood that you expected, remember that the transition to parenthood is a very trying time, but it's also a temporary one.

Following are tips for fighting the blues:

1. Know that you are not alone. Talk to other moms and your doctor about your feelings.
2. Accept help when people offer it. If your friend brings you dinner and your husband changes the diaper, welcome their aid with open arms. You don't have to do everything yourself.
3. Sleep whenever you can, wherever you can.
4. Get fresh air by going for a walk with your baby in the stroller every day.
5. Eat healthily. Loading up on junk food with empty calories will leave you lethargic and bloated.
6. Give yourself time to adjust to motherhood. You don't have to be a perfect mother and have everything figured out on day one. Being a mother is a learning experience.

7. Don't stress about the details. It's okay if your baby's outfit doesn't match, or you haven't sent thank-you cards for baby shower gifts yet. These little things can wait.

8. Take time to appreciate what you have already accomplished.

Postpartum Blues versus Depression

Because postdelivery emotional volatility is so common, distinguishing normal baby blues from chemical changes that can evolve into full-blown postpartum depression can be difficult. Most women harbor secret doubts about whether they're going to be good mothers, and many also worry that their baby may not love them. Every new mother has to go through a transition to feel comfortable with the concept that, sometimes, babies cry no matter what you do.

Postpartum blues, or the baby blues, is a transient phase of depressive mood that can include tearfulness, anxiety, irritation, difficulty concentrating, and restlessness. The baby blues can start two to three days after delivery and last up to six weeks. This condition differs from depression in its intensity, severity, and duration.

Postpartum Depression Diagnosis

Postpartum depression (PPD) is underdiagnosed because many women feel ashamed and afraid to talk about their feelings with their family, friends, or doctors. These feelings are so at odds with what society implies that they should be feeling—constant bliss at the miracle of their bundle of joy—that the lack of interest in their babies, the sadness, and the inability to cope with motherhood fills them with guilt. The depressed mom may begin to feel that she will never be a good mother.

Family members and friends may mistake PPD for the normal adjustments to motherhood. The diagnosis may be missed unless the doctor specifically and routinely questions the new mother about her mood. The new mother herself may not volunteer this information.

Depressive symptoms that intensify as the weeks go by are a signal that full-blown depression may be developing. *Postpartum depression* is defined as intense feelings of sadness, anxiety, or despair in the postpartum period, feelings so intense that they interfere with the mother's ability to function and don't resolve on their own. Untreated postpartum depression can result in serious harm to the mother or the infant. From 10 to 15 percent of women encounter postpartum depression, and nearly half have symptoms that persist for more than six months.

Doctors have a specific set of criteria to diagnose postpartum depression. First, one of the following must be true:

Depressed mood for most days for at least two weeks
Anhedonia (loss of pleasure or interest in usual activities)

Plus, the person must have four of the following symptoms or three if both preceding symptoms are present:

Weight loss or loss of appetite
Difficulty sleeping or sleeping too much
Feeling agitated
Loss of energy
Feelings of worthlessness or excessive guilt
Decreased ability to concentrate
Recurrent thoughts of death, suicidal ideas, or attempted suicide

Severity of postpartum depression

You can't just tell a mom with postpartum depression to cheer up and snap out of it—real postpartum depression is nothing to be taken lightly. With this type of depression, the mom almost always has unrelenting, terrible feelings about herself. The mother might also harbor ill feelings toward her baby. The depression may present as dramatic and severe, but it may not always show on the surface, especially if the mother is hiding her feelings or is ashamed to share her feelings. Guilt, shame, and isolation often become factors in postpartum depression, and can make a bad situation even worse.

▶ ▶ ▶ YOU ARE NOT ALONE

My patient, Misha, was always a sunny, positive person. She is a woman of great strength, character, and courage, keeping an upbeat attitude as she struggled through two ectopic pregnancies and two miscarriages before she was finally able to deliver her first child; a healthy baby girl. Misha sailed through her postpartum period with ease, but then she unexpectedly found herself pregnant again when her infant was only a few months old. Misha was elated. I delivered another beautiful, healthy girl, and had no reason to think she wouldn't go forward again with the same cheerful demeanor I'd always seen her exhibit, even during tough times.

However, this second postpartum period was very different for Misha. Sleep deprivation and stress evolved into the blues, which evolved into serious depression. Compounding Misha's anguish was how much she was beating herself up for not feeling joyful all the time. After all, hadn't she wanted to have a baby more than anything? Now that she had everything she had always wanted, why didn't she want to get out of bed in the morning? Misha tried talking about her feelings with some close female relatives—also moms—who gaped at her in disbelief. They couldn't relate to what she was desperately trying to describe. Misha felt like an outcast, terribly guilty, and very much alone. She was judging herself unmercifully and was sinking deeper and deeper into despair.

Fortunately, Misha reached out to me during her postpartum care. I assured her that she was not alone in these symptoms, despite the fact that her own family hadn't experienced them. We first worked on getting her some solid sleep. Her husband agreed to take the night shift for several nights to let her catch up. The next step was starting her on an antidepressant. I suggested she talk to our colleague Taryn (mentioned previously in this chapter), who had made it through the same experience. By supporting her needs and ending her isolation, we were able to get her through this dark time.

No woman can predict how she will feel after her baby comes or how it will affect her emotionally. Just because you are happy that you are pregnant and excited about your baby doesn't mean you are immune to depression. But you don't have to be alone!

—Yvonne ◀ ◀ ◀

Risk Factors and Treatment for PPD

Some women are predisposed to postpartum depression. The risk factors include young age, multiple life stresses, divorce, and previous history of depression. However, only about 40 percent of women with PPD will have one of these risk factors.

Treatments for PPD include a combination of therapy and antidepressants. The therapy is used to confront any underlying stresses, and the medications alter brain chemistry. Most antidepressants can be taken safely while breastfeeding. Although relief is not instantaneous, studies show that antidepressants can reduce symptoms by 50 percent within four weeks.

What Friends and Family Can Do

If you think your partner, sister, or daughter seems to have postpartum depression, offer her help. She may be afraid to express what she is feeling. Depression that is untreated or ignored can have serious consequences for her and the baby. Do not suggest that the new mom "snap out of it," and do not make her feel bad or deviant for having these feelings. Just because you and other women you know didn't experience depression doesn't mean that it is abnormal.

WAYS TO HELP A MOM WITH PPD

- Understand that she is experiencing a chemical reaction that is out of her control. PPD is not a choice.
- Help around the house, do the laundry, cook some meals, put away the dishes—anything to relieve her burden.
- Let her talk about her feelings.
- Limit visitors to those who are there to help. Sometimes a new mom may become exhausted trying to entertain guests.
- For a new dad, tell your wife you love her and love your baby. Tell her she looks beautiful. Be affectionate.

PPD with Another Pregnancy

Just because you had postpartum depression in a previous pregnancy does not mean you will have it again. Every pregnancy and every baby is different. The first time can be so overwhelming that the mom may be more prone to depression. With experience, she may know what to expect and may not feel quite so overwhelmed, which may decrease her chances of developing depression in a subsequent pregnancy.

If you have had preexisting depression before becoming pregnant or a history of postpartum depression, we recommend that you watch for the warning signs and contact your provider early if symptoms are developing. Early diagnosis and treatment can greatly decrease the effects of this condition.

▶ ▶ ▶ MATERNAL INSTINCTS AND BONDING

My patient Krystal and her husband Paolo were dedicated to having a healthy pregnancy even before it began. Two years before she conceived their first child, Krystal, a high school guidance counselor, was diagnosed with high blood pressure. She did everything she could with diet and exercise, but in the end, she needed to take blood pressure medicine as well. Before she got pregnant, she saw her doctor to change her medicine to the safest possible drug.

Everything went well during the pregnancy. Krystal was diligent about keeping her blood pressure under control, even monitoring it between classes at her school. She had serial ultrasounds to make sure the baby grew well, and underwent nonstress testing twice a week. As her due date approached, we discovered her baby was breech, so I delivered her by cesarean. Krystal and Paolo left the hospital with their son Antonio after three days, excited to begin the next chapter in their lives.

After they got home, everything changed. Antonio had a difficult time latching on to breastfeed, Krystal's incision hurt, and no one was getting any sleep. Krystal began feeling that she must be doing something wrong, and found herself tearful and frustrated most of the time. Each day seemed like an eternity.

Krystal and Paolo came to their two-week postpartum visit, concerned that Krystal was developing depression. Her biggest concern was that she did not feel bonded to her son. Although she felt the instinct to protect him and care for him, the baby seemed like a stranger. She didn't know anything about him and couldn't figure out what his cries meant, what he needed, or how to soothe him. Krystal would sometimes just stare at the baby, not knowing what to do next. She felt resentful. And she was scared that she would always feel this way about Antonio.

By her six-week postpartum visit, the tide was finally beginning to turn. Baby Antonio had smiled at her for the first time, and while it may have just been gas, Krystal felt like they had finally made the connection she was longing for. Krystal confided to me that the previous six weeks had been some of the hardest of her life, especially trying to come to terms with the fact that she didn't seem to have the same instant maternal bond that some of her other friends had described. She and Paolo left the visit hopeful and optimistic that those early seeds of bonding would continue to strengthen and grow.

Maternal instinct is different for every mom. Many women fall in love from the first moment they see their baby, but others struggle with their feelings. If, by the luck of the draw, their babies happen to be particularly irritable, poor sleepers, fussy feeders, or difficult to soothe, some new moms may feel angry, frustrated, resentful, or defeated. They may also feel very alone if their friends or family can't identify with their experiences. Thankfully, for almost all women, the bond eventually forms. A smile, a coo—these small miracles of life are the threads that time weaves to form the rich tapestry of a real mother-and-child relationship. Just when they thought it would never happen, these women, like Krystal, find that the deep, fulfilling love they'd always hoped for begins to flood into their lives.

—Allison ◀ ◀ ◀

Getting Back to "You" Again

Now that you've become accustomed to your new life and routine with your baby, being a mom begins to feel like your natural state of being. As your life begins to take on a new kind of normalcy, however, you may suddenly pass by a mirror and wonder if you will ever look and feel like the old "you" again. The truth is, your body has gone through tremendous changes during your pregnancy in preparation for your baby's birth and is continuing to change postpartum. For most women, both time and patience are required before they return to their prepregnancy physical state.

Your Postpartum Body

You will have a postbirth visit with your provider about six weeks after your baby is born. At this checkup, we perform a physical exam to make sure you have healed adequately after the delivery. We check that the uterus has decreased to normal size and the vaginal lacerations or episiotomy has healed properly.

If you are still feeling uncomfortable about your body six weeks after baby, relax and know you're normal. Only about 30 percent of women will have returned to their prepregnancy weight by the six-week postpartum visit. In addition, many still look like they are four months pregnant because the muscles and the skin have been stretched by the growing baby and uterus. Regaining that muscle tone takes time. Doing core exercises—such as yoga or sit-ups—helps, but you have to work long and hard to get back your prepregnancy appearance.

If everything appears to be healing well, you can return to most of your normal activities after the six-week mark. You can have sex, swim, take baths, and start exercising more vigorously.

With exercise, we recommend that you ease back into your routines slowly and don't attempt to go full force the first day back at the gym. Understandably, many women recovering from pregnancy find that they have lost their stamina. During the last stages of pregnancy, most women aren't working out much. Adding to that the residual exhaustion of getting through those first weeks of their babies' infancies, it makes sense that their bodies get fatigued easily when they return to their exercise routine.

One other caveat regarding exercise: During pregnancy, the *pubic symphysis*—the joint that unites the two pubic bones—naturally separates. The joints of the hips and pelvis also loosen to accommodate the passage of the baby. In the postpartum period, these joints may remain lax, causing some women to feel unsteady when they start running and doing higher-impact aerobic exercises. Therefore, you should listen to your body, be careful, and use common sense about how hard and how often to exercise.

Postbirth Contraception

Finally, during this six-week visit, we will discuss contraception options. You cannot take contraceptives containing estrogen—such as combination birth control pills (with both estrogen and progestin components)—while nursing because they decrease your milk supply. Breastfeeding moms who want to use a hormonal method must use a progestin-only medication such as the minipill, Depo-Provera (a long-acting injectable form of progesterone that is given every three months), or a progesterone-releasing IUD (Mirena). If a mom wants to use a nonhormonal form of contraception, she can use condoms, a diaphragm, or a copper T IUD (Paraguard). Another option, if she and her partner feel they are finished growing their family, is permanent sterilization—tubal ligation or vasectomy.

Tubal ligation is a procedure performed on women wherein the fallopian tubes are either burned (coagulated) and cut, or tied, cut, and coagulated. This procedure prevents the egg and the sperm from uniting in the fallopian tube and prevents conception. The type of surgery depends on whether or not it is performed immediately after the baby is delivered or sometime later, through a procedure called a laparoscopy. The tubal ligation procedure requires a spinal or general anesthesia.

A vasectomy is a procedure performed on a man in which the vas deferens in the man's scrotum is ligated and transected to prevent the sperm from being ejaculated during intercourse. This procedure is performed in an office under local anesthesia.

Losing Your Baby Weight

Most women never return to their prepregnancy weight, holding onto about three to five extra pounds after one year. The best predictor of your ability to lose your pregnancy weight is how much you gained during the process. Especially for women who gained excessive amounts of weight (more than thirty-five pounds), the weight may never come off unless you put tremendous effort into your diet and exercise regime. Women who gained more than thirty-five pounds were on average eleven pounds heavier than their prepregnancy weight after one year. For women who gained a normal amount of weight (twenty-five to thirty-five pounds), most will finally reach their goal by about eight months after delivery.

Women who nurse and those who don't experience relatively similar weight loss.[2] Although you expend about 800 extra calories a day producing breast milk, nursing moms may find they have an increased appetite, so weight loss between the nursing versus the non-nursing moms often remains the same. If you keep your calorie intake moderate while you are nursing, you may shed the extra pounds quite easily. Ultimately, you need to go back to the basics: eating a sensible diet and initiating a good exercise program.

When you have a newborn, finding both the time and the energy to exercise is only a part of the problem. It's hard for a woman to get out to a gym unless it provides a day care center for infants—most don't, especially not for newborns. A more practical option is to just get outside with your baby and take a walk or a jog with the stroller for thirty to forty minutes each day. It's good to expose babies to new environments, and the fresh air is great for mom's stress, as well.

▶ ▶ ▶ EXERCISING WITH OUR NEWBORNS

Most of us who have to go back to work don't know how we will ever fit exercise back into our schedules. If you're like me, you'll also have those unavoidable feelings of guilt: "If I've been away from my baby all day at work, how can I possibly return home a whole hour later so I can squeeze in some exercise?" I finally found a good solution. I would come home, wrap Kylie in my Moby wrap—a giant piece of fabric that works as a baby carrier—and walk three miles a day. She would sleep against my chest, which made me feel close to her, and I was able to exercise at the same time. The more she grew and the heavier her weight, the better the exercise was for me! I found that she would be happier and sleep better on the days that we did our ritual walks. The frequency that she fussed during the "bewitching hour" definitely decreased on walk days.

These walks also gave my body time to get back into the swing of exercise. I had had a cesarean with her and was on bed rest—which meant exercise rest!—from the time I was twenty-four weeks pregnant until delivery. The wonderful thing about a long walk with your baby is that you don't need a gym or a babysitter to do it! I found my daily walks with my baby, along with the extra calories I burned breastfeeding worked together to eventually help me lose my baby weight.

—Yvonne ◀ ◀ ◀

Finding the time with a newborn and a four-year-old to exercise is difficult. So I followed Yvonne's example after my second was born, always exercising with my Max in tow. Max was an early riser like me, so rather than awaken everyone else in our home, I would take Max in his stroller for a walk around a high school track near my home. My husband and older son were able to get more sleep time while Max and I had our exercise—and a special chance to bond, too.

—Alane ◀ ◀ ◀

Having Sex Again

One of our jokes with patients is that breastfeeding is nature's birth control. Beyond the fatigue and crazy schedule, if a woman is breastfeeding as well, her estrogen drops to a very low level. This drop causes the vaginal walls to dry and thin. Not only do you not produce much natural lubrication, but the vaginal tissue also loses its elasticity. We often say "your vagina is in menopause." So sex in general just does not feel great. To counter it, we recommend that you use an artificial lubricant and take your time. After your menstrual cycle returns as you nurse less frequently, your estrogen levels will be back to normal and the dryness should go away.

Many of our patients come in and ask, "Is this how it's going to be from now on?" We reassure them that this situation is normal and resolves with time. Even though sex is uncomfortable, it doesn't mean there's something wrong with you.

Many women also find that their libido takes a vacation for those first few months. When you are tired and stressed, sex is the last thing on your mind. In addition, when you are with your baby all day, especially if you are nursing, you are having constant physical contact with him or her. So when the baby is asleep, often all you want is some space, and even your partner's touch can seem like the straw that broke the camel's back. Be sure to explain to your partner how you are feeling and what you need during this phase, which—we can assure you—is purely transitional. Like everything else about the early weeks and months with a newborn, the lack of libido will pass with time too.

Hair Loss

"My drain is clogged and my brush is full of hair." The postpartum period leaves many women wondering what happened to their lustrous locks. About 10 percent of new moms will experience a crazy amount of hair loss after delivery, starting at about three months after birth. This is called the postpartum effluvium. Some women associate this hair loss with breastfeeding or low vitamin levels, but actually it is a result of the pregnancy itself.

Hair grows in ninety-day cycles. When you are pregnant, more hair is in the anagen, or growing, phase, which is why a pregnant woman's hair becomes thicker. Due to the physical stress of labor and delivery, hair will switch from the anagen phase to the telogen, or resting, phase. And about ninety days after delivery, you will have a noticeable loss of hair when combing or in the shower. This situation is shocking and upsetting for most women. But do not worry: Your hair will revert to its normal growth cycles soon, and in most cases, postpartum effluvium will completely resolve by fifteen months after delivery.

Reentering the World

◗ ◗ ◗ A NEW DAD'S DIARY: THE MIRACLE OF A MOM

I am amazed with my wife and how she cares for our baby. No matter how much Jacob screams, she is so nurturing and caring. I realized something about women versus men—although women can be just as driven to perform, men are probably more one-dimensionally so. When my baby screams his head off and gets red in the face, to me it sounds like he's criticizing my abilities as a dad. I know that sounds irrational, but that's what it sounds like to me. And I get frustrated and annoyed really fast, something I'm learning to overcome. But my wife, from the very start, has not been annoyed by our baby's screams—they are communication. To her, they always just sound like need.

—Dominic, Alane's patient ◖ ◖ ◖

We are all working mothers, and trust us, we know how hard it is to transition back from full-time motherhood to a busy professional schedule. It seems as if the whole world is counting on you. We tell our patients that they shouldn't be afraid to ask for help: from us, from their pediatrician, from their partners and families, and from outside professionals.

Getting Extra Help

In the early days after bringing your baby home, new moms are shocked to find that they don't have time to shower, cook dinner, or finish much of anything. Just as you start a simple task, the baby wakes up and you have to change or feed him. You never get to complete anything, which can be incredibly frustrating.

Although we're always supportive of our patients who pay for a doula or a birthing coach to help them through delivery, for some new parents, we've noticed that the money would be just as well spent finding professional postpartum assistance. For about the same cost, a couple could have a nanny or housekeeper come in for four hours a day for the first month. Until you have a new baby at home, you can't begin to value the worth of a person who can straighten up your house, wash your clothes, make you something to eat, and help with so many simple things that can become big issues while your entire focus is on your new baby. Don't be afraid to ask for help!

● ● ●

Mothers who are on their second babies find that everything feels easier this time around because they lived through it once already. They know what life with a tiny infant is like and can accept the inevitability that the majority of their focus during those first few weeks will be on their children. An experienced mother knows how to redirect and reprogram her priorities; to psychologically prepare herself to just get in there and get it done. We've all found that the time seems to fly by much faster, too, now that you're aware that your baby will be an infant for only a sliver of time.

Going Back to Work

Not all our patients are willing to share with us certain fears. As the birth day approaches, some women feel vaguely anxious and overwhelmed about the reality of parenthood. They begin to ask themselves, "How am I going to take care of this baby after I return to work? What kind of parent will I be? How am I going to deal with the sleep deprivation when I have a full-time job during the day? What am I going to do for child care when I go back to work? Will I be prepared for this child, for which there are no instruction manuals?"

Remember that you are not alone. In the United States, 72 percent of mothers do some kind of work outside the home during pregnancy and may need to continue for financial reasons after the baby is born.[3] However, child care costs are often so high that even a two-income family can't swing them, and the idea of leaving a small child in day care raises issues about both physical and emotional health risks down the line. Even women who can safely afford a nanny don't always feel comfortable leaving their child with a nonfamily member all day.

All three of us are working moms. We have to be good at multitasking because we have a lot of different balls in the air at the same time. We do our best to keep things under control, but invariably, we drop a ball or two. Remember that it's okay not to be perfect one hundred percent of the time. We won't lie to you—all the juggling can be tough. But millions of women do it and manage to do it well. A lot of women have to work, and like us, they must learn how to keep the balancing act going.

That mother's guilt you hear people talk about? We definitely have that going on. We want to be there for our children and not miss a moment of their growth. On the other hand, we struggle with the fact that our many years of education and training were undertaken for a purpose—to help other women and fulfill what we feel is our mission in life.

Our children range from less than two to nine and a half, so we have some years of experience and experimenting under our belts. Our patients often ask us, "How do you do it?" We realize what may work for one working mom may not work for another, but we'd like to share some of the hard-earned pearls that helped us to transition back into work, each with a child or children at home. It's always a work in progress.

Here are some of the things we tried to help us ease back into work. We hope our experience can help. Some of this advice comes from our patients, too, who always share with us the ups and downs of their own adventures in working motherhood:

1. Go back to work on a Thursday or Friday. Returning to work on a Monday can seem a bit daunting, and starting later in the week makes the return a little less overwhelming.

2. If you are a working mom, it is impossible to breastfeed exclusively. However, it is possible to give your baby a diet of 100 percent breast

milk by pumping and breastfeeding. Pumping is hard work, but definitely worth it. After you establish a breastfeeding pattern, you should also give your baby pumped milk in a bottle so that whoever cares for your baby while you are at work has an easier transition feeding him or her. It will be much harder to transition to bottles if your baby has been exclusively breastfed for three months, and you wait until the day before you return to work to surprise him or her with that very first bottle.

3. Practice pumping in work-like conditions before you return. Try pumping at home a few times while pretending that you're at work so that you can make sure you have everything you need at your fingertips when you return. For example, one of our patients realized during a dry run at home that she would need some type of brown paper or plastic bag in which to carry the pump parts from her office to the mother's room, where she could wash and sanitize them. "Had I not brought that bag," our patient recalls, "I would have had to throw them in my purse (ew!) or walk through the office with my arms full of pump parts." Office pumping is awkward enough, so the more prepared you can be, the better. You will need your pump with tubing, bottles, nipple shields, milk storage bags, and a small cooler to store the milk during the day. You should also get a bottle brush and drying rack.

4. Print some pictures of the baby for your office when you return.

5. Whether you decide on a nanny or day care, make sure you do your research a few months before your due date. Check out a few different day care centers so you get a feel for the environment in which your child will spend part of his or her days. If you plan to have a nanny, interview several of them well ahead of time.

6. If you do have the option to hire a nanny, have her start a few weeks before you go back to work. Make out a formal daily schedule in which the nanny can chart your child's naps and food intake for each hour of the day, as well as any big development milestones or events that you should know about.

7. Think about a backup child care plan. What happens if your mother or nanny is sick? Who else can you count on for help? Make a short list of reliable friends or family members who could lend a hand in an emergency.

8. Talk to your boss about your return. If you need to modify your hours to accommodate a day care schedule, let your boss know early. Perhaps he or she can make arrangements that will fit both of your needs.

9. Discuss your breast pumping needs with your boss. Is there a private room you can use? Can you take a few minutes every three hours to do it? How can it fit into your work schedule?

10. Find a way to stay connected to your baby during the day. If you have access to a Skype or Facetime phone, use it to check in regularly.

11. Give yourself a break. You do not have to be Superwoman: perfect mom, perfect partner, and career woman all the time. We all do the best we can.

12. Let go of the guilt that you may feel by leaving your baby at home. Financially, you may need to work to support your family. In addition, you may actually enjoy your job. Remember that it is still okay to find pleasure outside motherhood.

13. Remember to take care of yourself. You cannot be there for everyone if you neglect yourself. Get yourself a cup of coffee, take a nice walk, do yoga, go for a run, or have a well-deserved pedicure once in a while. These activities help to boost your spirits and make you more calm and relaxed. Sometimes, the best thing you can do for your baby is to take better care of yourself.

The Fourth Trimester Is Not Forever

Even though the transition through the fourth trimester is often rough—for us, this period was much harder than labor, in fact!—the rewards on the other side far outweigh all the pain and stress we have to go through. In the blink of an eye, your baby will be crawling, then walking, then running. You will look back at pictures of your tiny infant in a few months and marvel that your baby was ever so small.

Where did that time go? In the day-to-day struggle of it all, it may seem like the postpartum phase lasts an eternity, but we promise that you'll marvel at how quickly it passed. Enjoy the two- to three-hour naps because they will shortly disappear and your toddler will be climbing, falling, and putting raisins or marbles up his nose. You might even laugh at yourself for suddenly feeling nostalgic for those simple days when all you had to do was feed your baby and put him to sleep. Try to think of every phase of the journey as an important one because it all really does pass by far too quickly.

chapter eight

COMPLICATIONS IN EARLY PREGNANCY

Fertile or Infertile?

Many of us take for granted the ability to have a child. After all, just like they warned us in middle school health class, egg meets sperm and boom! You should get a positive pregnancy test just a few weeks later. The reality is that even for young, healthy couples with no known fertility issues, the monthly chance that they will be able to conceive is only about 20 percent per menstrual cycle. As a result, we counsel our patients not to fret if they do not get pregnant after their first try. For many couples, conception will take some time—sometimes six to twelve months—to see the plus sign pop up on that pregnancy test stick.

Unfortunately, about 10 to 15 percent of women less than thirty-five years old will face infertility. And for those older than thirty-five, one in three may potentially face difficulties conceiving. A diagnosis of infertility is made after a couple has had unprotected intercourse at the time of ovulation for twelve consecutive months and still has not become pregnant. At that point, we usually recommend that the couple

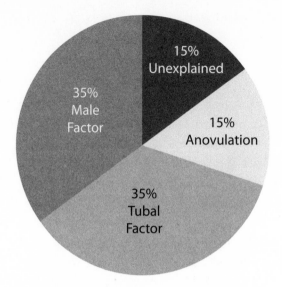

Figure 8-1: Common Causes of Infertility

see a fertility specialist. However, if a woman is close to age forty, we recommend that she has a fertility consultation after only three to six months of trying. People shouldn't feel that they failed because they need the services of a fertility expert. Due to spectacular strides in medicine, thousands of women who, just a few years ago, would have been considered infertile without any hope are now able to get pregnant—even more than once—and fulfill their dreams of motherhood. The common causes of infertility are shown in Figure 8-1.

Tubal Blockage

Tubal factor infertility, which accounts for 35 percent of couples not being able to conceive, occurs when a blockage in the fallopian tube prevents the egg and sperm from meeting. If a woman has had prior pelvic infections such as pelvic inflammatory disease caused by chlamydia, she may have blocked or damaged fallopian tubes. Similarly, having a history of endometriosis, ruptured appendix, ectopic pregnancy, or prior pelvic surgery can lead to tubal damage. When we suspect tubal factor, we perform a special X-ray called a hysterosalpingogram (HSG). If a tubal blockage is found, a woman can have surgery to repair the tubes or use in vitro fertilization, where the embryo is implanted directly into the uterus, bypassing the fallopian tubes. (See page 352 for information about IVF.)

Male Factor

Male factor infertility explains about 35 percent of infertility cases. One reason for male factor infertility is sperm abnormalities—the sperm count is low, the sperm do not move well, or the shape of the sperm is abnormal. The diagnosis is made with a semen analysis after three to five days of abstinence. Another cause of male infertility is obstruction in the genital tract, preventing the sperm from coming out. Varicoceles, which are dilated varicose veins surrounding the testicles, can cause overheating of the testicles, which in turn may damage sperm. Other reasons for male infertility include hormonal imbalances, history of trauma, stress, drug use, frequent intercourse, history of testicular surgery, and smoking. When an abnormal semen analysis is found and male factor infertility is suspected, the man is referred to an urologist, who can determine the cause and suggest treatment options.

Anovulation

For a woman to conceive, one of the first things that needs to happen is the release of an egg from the ovary, or ovulation. If you do not ovulate—the technical term is *anovulation*—you can't get pregnant because there is no egg to be fertilized. Anovulation is the cause of infertility in approximately 15 percent of infertile couples.

Most women have regular menstrual cycles every twenty-one to thirty-five days. Women who don't ovulate have cycles that are less frequent—every two to three months or longer. We can detect ovulation with an ovulation predictor kit (discussed on page 38) or by checking for the presence of progesterone (a hormone produced only after ovulation) in the blood in the last third of the woman's cycle.

The most common cause of anovulation is a hormonal imbalance that interferes with the natural rhythm of monthly egg release. Women with

WITH UNPROTECTED TIMED INTERCOURSE ◀ ◀ ◀

In 3 months: 50 percent of women will be pregnant

In 6 months: 75 percent of women will be pregnant

In 12 months: 85 percent of women will be pregnant

polycystic ovarian syndrome (now known as hyperandrogenic chronic anovulation), anorexia, excessive weight gain or loss, thyroid problems, excessive stress, women who travel frequently, or women who are breastfeeding may experience anovulation.

Unexplained Infertility

If a woman ovulates, has normal ovarian function determined by her FSH (follicle stimulating hormone), and no uterine or tubal problems and if her partner's semen analysis is normal, she has unexplained infertility. Unexplained infertility is diagnosed in 10 to 15 percent of infertile couples. Of course, infertility is always caused by something, but in unexplained infertility, health professionals are not able to identify its cause.

myth: My uterus is tipped so I won't be able to get pregnant.

FACT: All women are born with their uterus in a certain position within the abdominal cavity. Some tilt forward toward the bladder and others tilt back toward the spine. However, the position of the uterus does not influence a woman's ability to get pregnant.

Advanced Maternal Age

Yes, there really is a biological clock. Female fertility rates begin to decline when women are in their thirties. By age forty, the chance of conceiving naturally decreases to 7 percent per month. Even though women lose eggs every month throughout their lives, they retain 70 percent of their fertility potential through age thirty-five. However, by age forty, that number drops by half.

A blood test for FSH (follicle stimulating hormone) performed on the third day of the menstrual cycle can give a general sense of a woman's ovarian function. If the FSH is less than 10 in-

CHANCES OF LIVE BIRTH BY AGE

Less than age 35: chance of live birth is 20 percent per month

Age 35: chance of a live birth is 14 percent per month

Age 40: chance of a live birth is 7 percent per month

Age 45: chance of a live birth is less than 1 percent per month

ternational units (IU), the chance of making viable eggs is still good. If it is greater than 20 IU, the chance of producing viable eggs is almost zero. For women with FSH between 10 and 20, the chances are reduced but pregnancy is still possible.

Fertility Treatments

We see many patients who never imagined they would encounter fertility problems. An infertility diagnosis can rock many couples to their core.

The good news is that the range of treatments is vast, running the gamut from basic insemination procedures, to ovulation induction, to in vitro fertilization, to egg donation and surrogacy. With the advancement in fertility science, it is possible that no matter what your issue, a fertility doctor can help you get pregnant.

Depending on the reason for infertility, doctors usually begin with the least expensive and least invasive form of treatment.

Ovulation Induction

If anovulation is the cause of your infertility, we can use *ovulation induction*: medications to stimulate the ovaries to release the eggs. The first-line treatment is Clomid (or clomiphene citrate), a hormone pill that causes the pituitary gland in the brain to release more FSH, which eventually leads to egg release. Another oral medication called metformin, a drug used to treat diabetes, has also been found to cause ovulation in about 75 percent of previously anovulatory women, specifically if the woman has PCOS.[1] If these two drugs are ineffective, the patient can move on to injectable forms of FSH, which directly stimulate the ovary to release eggs.

These medications increase the likelihood of multiple gestation pregnancies. Without ovulation medicines, the chance of becoming pregnant with twins is 1 percent. On Clomid, the chance is increased to 5 to 10 percent, and with the injectable medications, it can be up to 25 percent. In addition, the monitoring and the cost of these drugs may be difficult for some patients to manage. Thankfully, anovulation is the easiest form of infertility to treat, with approximately 60 to 75 percent of women conceiving within six months of therapy. [2]

A reminder of something we've already pointed out: If you are over-weight or obese, a weight loss of approximately 5 to 10 percent can help you resume normal ovulation without the use of any medications.

Intrauterine Insemination

If male factor infertility is diagnosed, insemination is the first-line therapy. With this treatment, a woman checks for ovulation with an ovulation predictor kit. When the test is positive, she and her partner go to the fertility office. A semen specimen is collected and washed to separate the sperm from the semen. The sperm is then injected di-rectly into the uterus, using a small catheter that we insert vaginally through the cervix.

When sperm problems are more severe, the couple may opt for in vitro fertilization, described next, with ICSI (intracytoplasmic sperm injection). In this treatment, each egg is individually injected with a sperm in the lab to confirm that fertilization has taken place.

In Vitro Fertilization

The first birth from in vitro fertilization was in 1978, and now the technology accounts for about 1 percent of all births in the United States yearly.[3] *In vitro fertilization* is used as a treatment when there is tubal blockage, unexplained infertility, or advanced maternal age.

With IVF, the first step is to temporarily shut down the woman's natural reproductive process with hormones so that egg growth and development can be controlled from the outside. After the natural system is shut down, the woman uses daily injections to stimulate her ovaries to produce multiple eggs that grow at a similar rate. She is monitored every two days with blood tests and ultrasounds while on these injections to make sure that her body is responding appropri-ately to the hormones. The dosage of the medications is then altered depending on the ovarian response. If not enough eggs are produced, the success rate is lower. If the ovaries overrespond, the woman can get ovarian hyperstimulation syndrome (OHSS). In this serious med-ical condition, the ovaries enlarge and the woman swells, feels bloated, and may have abdominal pain. In severe cases, electrolyte imbalances may occur, requiring hospitalization. OHSS is seen in 10 percent of women undergoing IVF.

Figure 8-2: IVF Success Rates

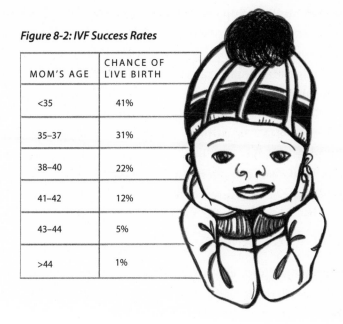

MOM'S AGE	CHANCE OF LIVE BIRTH
<35	41%
35–37	31%
38–40	22%
41–42	12%
43–44	5%
>44	1%

After the eggs are mature and of an appropriate size, doctors re-move them from the woman by inserting a needle into the ovary through the vagina (under anesthesia). The eggs are then mixed with her partner's sperm, grown in the lab for a few days, and then trans-ferred back as embryos to an optimal position in the uterus. The num-ber of embryos transferred depends on the age of the woman and the quality of the embryos. In younger women, fewer embryos are trans-ferred—usually just one or two. For older women, many more embryos are transferred. If extra embryos remain, a couple can freeze them for future IVF attempts. If male factor infertility is identified, the doctor may use ICSI to fertilize the eggs.

Figure 8-2 shows the most recently published success rates for IVF using fresh, non-donor eggs from the 2008 edition of the "Assisted Reproductive Technology Report," which is published annually by the CDC.

GIFT and ZIFT

Gamete intrafallopian transfer, or GIFT, is a process by which several eggs are removed from the patient as in an IVF cycle. However, they are not fertilized in the lab. Instead, they are washed in a special solution and surgically placed into the fallopian tubes along with the partner's sperm, in the hopes that normal fertilization will take place within the tube.

In zygote intrafallopian transfer, or ZIFT, IVF is performed as explained in the preceding section. However, instead of transferring the embryos into the uterus, they are surgically placed into the fallopian tubes. To have ZIFT, a woman must have normal, open fallopian tubes. In some studies, ZIFT has a higher success rate than traditional IVF.[4] Because the embryos are placed into the fallopian tube, ZIFT more closely mimics what happens in natural cycles.

▶ ▶ ▶ MY IVF EXPERIENCE

My first baby, Ryan, was conceived naturally on our first attempt. After my husband and I decided to have a second child, I had two miscarriages. I was turning forty years old, and I felt that if I didn't have a baby soon, I was going to lose my opportunity, so we decided to go forward with IVF. Each attempt takes about three months from the time you start—when you give yourself the drugs—until you learn the outcome. I went through the process three times.

The first time, I was given birth control pills to suppress my natural cycle, but it didn't work. My follicles developed at different rates so I had to stop the process midway. The second time, my fertility doctor tried a different drug called Lupron to suppress my follicles and this was effective. We transferred five embryos into my uterus and I got pregnant, but the pregnancy didn't grow, resulting in another miscarriage. In my third attempt, we did the same drug protocol as the second time, but I did ZIFT instead of intrauterine transfer. Four embryos were put into my fallopian tubes and one stuck—and is now my baby girl, Kylie.

I conceived so easily and naturally the first time that it was hard to compare my first pregnancy to the stressful and emotionally challenging experience of the IVF procedures. The entire experience helped me to be a better doctor and to empathize with patients who struggle to conceive. Now I can share with them my experiences with IVF. In the end, despite the hardships of the process, I am grateful that current medical technology allowed me to have a second baby.

—Yvonne ◀ ◀ ◀

The IVF process can perform miracles but is expensive, usually costing $8,000 to $12,000 per cycle. The fertility drugs are an additional $1,000 to $4,000 per cycle, depending how much medication is required to stimulate your ovaries. Because most IVF is not covered by insurance, many people simply cannot afford IVF.

In addition to being expensive, the IVF process is time consuming. Every step must be calculated and timed, and at every step something can go wrong. The daily hormone injections can be painful. When the ovaries are stimulated, they can grow very large, causing discomfort and bloating. The experience is also a marathon of unsettling emotional ups and downs.

We counsel our patients to prepare mentally for this emotionally demanding experience. You'll be injecting yourself with medication and seeing the doctor every other day for blood tests and ultrasounds. You will be monitored in depth to see *if* your eggs are forming, whether *enough* eggs are forming, or whether *too many* eggs are forming. Meanwhile, the male partner is placed in the uncomfortable position of having to deliver sperm on demand. The ordeal was an emotional roller coaster even for Yvonne, who had a medical background and understood all the intricacies of the process.

On the other hand, Yvonne is also a vocal advocate for the miracle of fertility treatments. "Having had both experiences—an easy conception and a difficult one—I can empathize with people who are struggling with infertility," she says. "Sure, it was a long struggle to go through the treatments and all the disappointments, but when you hold your baby in your arms, you forget all that and are simply grateful."

Despite the psychological strains and financial demands of infertility treatments, remember that thousands of couples are more than willing to do whatever is necessary to get that positive pregnancy test result. All our patients who do conceive this way tell us that the end of the journey is well worth the struggle they took to get there.

Donor Eggs

As we discussed, when a woman enters her forties, her ability to produce eggs that can be fertilized and formed into a normal embryo is significantly decreased. We see major declines in fertility success rates by the age of forty-two. If a woman wants to have a baby and her ovaries are not making quality eggs, she can use an egg from another woman to help her conceive. Usually, egg donors are between the ages of twenty and thirty, and are anonymous. In some cases, however, a woman may use eggs from a sister, a friend, or another relative. The donor egg is retrieved as in IVF and fertilized with her partner's sperm, and then the embryos are placed into the recipient's uterus. She carries and delivers the baby, but the baby is not genetically her own. The success rate for this procedure depends on the age of the donor, and usually is quite high, about 55 percent per cycle.

▶ ▶ ▶ A DIFFERENT PATH

When I got married at thirty-seven, I knew that my clock was ticking away. My husband and I assumed that we had the next five years to start a family. We started trying immediately, but after eleven months, I decided to see a fertility specialist. A round of diagnostic tests determined that my egg quality was diminished and I had a uterus full of fibroids. I was shocked. Even though I was seeing a fertility specialist, I never imagined that my eggs would be the issue—I thought we needed a little help. The women in my family have lots of babies as well as babies late in life.

My FSH was high but within a range that the specialist was comfortable with. I had surgery for my fibroids and after I healed, the testing began again. Now, however, my FSH had doubled and was too high. They say you're only as fertile as your worst FSH, and mine was 29.

I tried alternative therapies (acupuncture, yoga, and nutrition) to try to get my FSH levels down and succeeded twice. The first IUI attempt resulted in a chemical pregnancy. After the second attempt, I took a home pregnancy test (on Valentine's Day) and it read positive. The next day at the doctor's, I had a blood test but it came back negative. I am the rare person who had a false positive. I was devastated.

When I finally realized that I couldn't conceive with my eggs, I became depressed. I had to allow myself to grieve the loss of my eggs, the child who would not look like a mix of me and my husband, and the end of my family's lineage. Through this process I realized that this is my journey, like it or not. I would still have babies but not in the way I had imagined or wished. We revisited our options and decided to try egg donation.

After we made the decision, the process moved quickly. We registered with a few agencies and began to browse the list of potential donors, which felt like online dating for the genetic mother of your child. The process can be creepy and a little voyeuristic, which is why you have to find the right agency. For us, it was important to meet the woman for at least a few minutes, not because we wanted to have a relationship with her, but to get a feel for who she was. After meeting several women, we met another donor for coffee and made the decision on the spot. Within two months we were in the process of doing a donor egg transfer. I became pregnant the first time, and with twins!

I never think of these babies growing inside me as anything but my own. I think fondly of the amazing woman who helped us create our future family and wonder what traits of hers my children will have. I don't regret any of it—the surgeries, shots, setbacks, and grief. I believe that this is the path I was meant to take, and I think that I am in a better place because of it.

—Helen, Allison's patient ◀ ◀ ◀

Donor Sperm

In some cases, the man's sperm count is so low that he is not a candidate for IUI or IVF with ICSI. Another option is to use donor sperm from a sperm bank. The couple can choose a donor who has similar features to the partner, and then undergo IUI with the purchased sperm. In addition, same-sex couples or single women without a partner may choose this route to conception.

Surrogates

Another miracle of modern fertility science is that a woman who has a chronic disease that will not allow her to carry a pregnancy or a woman who has had a hysterectomy can still become a mother. Through IVF, her eggs can be removed, fertilized with her partner's sperm, and the embryos implanted into a surrogate. A surrogate is a woman who carries a fetus on a couple's behalf, gives birth to the baby, and then gives the baby to the biological parents. Sometimes she may be a close family friend or relative, but most women are hired for this service through a surrogacy agency.

▶ ▶ ▶ TWICE IN A LIFETIME

When I first met Gretchen, she had just been through the most trying years of her life.

A twenty-nine-year-old librarian living in Boston, Gretchen and her husband, Dexter, a college professor, had been married for five years. During that time, she'd been pregnant twice. Her first pregnancy ended at twenty-two weeks when, without any warning, she lost the baby due to cervical insufficiency. (For information on this disorder, see Chapter 9.) She and Dexter were devastated, but after taking a year to grieve, they felt ready to try again. This time, Gretchen had a cerclage (a stitch that keeps the cervix shut) as a preventative measure when she was sixteen weeks pregnant. Despite their best efforts, the cerclage stitch did not hold and Gretchen's cervix started to open at twenty-two weeks. She was able to keep the baby inside until twenty-five weeks, but then her water broke and her daughter Evie was born, weighing only one and a half pounds. After only two days, Evie passed away from complications of her severe prematurity.

Again, Gretchen and Dexter struggled through the crushing grief of losing a child. Yet through it all, they never lost the overwhelming desire to be parents. The couple first came to me for a consultation shortly after they'd moved to Los Angeles, where Dexter had taken a new teaching position. We talked about their pregnancy history and the various options for carrying the baby. Gretchen felt that she could not go through the stress and fear again, and had read about the option of having another woman carry her baby for her.

I explained the surrogacy process, describing the fertility drugs required and the method of transferring the embryo to the recipient. Finally, we talked about how to go about choosing the right surrogate. Gretchen and Dexter left my office full of information—and confusion.

Six months later, this determined couple returned to my office beaming with excitement, bringing with them Gretchen's mother, Diana. After a long deliberation, they had asked Diana to be her own daughter's surrogate. Diana, frustrated by years of helplessly watching her daughter suffer through the loss of two babies, was happy to agree. She was a healthy woman, fifty-two but appearing much younger, who had given birth to four babies without any problems. The couple had gone through fertility treatment, and Grandma Diana was implanted with Gretchen and Dexter's embryos. On the first try, one of the embryos took, and Diana was twelve weeks pregnant with a healthy baby.

I took care of Diana during the pregnancy, which went without a hitch. At thirty-nine weeks, her water broke and she went into labor, giving birth to her own eight-and-a-half-pound grandson. I watched as Diana handed the baby to her daughter and wondered, "How many mothers have the opportunity of giving their child the gift of life twice?" Every one of us in the room that day felt awed and touched by the power of the miracle we'd just witnessed.

—Allison ◀ ◀ ◀

The Odds of Multiples

Today's newspapers are speckled with human-interest stories of infertile couples who end up with high-order multiples—from triplets and quads to even octuplets! Most fertility treatments involve stimulating the growth of multiple eggs or placing multiple embryos inside the mom-to-be. With these treatments, the chance of multiples is about 25 percent. Physically, the uterus is not made to carry so many babies at once. Multiple gestations have the increased risk of complications such as diabetes, preeclampsia, and preterm delivery. In addition, many parents simply are not financially prepared to care for an instantly large family. For these reasons, fertility specialists monitor cycles closely to ensure that the couple ends up with a pregnancy that is safe and reasonable for them.

We know that some readers may regard fertility treatments as being contrary to what nature had in mind for us when it comes to reproduction. Being mothers ourselves, however, we also understand at the deepest level what a great gift it is to be able to have children and raise them. Did nature provide us with all the necessary tools to conceive on our own? Yes. But if the standard biological equipment fails us, nature has also provided us with the assistance of intellect and science to compensate for what we might lack.

▶ ▶ ▶ **A FERTILITY SPECIALIST SPEAKS**

I'm a reproductive endocrinologist, better known as a fertility specialist. In medical school, I studied obstetrics and gynecology, but what really excited me was the science of reproduction. I completed two additional years of training to become one of the scientists who helps to create what used to be called test-tube babies. We now use the term in vitro fertilization (IVF). Four million babies have been born using IVF since the birth of Louise Brown in 1978.

These days many of my patients are single professional women in their mid- to late thirties who feel the pressure of the fertility clock and who consider motherhood as one of their important life goals. These women now can turn to egg freezing to preserve their fertility. I explain egg factor infertility to them, which is how aging influences the ability of the egg to create a chromosomally normal embryo. The chance of having a baby drops by 65 percent at age forty and by 95 percent at age forty-five.

My medical recommendation for my younger, single patients is to get pregnant as soon as possible using their fresh eggs, regardless of the sperm source. Most women, however, are hesitant to become single mothers and still hope to find a partner and build a family. The idea of freezing eggs or embryos for future use is usually more appealing to them.

At age forty, the chance for a live birth from IVF is only 20 percent per attempt; by forty-five, it drops to less than 5 percent. In the news, we often hear of celebrity mothers in their late forties giving birth to healthy babies and in some cases twins, but the majority of these pregnancies are the result of egg donation. Because that fact is rarely revealed publicly, women get the message that pregnancy is possible and even easy well into the fifth decade of life. As a fertility specialist, I have to break a lot of hearts when I shatter this myth.

Many of my patients who choose egg donation go through a period of grieving over losing the opportunity to birth a genetically related child. However, the experience of pregnancy, the miracle of childbirth, and the joy of parenting soon overcome the feelings of loss.

My field is growing and changing every day, with amazing, cutting-edge reproductive technologies available. In the past, the strategy of IVF was to increase the odds of pregnancy by creating multiple embryos. Now, newer technologies focus on creating healthier embryos, using microchips embedded with thousands of genes, and nanotechnology-based systems to create better laboratory microenvironments.

It's a privilege to be at the fulcrum of the creation of life, and to have the opportunity to take this intimate journey with my patients as they fulfill their dreams and build their families.

—John Jain MD, reproductive endocrinologist ◀ ◀ ◀

When a Pregnancy Doesn't Take

As doctors and as mothers, we understand that as soon as you see a positive result on the pregnancy test stick, you begin to feel and act differently. You are more aware of what you are eating and drinking, and smoking no longer holds any appeal. You may wonder why you did not exercise more or pay more attention to your health before you got pregnant. Suddenly, you know that what you do with and to your body matters. Even though you may not see a fully formed baby yet on the ultrasound, and even though your belly is not curving over the top of your jeans, we understand that you are already beginning to feel like you are a mom.

We always want to be bearers of good news. So when we do that first ultrasound and don't see a normal pregnancy, it's hard on us, too. Letting a patient know that we are concerned that her pregnancy isn't healthy is one of the hardest parts of being an obstetrician. When a pregnancy has a problem early on, the reason is most likely a genetic abnormality, and therefore, a healthy baby was not developing. Sometimes we have to trust nature and let it do its job. We know that in most cases, you will have a healthy pregnancy—if not this time, the next time.

▶ ▶ ▶ **THERE NEVER WAS A BABY**

"What do you mean, Doctor? What happened to my baby?"

Rosa was staring at me as if I was from outer space. A thirty-year-old second-time mom, she had confirmed for herself at home that she was pregnant, and then came to see us for the first time at eight weeks .

I had completed a thorough ultrasound, and all I could see was a large empty sac. Gently, I tried to explain that this was an abnormal pregnancy; that her baby didn't form and she would experience a natural miscarriage.

"I don't understand," she kept repeating. "But where is the baby?"

I tried my best to clarify the situation, to tell her that the fetus hadn't formed, most likely because something wasn't genetically right with the pregnancy. I recommended that Rosa take some time to process this news and come back for a follow-up ultrasound in a week to confirm the diagnosis.

Sometimes patients need a second look to be sure for themselves that things are really abnormal.

Rosa left our offices in disbelief. Despite my best attempts to explain, she couldn't grasp this concept: the idea she could be pregnant but not have a baby. Her confusion is common. Most new moms are unaware that you can have a positive pregnancy test, feel pregnant, yet not have a normal fetus growing inside.

—*Allison* ◀ ◀ ◀

Miscarriage

We've seen thousands of miscarriages in our years as doctors, and we're here to share with you this fact: Miscarriages that occur in the first trimester usually happen because of genetic problems in the fetus. Still, as often as we might repeat this, some of our patients insist on searching for some external reason why their pregnancy didn't take. A lot of women who have had miscarriages blame themselves. "Is it the one glass of wine that I drank?" "Is it because I've been stressing out at work?" "Is it because I carried something heavy?" We tell our patients it's not because of something they ate or did. If a woman consumes a small amount of alcohol before she realizes that she's pregnant, that won't cause her to miscarry. A miscarriage occurs when the cells within the early embryo are not growing and dividing normally. Our bodies are often smarter than we are, and nature is programmed to weed out the potentially bad pregnancies before they can progress very far.

At least one in five pregnancies—or 20 percent—result in a miscarriage. And the reason for the miscarriage in 50 to 60 percent of cases is chromosomal abnormalities in the fetus, meaning the fetus was not normal or healthy.[5]

The pregnancy can miscarry at several different times during the development of the fetus.

Chemical pregnancy: A common scenario resulting in miscarriage is a *chemical pregnancy,* one that ends shortly after conception occurs. Little fetal tissue develops and the level of the hormone of pregnancy (hCG) doesn't rise high. The woman will experience bleeding for five to seven days that resembles a moderate period that comes late.

Anembryonic gestation: Another common cause of miscarriage is an *anembryonic gestation*, or blighted ovum. An anembryonic gestation can be diagnosed through ultrasound at seven weeks of gestation when an empty sac is seen without an embryo. The sac may grow quite large and persist for many weeks.

When an egg is fertilized, it makes its way to the uterus, implants in the wall, and starts to grow. From here, in a normal pregnancy, some of the cells divide to become the amniotic sac and the placenta, and some grow to become the baby. But if the cells don't divide according to plan, everything becomes the sac and nothing becomes the baby. Pregnancy tissue is present, causing hCG to rise and setting off a positive pregnancy test, but the embryo never grows. Eventually the body recognizes this and the hCG levels will drop, inducing cramping and bleeding resulting in miscarriage. However, this process may take as long as four to six weeks after the sac develops.

Women with an anembryonic gestation can feel pregnant because the hCG is present. They feel sick, their breasts hurt, and they're tired. However, sometimes in these cases, the symptoms are not as severe because the hormone levels don't rise as high as in a normal pregnancy. When a patient comes in and says, "I don't feel anything," or "I was sick two weeks ago but now I feel fine," it can be a red flag that the pregnancy isn't progressing. Since some women have minimal early pregnancy symptoms or nausea, the lack of symptoms doesn't necessarily mean something is wrong. Maybe they are just the lucky ones.

Fetal demise: In a normal pregnancy, at five weeks of gestation, we can see a sac and a yolk sac, which provides nutrients for the fetus. At six weeks, we should see a fetus with a heartbeat. After the baby has a heartbeat, the chance of miscarriage drops dramatically, from 20 percent to between 3 and 5 percent. After confirming the presence of a fetal heartbeat, your doctor will probably ask you to return in two to four weeks, as long you don't have cramping or bleeding. If the fetal heartbeat is not detected in future visits, this is an indication that the fetus has died. We refer to this sad condition as *fetal demise*. Fortunately, fetal demise is rare and usually occurs in the first trimester. But on occasion it can happen later in the pregnancy as well.

If a fetal demise happens before twelve weeks, in 50 to 60 percent of cases, it is because something was genetically wrong with the baby. As with the anembryonic gestation, the hCG levels will begin to decline, which may lead to spontaneous cramping and bleeding as your body expels the pregnancy tissue. This process can take a long time— between four and six weeks after the demise occurred.

Managing an Abnormal Pregnancy

An abnormal pregnancy can feel devastating, like a small earthquake or a death. But take a step back and look at the big picture. With all the things that have to happen perfectly for a baby to be formed, it's not surprising that 20 percent of the time the baby's development doesn't happen exactly right. The way the tissues have to grow is incredibly complicated, and when the system has a glitch, the body knows when to step in and prevent a potential mistake.

When we are absolutely certain that you do not have a normal pregnancy, you have several options in terms of how to manage the situation.

Expectant Management

Your first option for managing an abnormal pregnancy is to wait for nature to take its course and expel the pregnancy tissue. In a spontaneous miscarriage, you will experience moderate to severe cramping and bleeding and will see passage of some pinkish-white tissue and blood clots. After the tissue passes, you may have more bleeding that resembles a moderate period for about a week. The waiting time for this natural process to occur is up to four to six weeks after the failed pregnancy is recognized.

D&C

A D&C (dilation and curettage) is a surgical procedure in which we remove the pregnancy tissue. We first dilate the cervix, and then we insert an instrument into the uterus to clean out the pregnancy tissue by suction. We then gently scrape the inside of the uterus with an instrument called a curette. This is a minor surgical procedure performed under IV sedation or general anesthesia so you don't feel any pain. However, some gynecologists do this procedure with a local anesthetic only. Risks involved with D&C are rare but include infection, bleeding, and perforation of the uterus. Risks are higher the further along you are in the pregnancy.[6] The advantages to having a D&C are that you don't have to wait to have a natural miscarriage, the procedure is fairly quick, performed on an outpatient basis, and the success rate is almost 100 percent.

Medical Management

We can also use a prostaglandin medication called misoprostol to induce bleeding and miscarriage. Misoprostol can be taken orally or placed vaginally by your doctor, and is 80 to 90 percent effective. The advantage is that the medication allows you to avoid surgery. The disadvantage is that you will need a D&C if the medication doesn't work. The pain and bleeding associated with the medication are similar to that of a natural miscarriage. For women who do not fare well with pain or the sight of blood, the D&C may be a better option.

Recurrent Miscarriage

A recurrent miscarriage is three or more consecutive miscarriages at twenty weeks or less. When miscarriages recur, further workup is indicated to see if there may be an underlying cause. We perform a variety of blood tests to look for potential causes, including parental chromosomal abnormalities, abnormal blood clotting problems, hormonal factors (such as uncontrolled diabetes and thyroid diseases), and autoimmune diseases.

The Emotional Toll of Miscarriage

In general, we find that people are never expecting to have a miscarriage. Women don't usually walk into their first OB appointment thinking, "Maybe this pregnancy isn't normal." The ones who think that a miscarriage is a possibility are the ones who've been through it before. Trying to become pregnant again may be scary, especially for those women who lose their first pregnancy, but don't be afraid. Continue to take good care of yourself, and the odds are that you'll have a normal pregnancy the next time.

▶ ▶ ▶ MOVING ON FROM MISCARRIAGE

I recently had an experience that touched a chord deep within me, reminding me of how agonizing even an early miscarriage can be for a woman. Rebecca was a first-time mom, twenty-eight weeks pregnant with a little girl.

I guided Rebecca through the normal components of an average twenty-eight-week exam: I checked the baby's heartbeat, measured the baby, and recorded her weight and blood pressure. All systems were go—everything was happening right on schedule. Throughout the visit, however, Rebecca had a pained, stoic expression on her face, as if she just did not trust that everything was really okay. She asked if she could get another ultrasound to check the baby. I asked if she was worried about something specific.

Much to my surprise, Rebecca put her head in her hands and began to quietly sob. She confessed that she was terrified that something was going to go horribly wrong with her baby. The year before, she had lost a pregnancy at eight weeks and was completely blindsided by that experience. She was angry at herself for being so naïve, not realizing how common miscarriage was, and not knowing that it could happen to anyone. "Last year, when I first got my positive pregnancy test back," Rebecca admitted, "I was already twenty years down the road with my child—where he or she would go to college, what I would wear to his or her wedding. It never even dawned on me that the pregnancy might not make it."

After she recovered from the loss, Rebecca and her partner cautiously tried again, and she conceived right away. But she didn't bond to this pregnancy because she was just too afraid of getting hurt again. "The worst part is," she told me, "I feel so guilty that I'm not letting myself get attached to my daughter. I haven't done anything, haven't made any plans or bought anything for the baby yet." Rebecca was keeping herself at arms length emotionally, fearing that, at one of these appointments, she will find out that something is terribly wrong.

Rebecca and I talked for a long time. I let her know that it is okay to feel this way, and that her bonding may not truly come until after she is holding her baby in her arms. The trauma of her first loss robbed her of that beautiful, naïve glow of a first pregnancy, but I wanted Rebecca to understand that she is not alone in this experience. Unfortunately, like many other moms who have lost a pregnancy, the difficulty bonding in the next pregnancy is a fact of life.

—Allison ◀ ◀ ◀

▶ ▶ ▶ THIRD-TIME STRUGGLES

Wendy is a classic Irish redhead, a thirty-year old physical therapist, and a gung-ho mother of two. Growing up among many siblings herself, she always dreamed of having three children to complete her own family. After easy experiences from conception to delivery with her first two babies, her attempt to have a third was a different story. Her first endeavor ended in an anembryonic gestation at about six weeks, which was treated with a D&C. The next two attempts were fetal demises at eight weeks, also treated with D&Cs. When I saw her on her fourth go-round, we had the results from a workup for recurrent pregnancy loss: She tested positive for a condition called the antiphospholipid antibody syndrome, an autoimmune disorder. Wendy was treated by a hematologist and was prescribed Lovenox, a blood thinner. I was her treating physician at this point and because I had suffered two recent miscarriages myself, Wendy and I formed a bond that went beyond that of simply doctor and patient. I saw her every week until she was twelve weeks pregnant and then every two weeks until she could feel the baby move. Thankfully, this time she went on to deliver a healthy baby.

Until she held her son in her arms, however, she approached every visit with a secret dread. Wendy had been so traumatized by her first three losses that she couldn't believe everything was going to be okay. I also conceived shortly after Wendy did, and we would both cheer one another on in our shared hopes for successful pregnancies. I delivered Wendy one month before I gave birth to my own daughter, Kylie. Her story and my own reveal how devastating miscarriage can be, even for a couple of seasoned moms.

—Yvonne ◀ ◀ ◀

Ectopic Pregnancies

An *ectopic pregnancy* is one that develops anywhere outside the uterus (see Figure 8-3). The most common place for an ectopic pregnancy is within the fallopian tubes. That's why this type of pregnancy is often referred to as a tubal pregnancy.

Here's how an ectopic pregnancy can occur: After the sperm fertilizes the egg in the fallopian tube, the embryo floats from the tube into the uterus in three or four days. If there is a narrowing of the tube or scarring around the tube, the passageway can be narrower and the developing embryo can get stuck as it is trying to pass through. Endometriosis or pelvic infections such as chlamydia can create this kind of scarring, but many times the cause is not clear. Unable to burrow into the wall of the uterus as it is programmed to do, the fertilized egg latches onto the wall of the fallopian tube instead. This tube is paper-thin compared to the wall of the uterus and was not designed to host an embryo. Eventually, the growing embryo will rupture through the tube, possibly causing internal bleeding. If the bleeding is unrecognized, it can actually lead to maternal death.

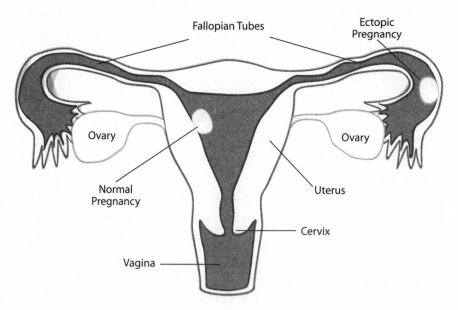

Figure 8-3: Ectopic vs. Normal Pregnancy

Statistics from the National Institute of Health show that 50 percent of women who experience ectopic pregnancies have had swelling in their fallopian tubes or a pelvic inflammatory disease (PID). The good news is, approximately 85 percent of women who have had ectopic pregnancies are eventually able to have a baby through normal means.

We are usually able to diagnose an ectopic pregnancy by ultrasound at six to seven weeks. Monitoring hormone levels can also aid in diagnosis. With tubal pregnancies, BHCG doesn't rise in the same pattern as normal pregnancies. So, we can often tell with a combination of ultrasounds and hormone blood tests whether a pregnancy is ectopic. More good news: ectopics occur only in 1 out of 100 pregnancies.

▶ ▶ ▶ THE MOTHER OF ALL ECTOPICS

We could hear Belinda's piercing screams echoing in the hallways of LA's vast County Hospital, where the three of us were doing our trial-by-fire residency. When we arrived at the examining room, we saw a clearly pregnant twenty-four-year-old woman with a face distorted by pure physical agony.

"What's the matter?" we asked her as we prepared the ultrasound machine, trying to get to the source of the pain. "Where does it hurt?" Was this premature labor? Round ligament pain? Appendicitis? Belinda's chart showed she hadn't had much prenatal care to this point, and her body looked as if she was well into her third trimester.

"The baby's kicking me!" she sobbed. We looked at one another and shook our heads. Most mothers can feel their babies' move, and sometimes it can be a little uncomfortable, but Belinda was groaning and gasping as if a professional boxer were jabbing her in the gut.

The ultrasound showed us a thirty-two-week fetus, but Belinda's uterus was its normal prepregnancy size. Finally it dawned on us: She had a nearly full-term fetus gestating not in her uterus but in her abdominal cavity! We pieced together what had happened: The fertilized egg had traveled the wrong way, out the far end of the fallopian tube, and ended up in her abdomen. The embryo then implanted and started to grow on the abdominal aorta, which is a large blood vessel. It settled in there and the baby had an unbelievably rich blood supply to draw on as it grew. It formed a placenta on top of the aorta and nobody realized it.

When the baby is inside the uterus as nature designed it to be, its mother is protected from the force of its kicks. But Belinda was literally getting punched in the liver, the spleen, and the ribs by her own baby. It really hurt!

Belinda's son was premature but viable, so we performed an emergency cesarean delivery. It wasn't even technically a cesarean because when we opened her up, the baby was right there and her uterus was normal size, with no baby in it. We couldn't remove the placenta because it had grown into the aorta.

This crazy story has a happy ending: We got the baby out, and because removal of the precariously placed placenta would have caused massive internal bleeding, we gave the mom a chemotherapeutic agent to dissolve it. This drug made the placenta stop growing, and it ultimately disintegrated and went away. The baby not only survived but thrived! He was born at thirty-two weeks, which is technically a preemie, but because of the incredible nutrients in the aortic blood supply, he was one big, hardy baby.

Belinda's extremely rare ordeal is a good illustration of how resilient and adaptable a growing fetus can be. When a baby really wants to be born, it's going to find a way.

Belinda's bizarre case, which we now refer to as "the mother of all ectopic pregnancies," is a wild exception, the only ectopic case we've ever heard of where the baby has gestated and been delivered. In all other cases, ectopic pregnancies cannot survive because they cannot be transplanted to the uterus. Their blood supply is already connected to the tube, and disrupting the supply will cause the embryo to die. As stated earlier, the baby cannot grow and develop in the tube because the tube is small and it will rupture when the pregnancy gets too big.

Ectopic pregnancies need to be treated as soon as they are recognized to avoid rupture and internal bleeding. The most common therapy for ectopics is surgery, which involves either removal of the pregnancy from the tube or removal of the entire tube. A second treatment is with a chemotherapeutic agent called methotrexate, which causes the pregnancy tissue within the tube to dissolve. In rare cases, the tubal pregnancy will resolve on its own. All decisions regarding mode of treatment need to be made with your gynecologist's guidance.

No amount of medical information that we can share with you here can change the fact that pregnancy loss can be devastating and frightening. Even with a successful future pregnancy, you may still be concerned that the loss will recur. The good news is, in our combined years of practice and in our own personal experiences, nearly all our patients who have experienced miscarriages have ultimately gone on to deliver healthy babies.

chapter nine

HIGH-RISK
PREGNANCIES

MOST OF YOU READING THIS BOOK will probably have no need to use this chapter. It contains some information that may make you feel nervous, but rest assured, even if you have been diagnosed with a high-risk condition, you don't need to be scared. During our years of training at the University of Southern California and Los Angeles County Hospital, there weren't many complications or conditions we didn't handle in that bubbling cauldron of chaos and emergency. During our residency training, we took care of almost exclusively high-risk pregnancies. The good news is that despite the crazy complications we've seen and managed, we ended up with healthy babies and healthy moms the vast majority of the time.

All three of us had some sort of complication during our own pregnancies that rendered us high risk. Allison had severe preeclampsia and preterm deliveries; Yvonne had placental abruption and placenta previa; and Alane had elevated blood pressure and growth issues with her second pregnancy. But here we all are. Between the three of us, we have six beautiful, healthy children from two to nine and a half. And we're all healthy and going strong, too.

This chapter is designed for those who have been diagnosed with any of these high-risk conditions or who just want to become educated on what to expect if any of these issues come up for you.

Again, the likelihood that any of these problems will arise for you is not high. If the risk does become a reality, be confident that your team of doctors will work with you to ensure a safe pregnancy and delivery for you and your baby.

So what makes a pregnancy high risk? Is it your age? Family history? A medical condition present before pregnancy or a variety of complications that develop during pregnancy can make a normal pregnancy riskier.

Having high blood pressure can increase the chance of a premature birth. A placenta that grows over the cervix can cause life-threatening bleeding. Uncontrolled diabetes can increase the chance of birth defects. However, your age does not necessarily put you in a higher risk category. Similarly, just because your mother or sister had a high-risk pregnancy doesn't mean you will too.

Monitoring High-Risk Pregnancies

One important advance in modern obstetrics is the capability to evaluate how a fetus is doing inside the womb to determine whether it is safe for the pregnancy to continue. In many high-risk situations, the uterine environment may *not* be the best place for the baby and delivery is necessary. To check the status of the fetus, some exams, called *antepartum testing,* have been developed. Antepartum testing is used in cases of high blood pressure, diabetes, fetal growth problems, post-term pregnancies, multiple gestations, cholestasis of pregnancy, and decreased fetal movement.

Many tests are available to assess your baby's well-being. In this chapter, we will review the most common method of antepartum testing used by many obstetricians, called the modified biophysical profile. This method has two components.

Nonstress test (NST): In a nonstress test, the mother is connected to an electronic fetal monitor that records the fetal heart rate and uterine activity during a twenty-minute period. This monitor is the same one used during labor. When the baby is receiving all the oxygen he or she needs, the fetal heart rate varies from beat to beat, and the recording of the rate will look like a jagged line. If the line is flat or dips down after a contraction, possibly the baby is not doing well. When the NST is normal, the chance of stillbirth within the next seven days is five out of one thousand.

Amniotic fluid index (AFI): The amniotic fluid index is an ultrasound measurement of the amount of amniotic fluid around the baby. Because the fluid is primarily fetal urine, a normal AFI tells us that the baby is producing ample urine and receiving adequate oxygen.

Preeclampsia

Preeclampsia is a form of high blood pressure that is caused by pregnancy. The condition was previously called toxemia because doctors thought a toxin in the blood caused mothers to become very sick. Affecting 5 to 10 percent of all pregnant women, preeclampsia is also responsible for 10 to 15 percent of all maternal deaths in the world.[1] Maternal mortality—deaths associated with pregnancy and childbirth—occurs in twenty-four per hundred thousand births in the United States. In parts of the developing world, however, maternal mortality remains as high as fourteen hundred per hundred thousand births.[2] Many theories exist about the cause of preeclampsia, including immune system dysfunction, abnormalities of the placenta, blood vessel damage, and genetic predisposition. However, none of these theories have been proven and the cause is still unknown. Preeclampsia occurs after twenty weeks of gestation, and 75 percent of cases will occur after thirty-seven weeks.

Risk Factors

Risk factors for developing preeclampsia include the following:

- High blood pressure before pregnancy
- History of preeclampsia in a previous pregnancy
- First pregnancy
- Age greater than thirty-five
- African American ethnicity
- Pregestational or gestational diabetes
- Pregnant with twins or multiples

- Autoimmune problems, such as Lupus
- Preexisting kidney problems
- Underlying blood clotting disorders
- Obesity (BMI of 30 kg/m^2 or greater)

Symptoms and Diagnosis

Preeclampsia is diagnosed when a pregnant woman has persistently elevated blood pressure and protein in the urine. It may also be associated with swelling of the feet, hands, and face, although these symptoms are often seen in normal pregnancies as well. At each of your prenatal visits, your doctor will check your blood pressure and urine for signs of preeclampsia. In most cases, a mom with preeclampsia will feel completely normal.

If a woman is found to have elevated blood pressure during an office visit, she will be observed over the next few hours and evaluated by blood and urine tests. If the blood pressure remains elevated for more than six hours, the diagnosis of preeclampsia is made.

Preeclampsia is categorized as mild or severe. The criteria for making a diagnosis of mild preeclampsia follow:

- Persistent SBP (systolic blood pressure, the number on the top) of 140 to 160 mm Hg, or DBP (diastolic blood pressure, the number on the bottom) between 90 and 110 mm Hg, or both. A normal blood pressure reading should be less than 140/90.
- Protein in the urine: more than 300 milligrams within a twenty-four-hour urine collection. A normal value is less than 300 mg.

The criteria for severe preeclampsia are as follows:

- Persistent SBP greater than or equal to 160 mm Hg, or DBP greater than or equal to 110 mm Hg, or both.
- Protein in the urine: more than five grams within a twenty-four-hour urine collection.
- Symptoms of headache, blurred vision, or abdominal pain in the upper-right quadrant or just below the breastbone.

- HELLP syndrome: HELLP stands for hemolysis, elevated liver enzymes, and low platelets. In this condition, blood cells are broken down, causing anemia and blood clotting problems. In addition, the liver swells, leading to elevation of liver enzymes in the blood.
- Decreased urine output.
- Eclampsia, which includes the symptoms of preeclampsia seen above, plus a seizure.

Management

Although numerous attempts have been made to prevent preeclampsia, none have been successful. Scientists have studied low-salt diets, calcium, magnesium, zinc, DHA, evening primrose oil, aspirin, blood-thinners, vitamins E and C, and traditional blood pressure medications. Unfortunately, none of them work.

The only cure for preeclampsia is delivery of the baby and the placenta. Because the cause of preeclampsia is different from that of traditional hypertension, blood pressure medications have little effect on preeclampsia. However, your doctor may use blood pressure medications to temporarily control your blood pressure until your baby can be delivered. In some cases, the progression of the disease can be slowed if the mom remains at strict bed rest. If a mom is diagnosed with preeclampsia at term, delivery is usually recommended at that time.

The situation is more complicated if the condition occurs earlier in the pregnancy. In these cases, we try to balance what is best for the baby—growing inside the uterus—versus what is best for the mother's health. When the risk to the mom outweighs the risk to the baby, we will deliver the baby. The worst time for preeclampsia to hit is in the second or early third trimester. At that stage, the baby, if delivered, could face many complications, but the danger to the mother's health may force the premature birth.

▶ ▶ ▶ MY PREECLAMPSIA

Never in a million years did I think I would become the poster child for preeclampsia. Before becoming pregnant, I had never had any medical problems, I ate well, and I exercised regularly.

When I was thirty-three, I became pregnant with my son Luke. I was working full time and had every intention of continuing until my due date. I thought I would be in the office, run over to the hospital, pop out the baby, and be back in the swing of things within a few weeks. Little did I know how my plans would change.

One day, as I entered my twenty-ninth week, I was driving to work and had a mild headache. By the time I arrived at the office, I was feeling a bit cloudy. I set off on my normal day, seeing patients in the office, answering phone calls, and delivering two babies. Toward the end the day, I could tell something wasn't right. My nurse checked my blood pressure and found it was 160/100. Immediately, I found myself in a wheelchair on the way down the hall to the hospital.

When I arrived, the nurse again checked my blood pressure. I gazed at the machine in disbelief as the numbers climbed over 160. How could this be happening to me? I asked the nurse to bring a different blood pressure cuff, as I was sure this one was broken. But to my dismay, the new machine showed the same result. The next thing I knew, I was receiving steroids in anticipation of a premature delivery.

For a short time, my blood pressure stabilized as long as I remained completely flat in bed. I stayed in the hospital like that for two weeks, getting up only to use the bathroom. Staying in bed for those weeks felt like an eternity, and some days I thought of sneaking out and going home. But I knew I wouldn't even make it down the hall without my blood pressure going up.

At thirty-one weeks, my blood pressure skyrocketed to 180/110 and I developed HELLP syndrome. My liver tests went haywire and my blood clotting ability started to drop. It was time to get the baby out. My labor was induced and went very quickly. I delivered my son, who weighed only three and a half pounds. I was able to see him just for a minute before he was whisked away to the NICU on a respirator.

During the labor and after the birth, I was given a medication called magnesium sulfate, which is used to prevent seizures in women with severe preeclampsia. This medicine made me feel horrible! I was dizzy, nauseous, and hot, and my vision was blurred. I didn't know if the symptoms were from the magnesium or if I was having a stroke. I was afraid to tell anyone how I felt because I didn't want to worry them, so I just closed my eyes and tried to sleep. More than twenty-four hours went by, and my blood pressure finally started to come down. As soon as the magnesium was turned off, I felt so much better. I was able to visit my son for the first time.

Even though I've been in the NICU a thousand times, nothing could prepare me for seeing my own child there. Luke was on a respirator, hooked to multiple monitors, and had IVs in his belly button and on his scalp. He was so skinny and red. I could stay with him for only a short time because my blood pressure would start to go up again when I was out of bed.

I went home after a few days and took blood pressure medicine for nearly two months until my numbers finally went back to normal. After an up-and-down course, Luke was discharged from the NICU after thirty-five days, weighing just four pounds, fifteen ounces. Thankfully, today Luke is a healthy eight-year-old with no consequences from his early arrival.

My experience educated me in a way that is different from reading about preeclampsia in a textbook. This disease changed my life. First, I was so grateful for prenatal care, knowing that in many parts of the world, my condition would have gone undiagnosed, and Luke and I may have died. In addition, having preeclampsia helped me understand that blank stare I get when I tell patients they have this condition. It truly is a disease that seems to come out of nowhere: no warning, no symptoms. I was in denial with the best of them.

—Allison ◀ ◀ ◀

As Allison's ordeal shows, often there are few or no symptoms before preeclampsia strikes. Many women feel fine even while they have preeclampsia and have no clue what's going on inside their bodies. A woman can hear her doctor tell her, "Your blood pressure is really high" and yet she feels completely normal. The next thing she knows, she's in the hospital having her baby.

The importance of consistent prenatal care cannot be overemphasized for this condition because it may be detected or anticipated by following your blood pressure trends. If we notice that your blood pressures are rising above your baseline, we may see you more frequently in the office or ask you to monitor your blood pressure at home. And by being vigilant, we may be able to prolong the pregnancy, keeping the baby inside longer before delivery.

Complications

If left undetected, the complications of preeclampsia are serious and include seizures, stroke, liver rupture, water in the lungs, and organ failure. Complications for the baby include placental abruption, decreased blood flow and growth problems, and low amniotic fluid volume. Luckily, after preeclampsia is diagnosed and the baby and the placenta are delivered, the symptoms usually resolve within a few days and the new mother is cured. On occasion, the elevated blood pressure persists, requiring the temporary use of blood pressure medications.

Diabetes

Diabetes is a metabolic disease characterized by high blood sugar. Normally, your body produces a hormone from the pancreas called insulin, which keeps blood sugar levels stable. If the amount of insulin is too low or if your body becomes resistant to its effects, your blood sugar will run too high, and you will develop diabetes. As you are probably aware, diabetes is currently an epidemic in the United States. According to the American Diabetes Association (www.diabetes.org), diabetes is the seventh leading cause of death and affects approximately 8 percent of our population, 23.6 million people in the United States. Of all women twenty years or older, 10 percent will grapple with this disease. Untreated diabetes is the culprit behind a plethora of health complications, including heart disease, stroke, blindness, kidney disease, nerve problems, and decreased blood flow leading to limb amputations.

Although diabetes can wreak serious havoc on your pregnancy if not well controlled, with careful prenatal care and commitment on your part, you should have a healthy pregnancy.

Pregestational versus Gestational Diabetes

Pregestational, or overt, diabetes refers to the diabetes you had before pregnancy. The majority of women with this condition know that they are diabetic before they come for a prenatal visit because they have previously been diagnosed by their primary care physician. Ideally, their blood sugar levels are under excellent control before conception. This may be accomplished with diet, medications, or insulin injections, always in concert with exercise.

On occasion, a woman will come to a prenatal visit with symptoms of diabetes, yet she has not formally been diagnosed. If you have symptoms of persistent thirst, frequent urination, or have a sudden unexpected weight loss, let your doctor know. These are warning signs of diabetes. You will be diagnosed by a test checking your blood glucose levels. If a random glucose level is more than 200 mg/dL or your fasting glucose (glucose before you eat anything in the morning) is greater than 125mg/dL, you likely have pregestational diabetes.

Gestational diabetes occurs during pregnancy. It affects approximately 4 percent of all pregnant women in the United States. Insulin from the pancreas is the hormone responsible for maintaining normal blood sugar levels. During pregnancy, a hormone from the placenta—human placental lactogen—makes insulin less effective. For reasons still unknown, some women are more sensitive to this duel between the hormones. They become insulin resistant—requiring more insulin to keep the glucose levels normal—and eventually develop gestational diabetes.

The risk factors for developing gestational diabetes are as follows:

- History of prior gestational diabetes
- Certain ethnic groups: Hispanic, African American, Native American, Pacific Islander
- Obesity
- Strong family history of adult onset diabetes
- Multiple gestation (twins, triplets, and so on)
- Chronic hypertension
- A previous large baby

Diagnosis

Because the placental hormone that instigates insulin resistance rises after twenty weeks, most women are screened for gestational diabetes between twenty-four and twenty-eight weeks. Some physicians screen all patients; others screen only women with risk factors. If pregestational diabetes is suspected, you may be tested on your very first visit. And if you screen negative during this early visit, you will be rechecked at the twenty-four- to twenty-eight-week mark. (See Chapter 4, page 162 for more about the screening test.)

Management

So what happens if you get the phone call to tell you that you have gestational diabetes? First, do not panic. However, your participation and commitment are required. We won't lie to you—maintaining your diabetes under good control is a lot of hard work—but we can reassure you that if you put in the effort, you will reap the benefits of a healthier you and a healthy baby.

After your diagnosis, you may be referred to an endocrinologist (a hormone specialist) and a nutritionist for a consultation. These specialists will educate you about your condition, explain the diabetic diet, and instruct you on how to monitor your glucose levels daily. Initially, you will be required to check your blood glucose levels four to five times a day with a blood glucose–monitoring device. To do this, you prick your finger with a small lancet, collect a drop of blood on a test strip, and insert it into the machine. We know that checking blood glucose levels is a drag, but it's important. Here's why: Glucose molecules are very small. As a result, they can freely cross the placenta and into your baby. If your blood sugar is too high, your baby's blood sugar will be too high, which can lead to complications.

Here are your goals for glucose levels:

Fasting:	<95 mg/dL
One hour after meals:	<140 mg/dl

Initially, you will attempt to maintain normal glucose levels with diet and exercise alone. Ideally, your diet should consist of 55 percent carbohydrate, 20 percent protein, and 25 percent fat. It's best to eat three meals and three snacks throughout the day. Remember that you still need to eat, and eat healthy. This is not the time to be going on a strict low-calorie diet.

Exercise is also important because it helps keep your glucose levels down. Try to do some form of exercise for thirty minutes daily. Walking immediately after meals is especially effective at keeping sugar levels low.

If diet and exercise are not enough to maintain normal glucose levels, you may need to take oral medication or start insulin injections. Insulin therapy has been the mainstay treatment for diabetes in pregnancy for many years, but today more studies are emerging on the effectiveness of using oral medications, such as glyburide and metformin. Please consult your obstetrician about which medication is right for you.

As you get further along in your pregnancy, you may notice that despite a good diet and exercise program, you have a harder time maintaining your glucose levels or you need more insulin or medication to keep the same control. This difficulty is common because the placental hormone levels continue to rise and you become more insulin resistant. Don't worry. Adjust your insulin or medication accordingly as instructed by your doctor. Or you may need to start insulin or oral medication if you were previously managing your glucose by diet and exercise alone.

In addition to blood sugar monitoring, you may also receive more ultrasounds to follow the growth of your baby. Moms with gestational diabetes are at higher risk of growing large babies, leading to complicated vaginal deliveries or a higher necessity for a cesarean delivery. For women who are on diabetes medication, you will also be monitored with modified biophysical profiles toward the end of your pregnancy to ensure a healthy, happy baby.

As you near your due date, please do not be surprised if your doctor recommends an induction. Because diabetes increases your risk of having a more difficult vaginal birth, your delivery will be more deliberately planned. You may need insulin through an IV that can be controlled during your labor, to help keep your glucose levels within the normal range at all times. The goal is to have a baby whose sugars will also be in the normal range. Often newborns of diabetic mothers need to be observed in the NICU for signs of low blood sugar.

We know that having diabetes in pregnancy may feel like a full-time job. Managing this condition takes enormous amounts of work and effort on your part. But go to your appointments and keep up with your diet, exercise, medications, and glucose monitoring, and you will see the fruits of your labor—literally—when you hold that beautiful, healthy baby in your arms.

Complications

Complications related to pregestational and gestational diabetes under poor control include miscarriages, preterm births, increased risk of birth defects (especially heart malformations), macrosomic infants (very large babies), and unexplained fetal deaths near term. Moms with pregestational or gestational diabetes are also at higher risk for developing preeclampsia.

Postpartum

If you work hard to manage your gestational diabetes, you will be pleasantly surprised to find that you no longer need insulin or medication after you deliver. Blood sugar levels often normalize the day after delivery.

Be sure to follow up with your general doctor or your endocrinologist after the pregnancy. They will perform a glucose test when the baby is three months old. Unfortunately, about 50 percent of women with gestational diabetes will develop overt diabetes some time later in life. The best prevention is to lead a healthy lifestyle by eating well and keeping up with your regular exercise.

Cervical Insufficiency

Cervical insufficiency is a condition in which the normally strong cervix weakens and dilates, usually resulting in a miscarriage in the late second trimester. Unnoticed and often underappreciated, your cervix is a remarkable part of your body. When you are pregnant, the cervix acts as the door to keep your baby in the uterus. Miraculously, the cervix knows how to keep itself closed until term. The cervix also knows just when it's time to open the door to let the baby out. It's amazing that the cervical canal, a pinhole in the middle of your cervix, can expand to 10 centimeters to let your baby out of your uterus during birth.

Normally, the cervix opens, or dilates, as the result of painful uterine contractions. Previously known by the rather insulting term cervical incompetence, cervical insufficiency occurs when there's a silent dilation of the cervix without contractions. Simply put, for exact reasons unknown, the cervical gateway opens too soon and your baby is delivered *way* before he or she is due. Usually, cervical insufficiency occurs between eighteen and twenty-four weeks, before the baby even has the ability to survive.

Cervical insufficiency is a heartbreaking event for the patient, her partner, and her family. Having been involved in many cases ourselves, it's hard on us doctors as well.

Cervical insufficiency occurs in about one in one hundred to one in two thousand pregnancies.[3] We know that's a broad range, but the numbers are so far apart for several reasons, including the difficulty in establishing a diagnosis, biases in reporting cervical insufficiency as the cause of miscarriage, and biologic differences among the study populations. On a personal level, it doesn't really matter how often it happens statistically: When it happens to you, it's devastating.

Risk Factors

You might be at risk for cervical insufficiency if you have any of the following conditions:

- Prior history of pregnancy loss in the second trimester
- History of multiple induced or spontaneous abortions
- History of procedures on your cervix (LEEP, cold knife cone, amputation of your cervix)
- Abnormalities of the uterus
- Multiple gestation

However, more often than not, none of the preceding risk factors are present.

Symptoms

Unfortunately, because cervical insufficiency is characterized by painless opening of the cervix, by the time symptoms are recognized, it's often too late to save the pregnancy. If you have any increased pressure in your pelvis, unusual amount of vaginal discharge, or vaginal spotting, call your doctor. If a woman complains of these symptoms in the fifteen- to twenty-four-week range, she will be evaluated by a vaginal exam or an ultrasound or both to make sure the cervix is closed.

Diagnosis

There's bad news and good news about cervical insufficiency. The bad news is that it's often not diagnosed until it's too late. The good news is that—if diagnosed early enough or if we know you've had cervical insufficiency in a previous pregnancy—the condition can be treated and you will have a very good chance of having a healthy term baby.

The key to diagnosing this problem is understanding your obstetrical history. If you have a second trimester pregnancy loss, be sure to keep your records and write down the details of what happened to share with your future obstetrician. The typical history is that you have a sensation of pressure in your vagina and lower abdomen with increased vaginal discharge or spotting or both. In some cases, the water bag breaks unexpectedly. The *cervix* is a cylinder-shaped organ that is actually the lowest part of the uterus. Normally it measures three to five centimeters in length and has a firm consistency. We can examine your cervix visually by placing a speculum into the vagina, similar to doing a Pap smear. We can also measure your cervical length with an ultrasound. For women who are at high risk for cervical insufficiency or have any of the symptoms, the *cervical length* is of utmost importance. If it is less than two and a half centimeters (about one inch), it may mean that the cervix has shortened and could potentially open prematurely.

Treatment

A cervical cerclage is an effective treatment for cervical insufficiency. A *cerclage* is a stitch placed around the cervix to hold it closed so it cannot dilate (see Figure 9-1). It is made of strong suture, like a fishing line. Envision your uterus as a bag with an opening at the bottom. The cerclage would be like the purse-string to keep the opening closed. Cerclages are placed under anesthesia either vaginally or abdominally. Vaginal cerclages are the simplest and have proven to be quite effective. They are placed preventatively at sixteen to eighteen weeks of pregnancy, before the cervix actually opens. Abdominal cerclages are usually reserved for those women in whom a vaginal approach has previously failed.

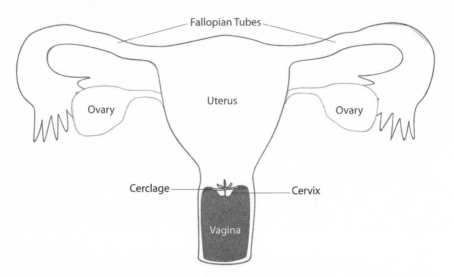

Figure 9-1: Cerclage—Weakened Cervix

Whether or not the incidental finding of a shortened cervix on ultrasound and subsequent cerclage prevents preterm births is the subject of conflicting studies. In our practice, we place a cerclage preventatively if we see a shortened cervix in a woman with any risk factors or symptoms of vaginal pressure.

In addition to cerclage placement, some women with cervical insufficiency may benefit from bed rest. Think of it this way: Suppose you had a bag with the opening at the bottom, closed shut with just a purse string. Now, however, imagine that the bag contains a watermelon. That purse string may not be strong enough on its own to keep the watermelon from falling out. However, if you laid the bag on its side with the purse string in place, you'd probably have a better chance of keeping the watermelon in the bag, because less pressure would be placed against the opening.

In some cases, a cerclage can be placed after the cervix has already opened. This is called an emergency cerclage. Unfortunately, placing the cerclage in this situation carries a higher risk of failure and complications, such as infection and breaking the bag of water.

As there is always art to medicine, your obstetrician may have a different approach to this condition. Talk to your doctor about what his or her practice may be.

▶ ▶ ▶ A CERCLAGE STORY

I adore Margarita. She has been my patient for almost ten years and loves to watch Korean soap operas as much as I do. We were pregnant at the same time with our first babies, except unlike me, she had a very hard time conceiving. Margarita had received fertility treatments in Mexico, involving a lot of money and even more emotional ups and downs.

One weekend when I was on call, Margarita phoned me, complaining of a lot of unusual pelvic pressure. I met her at the hospital for an evaluation, thinking that most likely everything was fine and she would be discharged home. To my dismay, I saw that her cervix had fully dilated. The amniotic bag was ready to come out—along with her baby. She was only twenty-two weeks along— the same as me—which meant there was no chance for her baby to survive. My heart sank. I held it together for Margarita because at that moment, she needed a doctor more than she needed a friend.

Margarita lost her baby that day. After I made sure she was stable and was able to be alone, I privately broke down. I felt so guilty that my pregnancy was going fine, but that Margarita had just lost hers after all her struggles.

Losing a baby from cervical insufficiency is devastating for any woman, but thankfully, it gives us the knowledge we need to prevent another incident in the future. Margarita has subsequently had two successful pregnancies in which we placed cerclages to prevent another miscarriage. When I got the call that she was starting labor—at term—with her third baby, I rushed to the hospital. By chance, she'd been admitted to labor room number 816. I knew that room well. Margarita had lost her first baby in the same room nine years earlier.

After delivery, when a beaming Margarita was holding her third child in her arms, a beautiful baby boy, I asked her if she remembered the room. She said, "Yes." This time around, the mood in that room was very different than it had been nine years earlier. Margarita had requested she have her tubes tied after this delivery. For both of us, it was poetic and satisfying that she ended her baby-making career on a positive note in LR816.

—Alane ◀ ◀ ◀

Cervical insufficiency is both unexpected and devastating. For a mother who has made it through twenty long weeks of pregnancy and has even experienced her baby moving, losing the child without warning is something out of a nightmare. Even though cervical insufficiency affects only one-half of one percent of all pregnancies, it's such a disastrous situation and so hard to predict that some doctors now routinely check the cervices of moms who don't yet have any symptoms. The truth is, a mom can have a normal looking cervix that can suddenly become dilated within a day or even within minutes. Thankfully, the treatment with a cerclage gives hope to mothers who would otherwise not be able to carry a pregnancy to full term.

Placenta Previa

Placenta previa describes a placenta that is near or covering the cervical canal and occurs in about one out of three hundred pregnancies. Because the cervix is the door out of the uterus during a vaginal delivery, a cesarean delivery is needed if the mom has placenta previa.

We describe placenta previas by their relationship to the cervical canal:

Complete placenta previa: The cervical canal is completely covered by the placenta

Partial placenta previa: The placenta is partially covering the cervical canal

Marginal placenta previa: The edge of the placenta is right next to, but not covering, the cervical canal

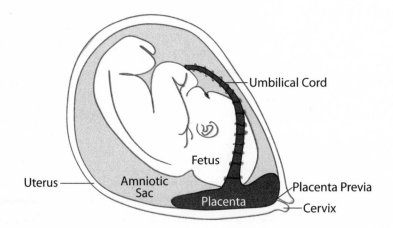

Figure 9-2: Placenta Previa

Low-lying placenta: The edge of the placenta is within one inch
of the cervical canal but not covering it

Often a placenta previa will be diagnosed at the twenty-week ultrasound. Typically, though, partial, marginal, or low-lying placenta
previas move out of the way as the uterus expands, pulling the placenta away from the cervix. However, complete placenta previas tend
to stay where they are, covering the cervix throughout pregnancy.

Risk Factors

Women at risk for placenta previa may have any the following conditions:

- Multiparity, meaning the woman has already given birth to at
  least one child
- Advanced maternal age
- Prior cesarean delivery
- History of induced abortion or miscarriage where a uterine
  curettage, or scraping, was performed
- Cigarette smoking
- Placenta previa in a previous pregnancy

▶ ▶ ▶ MY PLACENTA PREVIA

I woke up one Friday morning and went to the bathroom only to notice a toilet
bowl full of bright red blood. I was fourteen weeks pregnant with my second
child. I panicked. Could I be losing this baby I had tried so hard for? But something in my heart told me that my baby was still alive. I had exercised harder
than normal the night before—maybe that was the problem.

I rushed to the office and Alane was there, so I begged her to look at the
baby with me. The baby was alive, thank goodness, but that was the first time
we noticed that my placenta was completely crossing my cervix. I went to go
see Dr. Cliff Bochner, our beloved perinatologist. He noted that the baby
looked fine and thought it was technically too early to diagnose a placenta
previa. The bleeding stopped after a couple of days and I took the weekend off
to rest, then continued my prenatal care and hoped for the best.

At twenty weeks, I went in for my anatomical survey and found my placenta was still covering the cervix. I followed the general recommendation for anyone with a previa to stop sexual intercourse and reduce my activity. I eased off my hard exercise, switching to gentle walks, but I continued to go about my daily routine of work.

One morning, when Cliff was in our office doing scans for our obstetric patients, I asked him to look at my placenta again. Sure enough, at twenty-four weeks, my placenta hadn't budged and was still crossing the opening to my cervix. Cliff, being the wise and conservative doctor that he is, demanded that I stop work right away and go on bed rest. Even though I had had no further bleeding episodes since fourteen weeks, he didn't think that running around a busy hospital delivering babies every day was an appropriate job for a mom with such a high-risk condition. Excessive physical activity can lead to preterm contractions, and those can lead to unwanted bleeding and early delivery.

After much whining and protest, I took my doctor's advice and stopped work completely that day, not returning until my baby was thirty weeks and past the danger zone for severe prematurity. I then came back to a schedule of only four office hours per day until I delivered. Cliff backed me up with regular ultrasounds to ensure my baby was growing well. I had an amniocentesis at thirty-seven weeks to make sure my baby's lungs were mature, and shortly thereafter gave birth by cesarean to my beautiful daughter, Kylie. I did not have any other episodes of bleeding and was grateful to have made it through this potentially dangerous complication with no injury to me or my little girl.

—Yvonne ◀ ◀ ◀

Diagnosis

With today's access to ultrasounds, most placenta previas are recognized during prenatal care. In the past, patients often were diagnosed because of painless vaginal bleeding in the third trimester. Sometimes, symptoms of placenta previa might show themselves during the second trimester, as in Yvonne's case.

The most common symptom of a placenta previa is painless, bright red vaginal bleeding. The bleeding starts with no warning signs or pain. The amount of bleeding can vary—sometimes it is just spotting, but other times it is profuse with large blood clots that can prompt an emergency cesarean delivery and blood transfusion and, in the very worst case, cause both fetal and maternal death.

Management

After a diagnosis of placenta previa, patients are advised not to have sexual intercourse, exercise excessively, or have digital vaginal exams.

If light bleeding occurs and the baby is still preterm, the mother is usually hospitalized at bed rest until bleeding stops. If the bleeding is severe, the woman may be hospitalized for the remainder of her pregnancy.

For a mom with complete or partial placenta previa who doesn't have any bleeding, we recommend an amniocentesis at thirty-seven weeks to be certain the baby has mature lungs, and then a delivery by cesarean. We deliver a few weeks before the due date to decrease the chance that the mom goes into labor and bleeds profusely as the cervix dilates. For those moms with marginal or low-lying placentas, you and your obstetrician can discuss whether or not it's wise to attempt a vaginal delivery. Just be aware that if your doctor encounters excessive bleeding during your labor, you will need a cesarean right away.

Placental Abruption

Placental abruption occurs when the placenta separates from the wall of the uterus before the delivery of the fetus. Because oxygen and nutrition are passed from the mother to the fetus through the placenta, abruption can lead to oxygen deprivation, fetal distress, and even fetal death. The risk of fetal death with an abruption is nine times higher than in a normal pregnancy. Abruption occurs in one out of two hundred deliveries.

Risk Factors

Risk factors for placenta abruption include the following:

- Chronic hypertension
- Preeclampsia
- Preterm premature rupture of membranes
- Direct abdominal trauma (car accidents, falls, or kicks to the abdomen)
- Cocaine use
- Cigarette smoking

Symptoms

The symptoms associated with placental abruption include vaginal bleeding and abdominal pain. Often, the baby will show signs of distress on the fetal monitor. The majority of abruptions occur before the onset of labor.

Management

The management of placental abruption is determined by the gestational age of the fetus, the amount of bleeding, and degree of fetal distress. If the bleeding is excessive and the baby cannot tolerate the blood loss, immediate cesarean delivery is recommended. If the bleeding is light and fetal heart rate stable, a vaginal delivery may be attempted at term. If you are preterm, and the bleeding subsides, you may be able to prolong your pregnancy with bed rest, in the hospital or at home.

Complications

Complications of placental abruption can affect both mom and baby, and include the need for blood transfusions, problems with blood clotting, and decreased oxygen to the baby. Although these are potentially serious complications, if you are in a hospital with a team of doctors and support staff, they will take swift action to correct all these problems.

Placenta Accreta, Placenta Increta, and Placenta Percreta

Normally, after the delivery of your baby, the placenta detaches from the uterus easily. This occurs because of the natural separation between the uterine lining and the placenta. In placenta accreta, placenta increta, and placenta percreta, the placenta attaches to the uterine lining in an abnormal way. In *placenta accreta,* the placenta is directly attached to the uterine lining (see Figure 9-3). In *placenta increta,* the placenta grows into the muscle layer of the uterus. Finally, in *placenta percreta,* the placenta grows through the entire thickness of the uterine wall to the outer surface of the uterus.

The incidence of this condition is thankfully rare, and is about one in twenty-five hundred deliveries.

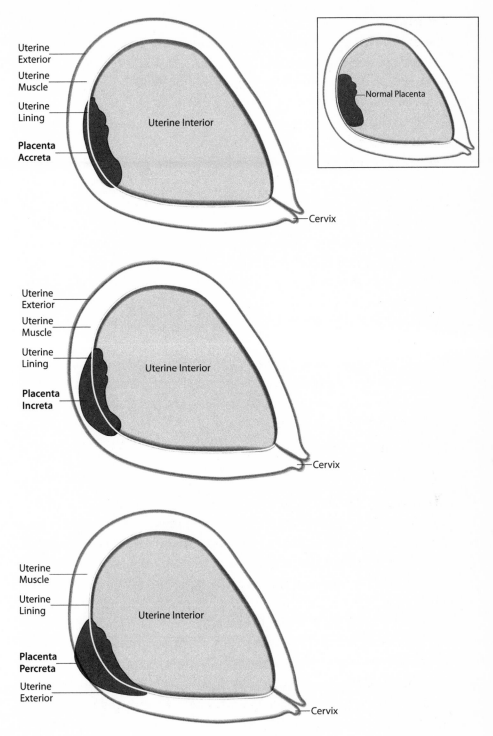

Figure 9-3: Abnormal Placentas

Risk Factors

Risk factors for placenta accreta, placenta increta, and placenta percreta include the following:

- Prior cesarean deliveries
- Prior uterine surgery
- Placenta previa

Diagnosis

Unfortunately, most women do not experience any warning signs of this condition prior to delivery. We usually make the diagnosis of placenta accreta, increta, or percreta at the time of the delivery when the placenta does not detach from the uterus in a timely fashion or we can get only portions of the placenta out. This inability to deliver the placenta in its entirety is often associated with hemorrhage because some or all of the placenta remains attached to the uterus.

If you have an increased risk—such as the presence of placenta previa with a previous cesarean—you may be evaluated before delivery. An experienced radiologist or perinatologist may be able to detect this condition in women during prenatal care, using ultrasound or an MRI.

Treatment

Most women with placenta accreta, increta, or percreta require a hysterectomy, or removal of the uterus, immediately after the baby delivers. However, in those women who desire more children and whose bleeding is controlled, more conservative treatment may be possible, such as sewing the sites of bleeding or blocking the arteries that feed the uterus.

Premature Rupture of Membranes

Premature rupture of membranes (PROM) means that the bag of water breaks before contractions have begun. At term, this occurs in about 10 percent of pregnancies. Before thirty-seven weeks, about 3 percent of moms will experience PROM. Most of these moms will go on to have a premature birth. In fact, premature rupture of the membranes is the most common reason babies are born prematurely.

Risk Factors

Similar to preterm labor, the cause of PROM is usually not apparent. Some risk factors include:

- Vaginal, bladder, or pelvic infections
- Smoking
- Previous history of PROM
- Poor maternal nutrition
- Multiple gestation
- Vaginal bleeding in the second or third trimester

Symptoms

Women with PROM will notice leakage of clear or pink-tinged fluid from the vagina. It may be a small, persistent trickle but usually comes in a large gush that can leave her standing in a puddle on the floor. Women may often initially think that they have lost bladder control. However, the leakage continues and the fluid has a distinctive odor that is different from that of urine.

Diagnosis

We confirm the diagnosis of PROM by examining the fluid from the vagina. Specifically, we can measure the pH of the fluid (which is greater than 6 in amniotic fluid) and identify a crystal pattern called ferning with a microscope. Finally, we can see low amniotic fluid levels on an ultrasound.

◗ ◗ ◗ A SHOCK IN THE NIGHT

My friend Katherine was twenty-eight weeks pregnant with her first baby, and everything was progressing smoothly and normally. After four frustrating attempts with IVF, she and her husband, David, were elated to finally be pregnant with their long-awaited son.

Then one night at midnight, my telephone rang. It was Katherine, telling me that she had just awakened from a sound sleep feeling wet. It was just a little bit of liquid, she explained; maybe she hadn't emptied her bladder fully before getting into bed. I told her to go back to sleep and call me back if anything changed. Two hours later, at 2 a.m., my phone rang again. Katherine breathlessly told me that her whole bed was now soaked. I told her to come to the hospital right away and I would meet her there.

Katherine and David arrived at the hospital at the same time I did. I took her in the exam room and found that her water bag was definitely broken. She had completely soaked through her clothes.

The couple looked at me in disbelief. They had been by my side a few years earlier as I took care of my own son, who was a preemie. Katherine had spent many evenings with me in the NICU, only to find that now she would most likely have a baby in there too. After many years of fertility treatments, they had thought the worst was behind them. They were disappointed and frustrated, and very scared.

The neonatologist came to their room to discuss consequences of the potential early delivery. Their heads were filled with statistics, possibilities, and the unknown.

Katherine received steroids to help the baby's lungs develop and antibiotics to prevent infection. Things were quiet for a few days, but eventually the baby started to show signs of impending infection. At that point, we decided it was time to deliver.

Katherine delivered little baby Blake that night, weighing just two pounds and fourteen ounces. He was taken to the NICU right away and received oxygen, antibiotics, and medicine to help his breathing. Blake may have been small, but he sure was a fighter. He did surprisingly well in NICU and was able to go home after only one month. Little Blake defied all the odds and has never had any complications from his early entrance into the world.

—Allison ◀ ◀ ◀

Treatment

The amniotic sac, which looks like a piece of stretchy cellophane, serves as the protective barrier between the baby and the bacteria that normally live in the vagina. After the water has been broken for more than twenty-four hours, the chance that an infection will get into the uterus is one in four. This infection can spread to the baby, causing newborn infections and fetal distress. For this reason, if PROM occurs after thirty-four weeks, we usually recommend delivering the baby immediately. For PROM before thirty-four weeks, we deliver the baby when signs of infection develop.

Umbilical Cord Prolapse

Umbilical cord prolapse occurs when the cord slips out through the cervix, before the baby, after the bag of water has broken. When cord prolapse happens, the baby must be delivered as quickly as possible. If the cord is pinched or squeezed between the fetus and vaginal wall, no oxygen is delivered to the baby.

Cord prolapse is more common when the baby is not in the head-down position. When the round head is covering the cervix, the cord usually cannot come out first. You can imagine that if the more irregularly shaped baby's butt or feet were over the cervix, the cord has more space for slipping through. Cord prolapse can also occur at the time of amniotomy (when the doctor breaks a patient's bag of water) if the head is not pressing down against the cervix firmly. Similarly, if excessive amounts of amniotic fluid, or *polyhydramnios,* are present, the head may not be positioned well against the cervix and a loop of umbilical cord can slip through.

With a cord prolapse, the best course of action is an immediate cesarean delivery.

▶ ▶ ▶ ON THE BED WITH MY PATIENT

As an ob-gyn, I find there's an art to doing cervical exams with your fingers—you are actually assessing a part of a patient's body without directly visualizing it. This skill comes only with experience—in our case, after thousands and thousands of exams. Along the way, you also become more proficient at knowing what part of the baby's body you are touching. It feels different to be touching a baby's head than a butt or an ear or an umbilical cord. Honestly, everything does feel kind of soft and slippery, but after enough practice, you can tell what's what.

During my first year in private practice, I remember a patient who came into the hospital in active labor after spontaneously having broken her bag of water. Suddenly, we could see on the monitor that the baby's heart rate was dropping rapidly . . . and staying down. When I did a cervical exam to see what was going on, I felt the baby's head, but I also felt a loop of cord along the side of her cervix, and I could tell it was about to slip farther down. I could feel the blood pulsing through the cord, so I was 100 percent certain that it was the umbilical cord.

I called out for an emergency cesarean delivery, then jumped up on my patient's bed and tried to keep the umbilical cord from slipping farther out by keeping my hands in her vagina, while the nurses ran down the hall, pushing my patient and me on the bed together toward the operating room. She may have been okay without my amateur heroics, but it was my first year in private practice and I acted out of instinct. At any rate, she definitely needed the emergency cesarean, and we ended up with a beautiful, healthy baby at the end.

—Alane ◀ ◀ ◀

Preterm Birth

Preterm birth is any birth that occurs before thirty-seven weeks. One in every eight babies in the United States is born prematurely. The consequences of prematurity include breathing problems, cerebral palsy, blindness, intestinal problems, and developmental delays in children. Prematurity is also the number one cause of newborn death.

Risk Factors

If this is your second pregnancy, we can estimate your risk of delivering early as follows:

- If your first baby was at term, your risk is 4 percent.
- If you first baby was preterm, your risk is 17 percent.
- If you've had two preterm babies, your risk is 30 percent.

Other risk factors for a preterm delivery include:

- Infections of the kidney, appendix, genital tract, or lungs
- African American racial heritage (the incidence of preterm births in African Americans is nearly twice that of Caucasians)
- An abnormally shaped uterus or short cervix
- Multiple gestation
- Smoking
- Poor nutrition
- Unexplained vaginal bleeding in the second or third trimester
- Use of fertility treatments

Note, however, that in more than half of the cases of preterm birth, the cause remains unknown. Preterm birth can affect any pregnancy at any time. Contrary to Internet rumors, no connection exists between preterm birth and sexual activity or stressful jobs.

Prevention

Prevention of preterm birth involves eliminating any known risk factors. For example, a woman can quit smoking. As doctors, we can aggressively treat any pelvic infections, or identify and correct uterine abnormalities in a patient before she becomes pregnant.

In February of 2011, the U.S. FDA approved the use of 17-Hydroxyprogesterone caproate (17-HP) for the prevention of preterm birth in women with a history of a previous preterm birth. 17-HP is administered as a weekly injection. Treatment may be initiated at sixteen to twenty weeks of pregnancy until thirty-six weeks and six days. The use of 17-HP decreases the chance of delivering prematurely by 50 percent.

Scientific studies have not shown any benefit to bed rest in the prevention of preterm birth. Subjectively, however, our patients tell us that they feel fewer and less intense contractions on bed rest compared to when they are doing normal activities. Clearly, bed rest is not harmful, but in cases of true preterm labor, it may not be beneficial.

Diagnosis

We make the diagnosis of preterm labor when a mom has uterine contractions that cause her cervix to open. These contractions are different from Braxton Hicks contractions, which often occur before thirty-seven weeks but don't dilate the cervix.

If we are unsure whether a patient is in true or false labor, we can test for the presence of a protein in the vagina called fetal fibronectin or we can check the length of the cervix by ultrasound. The results of these tests will help us determine who is truly at risk for delivering preterm.

Fetal fibronectin (FFN) is a protein made by the fetus that acts as a glue to attach the placenta to the uterus. It can be detected in the cervical and vaginal secretions of a woman experiencing preterm labor. Your doctor can test for FFN between twenty-four to thirty-four weeks with a Q-tip swab. If FFN is identified in the vaginal secretions, you have a 25 percent chance of delivering within the next two weeks. If the FFN is negative, the chance of delivery within the next two weeks is almost zero.

Measuring the length of the cervix using an ultrasound is another way we determine whether or not preterm labor is likely. The shorter a woman's cervix, the higher the likelihood that she may deliver preterm.

Treatment

Many drugs have been studied over the years as treatments for preterm labor. Unfortunately, these medications, called tocolytics, are usually not effective at preventing preterm birth, and a woman who truly has preterm labor will most likely deliver early. However, tocolytics can slow the process of labor to allow proper preparation for the delivery, such as transferring the mother to a hospital that has the proper NICU facilities to care for her newborn. In addition, we can give a steroid injection to the mother, which greatly reduces the risk of the most common complications in preemies—breathing problems, digestion problems, and bleeding in the brain. Finally, antibiotics can be given to decrease the risk of the Group B strep infection, which is also more common in premature infants.

Preterm Babies

The major goals of perinatal medicine are to reduce the incidence of premature births and improve the quality of life of the premature infants. Delivering a premature infant is always a risky proposition, especially if the birth occurs before twenty-seven weeks gestation. No matter how well designed and state-of-the-art our modern medical incubators may be, a mother is always a better home for a developing fetus.

According to a recent article in the *Journal of the American Medical Association*, the survival rates for preemies are as follows:

Twenty-two weeks: less than 10 percent
Twenty-three weeks: 53 percent
Twenty-four weeks: 67 percent
Twenty-five weeks: 82 percent
Twenty-six weeks: 85 percent
Twenty-seven weeks: more than 90 percent

The Neonatal Intensive Care Unit

▶ ▶ ▶ A PREEMIE DAD'S TALE

In the NICU, you can always tell the optimists from the pessimists. The pessimists see nothing but wires, tubes, and monitors, but the optimists are able to look beyond these things and focus on the baby. I was a pessimist.

Born three months early, my son Richard weighed just two pounds, three ounces, and bruises due to a rough delivery covered his arms and legs. When I first saw him, he was lying on his back, motionless, under bright blue lights. His eyes were taped shut and his tiny body was coated in a shiny lubricant. He struck me as half finished, as if the workers at the baby factory had gone on strike, turned off the machines, and left my newborn son on the conveyor belt. At two pounds, his twin brother Reeve looked like a hairless cat, skinny and stringy with painfully red skin. He couldn't breathe or eat on his own and had a Grade II brain hemorrhage. If it's true that "God only gives us what we can handle," I couldn't help but think the Lord needed to recheck His math—maybe He forgot to carry a 1 or something—because this, this I couldn't handle.

Then something extraordinary happened: My son Reeve—the half baby, half cat—opened his eyes. Intellectually, I knew his vision was not yet developed enough to see me, but emotionally, I knew there was no way I was going to let my boys fight for their lives without believing in them 100 percent. And in that instant, I became an optimist.

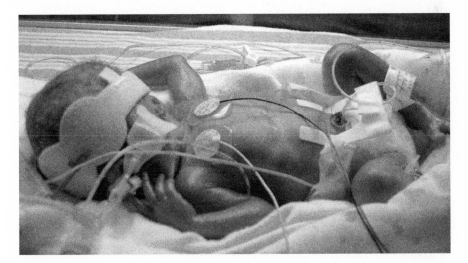

Figure 9-4: Baby Pearson

To this day, I'm not sure if my attitude adjustment had any effect on their long-term health, but I can tell you that it made my 108 days in the NICU much, much easier.

Optimism: I highly recommend it.

—Church Pearson, Alane's patient ◀ ◀ ◀

Premature infants, as well as full-term babies with medical conditions, are cared for in a neonatal intensive care unit, or NICU, by a pediatrician who is specially trained to care for the newborn, called a neonatologist. Not all hospitals have NICUs, and different NICUs may offer different levels of care. Therefore, sometimes a premature infant may need to be transferred to another hospital after birth if his needs can't be met where he was born.

If you have never been in a NICU, it may seem like another planet. Monitors are everywhere, staff members are in gowns and masks, and the babies are all sizes. If an early delivery is anticipated, a mother may visit the NICU beforehand, to familiarize herself with the staff and the potential medical issues that may arise. Often, this will make the transition less intimidating, leaving her more energy to focus on her newborn. We encourage our moms to ask questions: The NICU medical staff understands that you are asking questions about the most important thing in the world to you, your baby.

Problems with Preemies

In premature babies, the development of the brain, lungs, and intestines has not been completed. Therefore, the main issues confronted by preemies are their breathing, their digestion, and bleeding in the brain. Many of these babies are put on respiratory support, which can range from a full ventilator to oxygen supplied through their nose or mouth.

Digestive issues occur because the immature intestines cannot break down food easily nor move it through the gastrointestinal tract. In some cases, their intestines can even rupture. After they are able to digest food, they may need to be fed through a tube because their mouth muscles are not strong enough to suck well.

Infants born early have very little body fat, so they have a hard time controlling their body temperatures. For this reason, they are kept in a warm incubator until they can maintain their own warmth in the outside world.

Preemies are often hooked up to several monitors, which check their breathing, blood pressure, and heart rate. Because their nervous system is immature, they may stop breathing (apnea) or slow their heart rate (bradycardia). If either of these problems is detected, they are quickly remedied by the NICU staff.

Finally, premature babies are also very susceptible to infections, so they are often given antibiotics through their IV. Visitors are asked to wear gowns and masks to prevent exposure of infections to these sensitive infants.

▶ ▶ ▶ A PREEMIE STUDYING TO BE A NEWBORN

The moment that my baby, Alex, was delivered by cesarean, I felt his absence profoundly. I cried as I held my husband's hand. He was gone from me too soon. Born at only thirty-one weeks, I saw him being lifted, bloody and gleaming with amniotic goo, from the operating table.

I was still in the hospital during the first week of his stay in the NICU, recovering from my cesarean delivery. I felt so guilty. It was as if my body let me down and let him down, by releasing him into the world so early. I would get someone to wheel me up to the NICU every day after I furiously pumped out the little bit of milk I was producing, to bring it to the nurses to freeze so I could feel like I was contributing to his growth and recovery. I would go up there and I would cry while staring at this little beauty of a baby I was already so in love with.

I don't cry anymore when I visit him. I laugh, I talk to him the whole time, and I know he hears me. Then, after my husband and I stare at him for a few hours and comment on how cute and perfect every part of his little body is, we leave the kindhearted nurses to their work. We try to keep ourselves busy with housework, getting our place baby-ready for when he is ready to graduate from the NICU. But inside all I feel is a sense of emptiness, as if my heart has gone missing. And nothing anyone can say or do will fill this hole until I have my baby in my arms.

The NICU experience is one of complex and conflicting emotions. I am happy he is healthy and doing well. Alex hardly needed intubation and was breathing with only the help of prongs pumping oxygen through his tiny nostrils after one day. He is gaining weight, taking my breast milk through his feeding tube every three hours, and showing signs of being able to suck on the pacifier, which is as big as his face.

I can honestly say I long for poopy diapers, sleepless nights, and all the chaos and delight a new baby brings into the home. I can't wait. My husband and I stare at other couples with their babies a little too long. They probably think we are crazy, and right now we are. They all have their babies with them. Ours is a preemie studying to be a newborn at the NICU—the safest place for him to be until we can bring him home for good.

—Emily, Allison's patient ◀ ◀ ◀

Steps Forward and Steps Back in the NICU

When parents end up having a premature baby in the NICU, they tend to think of it as a linear journey, in which the baby will simply grow and improve as the days wear on. It can be a shock when they realize that their child's weeks in the NICU can be more like a roller coaster ride: Some days, it feels like two steps forward and one step back. One day, the baby may be doing fine, and then the next, the baby may end up with an infection and have to take antibiotics. Eventually, they get stronger and healthier, and most will eventually leave, but it can be emotionally exhausting waiting to get to that point.

Sometimes the NICU staff will ask a parent's permission to do procedures or tests to make sure that the baby's okay. When a parent gets a call and hears, "We need to do a lumbar puncture on your baby," or "Your baby needs a transfusion; are you okay with that?" it can be terrifying. Trusting that the NICU team is doing what is best for your baby may take a leap of faith. Always keep in mind that the NICU staff is there to ensure the health of your child. You will get to know many of the doctors, nurse practitioners, nurses, and secretaries as you make your frequent visits. They are there for your baby, and their goal is to send your baby home with you in as healthy a condition as possible.

Going Home from the NICU

A preemie needs to reach a number of milestones before he or she is allowed to go home. The baby needs to be able to breathe room air on his or her own and maintain his or her oxygen levels. He or she also needs to be able to eat and digest food without throwing it up.

Most preemies end up going home from the hospital right around the time that they would have been thirty-six weeks old, if they had stayed inside the uterus for the normal gestational period. So, if twenty-four of the weeks were spent inside the womb, often twelve weeks will be spent in the NICU. Allison's son was born at thirty-one weeks, and he went home almost exactly when he would have been thirty-six weeks.

Multiples

Even after all our years as obstetricians and the thousands of babies we've delivered, we are still amazed when we see a baby on an ultrasound. You can only imagine what we feel when we see two, sometimes three or more babies growing in the uterus! Multiple gestation describes any pregnancy with more than one fetus. Most commonly, these are twins (two fetuses) or triplets (three fetuses). However, due to ovulation induction agents and fertility treatment, or assisted reproductive technology (ART), pregnancies can be of even higher order.

In the old days of obstetric medicine, many twins were missed until a second baby made its unexpected appearance in the delivery room. Since the advent of the ultrasound, however, we are able to determine how many fetuses a woman is carrying as early as six weeks into the pregnancy.

The human uterus is designed to house one baby for forty weeks. When that same house has to be shared, complications are more likely to occur. Although many people may think "the more the merrier," this is not always the case. The addition of just one extra fetus increases the risk of all common obstetrical complications. For the fetuses, the risk of preterm delivery also increases over that of singleton pregnancies. The average time at which twins deliver is 35.3 weeks, for triplets, 32.2 weeks, and for quadruplets, 29.9 weeks. The earlier the fetuses are born, the higher the chance of permanent long-term disabilities. The risk of cerebral palsy, growth restriction, and unequal growth between the fetuses are all increased in multiple gestations.

Increased Incidence

The incidence of multiple pregnancies has skyrocketed since the increased use of ovulation induction agents and ART. Since 1980, there has been a 65 percent increase in twins and a whopping 400 percent increase in triplets or higher order births.

The chance of having identical, or monozygotic, twins (one egg is fertilized with one sperm and then splits into two embryos) *without* the use of reproductive technology is four in one thousand. For fraternal, or dizygotic, twins (two eggs are released and fertilized, each by a different sperm), the incidence varies based on age, race, parity (number of babies a woman has had previously), and fertility treatments. On average, they occur in one of one hundred births. In one tribe in Nigeria, the incidence of fraternal twins is—ready for this?—one in twenty births.

The use of Clomid (clomiphene), an oral medication to stimulate ovulation, increases the chance of conceiving twins to 10 percent. Injectable ovulation induction agents increase the risk to 25 percent. Older moms also have an increased chance of twins.

▶ ▶ ▶ **EARLY ARRIVAL TWINS**

Deeply in love, young, and healthy, Leslie and Jake couldn't believe it when they first had trouble conceiving. After years of testing and trying, they decided to undergo IVF to get pregnant. They were ecstatic the day they learned that the procedure worked and that Leslie was pregnant with twins.

The pregnancy itself, however, presented its own set of problems right from the beginning. Leslie developed a rare IVF complication called ovarian hyperstimulation, in which a woman accumulates enormous amounts of fluids in her abdominal cavity. Then, at twenty-one weeks, she started to have cramping fairly regularly. Twenty-one weeks is early for any woman to be having consistent uterine contractions. Because we noticed that Leslie's cervix was shortening, we had no choice but to admit her to the hospital for the long haul.

When we hooked Leslie up to a monitor in the hospital, we could see that she was indeed contracting regularly. We placed her on a machine called the terbutaline pump and gave her IV magnesium to try to stop the contractions. We called on an acupuncturist to give her treatments. We would see Jake by her side daily, holding her hand and supporting her emotionally.

Through her entire ordeal, not once did we hear Leslie complaining about any of it. Was she worried and scared? We're sure she was. Were we concerned that she would not make it to term? Yes, we were. But as a team, we were all working and hoping for the best, doing everything in our power to keep the twins inside their mom for as long as possible. Each day that passed by was a milestone overcome.

At twenty-six and a half weeks, however, Leslie went into active labor. Her cervix began to dilate, despite all the medications. We'd prepared as best we could—we'd been giving her steroid shots to speed up the babies' lung maturation, and the NICU team had already counseled her and Jake about what to expect after the premature infants entered the world. Our only choice now was to deliver.

Leslie's beautiful twin girls, Chelsea and Skylar, went straight to the NICU from the delivery room. It took months, and the usual ups and downs, before they were strong enough to come home, but today they are bright, active, happy four-year-old girls.

Management

Multiple fetal pregnancies are usually monitored by ultrasound to confirm that all the fetuses are growing equally. Growth of the fetuses is measured every three to four weeks after twenty weeks. We watch these mothers and babies closely, looking out for cervical insufficiency, preterm labor, preeclampsia, diabetes, and growth restriction—all of which are more common with multiples. We may restrict physical activity for moms with multiples because of the higher likelihood of preterm labor. If a preterm delivery is eminent, we use steroid therapy to speed up the development of the fetal lungs. If the babies do not grow well or one grows at the expense of the other, early delivery may be necessary.

Complications

Delivering multiples, whether vaginally or by cesarean, is more complicated than delivering singletons. You should be in a hospital setting with a skilled, experienced team of doctors, nurses, and support staff in case emergencies arise.

As mentioned, multiples tend to deliver preterm. But the goal is still to get you and your babies to term, or thirty-seven weeks, if possible. How your babies are positioned within the uterus is the most important factor that will determine the manner in which you will deliver. If both babies are head down, you may attempt a vaginal delivery. If the first twin is head down but the second is breech or transverse (lying on its side), a vaginal delivery may be attempted if the obstetrician is experienced with these deliveries. In some cases, the first twin delivers vaginally, and the second may require a cesarean delivery. If the first baby is breech, or if you have triplets, cesarean delivery is recommended. Most doctors would not attempt VBAC with twins, but consult with your obstetrician.

You have no control over whether you naturally conceive twins or triplets. However, if you are under the care of a fertility specialist, make certain you ask lots of questions and understand how many babies you may end up carrying. Multiples are amazing in so many ways, but they are also more complicated in terms of your care and the care of your babies.

Your best bet for minimizing the complications associated with a multiple pregnancy is closely monitored prenatal care and your cooperation in decreasing your physical activity level, should complications arise.

▶ ▶ ▶ TRIPLE THREATS

Olivia, the accountant for our practice, suffered from chronic anovulation (the lack of regular menstrual cycles), caused by the body's failure to release an egg every month. Using Clomid, a fertility drug, I assisted her in achieving her first pregnancy, resulting in the birth of a beautiful, healthy son forty weeks later.

When Olivia was ready to conceive a second time, however, she did not respond to Clomid, so I referred her to a specialist for infertility treatment. IVF therapy worked, resulting in three healthy fetuses: two girls and one boy. We discussed selective reduction from triplets to twins to reduce the risk of serious complications, but Olivia decided to proceed without any medical intervention for religious reasons.

I worried about Olivia for personal reasons: Just before Olivia's conception, Stefanie, another patient in our practice carrying triplets, broke her water at twenty-six weeks and gave birth to three boys at twenty-eight weeks. Despite heroic medical intervention, one of the boys just wasn't strong enough and died shortly after birth. Still saddened by this occurrence, I was determined to watch Olivia like a hawk. When, at thirty weeks, she began to have preterm contractions and cervical shortening, I placed her on strict bed rest and gave her steroid therapy to enhance fetal lung development. Olivia carried her triplets to thirty-four and a half weeks and delivered three healthy babies. They had a short NICU stay, but all went home healthy.

Olivia's story is a happy one. Even though her babies were premature, they were delivered after thirty-two weeks, which is the average gestational time for most triplets. Olivia also avoided any maternal complications. Still, as Stefanie's sad loss indicates, many other such cases do not always go as smoothly.

—Yvonne ◀ ◀ ◀

Postpartum Hemorrhage

Obstetrical hemorrhage, or bleeding within the first few hours of delivery, remains the number one cause of maternal death in the world, accounting for 25 percent of all cases. In developed countries, however, advances in modern techniques to control bleeding have made the risk of death due to postpartum hemorrhage extremely low (one out of one hundred thousand).[4] The true incidence of postpartum hemorrhage is difficult to determine because of a variety of factors, including how we define hemorrhage. In one method, we say that a postpartum hemorrhage is blood loss of more than 500 milliliters, which is equivalent to about one and a half cans of soda. But determining the blood loss at delivery is an estimate. In another approach, doctors identify a postpartum hemorrhage by whether or not a patient feels symptoms of dizziness or weakness or has a drop in her blood count by 10 percent or more.

▶ ▶ ▶ A NURSE CAN TELL

A registered nurse, Michelle was pregnant with her first child, and it was important to her to make an attempt at a natural, unmedicated childbirth. She carried to term and went into labor spontaneously, but after more than thirty hours of hard labor with no end in sight, she needed a little rest and requested an epidural. Michelle also had a low-lying placenta, where the placenta was near but not covering the cervix. Most women with low-lying placentas are still able to have normal vaginal births, as long as there are no signs of excessive bleeding during labor.

After more than forty hours, Michelle finally pushed out a beautiful baby boy. The new mom was elated but also exhausted from her hours of toil. It's always normal to have some bleeding during the labor and after the birth. Typically, after the baby and the placenta are delivered, the uterus begins to contract on its own, to help stop the bleeding. Unfortunately, Michelle began to bleed profusely, at a time when the bleeding should have begun slowing. I followed all the steps that we normally take when we encounter excessive bleeding: massaging of the uterus to help promote contraction, IV Pitocin, careful examination of the vagina and cervix to be certain there were no lacerations, inspection of the placenta to be certain there were no fragments left behind, and an injection of methergine, a medication to help the uterus contract. But even after all these steps, Michelle still continued to bleed.

It's important to maintain a calm, professional atmosphere in the delivery room no matter what the emergency. But Michelle, as a trained nurse, quickly noticed something out of the ordinary was going on. When she heard me ordering a second IV line and urgent lab tests, calling out for her vital signs, and asking the nurse to get two bags of blood ready, she looked up with her baby in her arms and, with a tremor in her voice, asked, "Dr. Park, thank you for being calm, but am I going to be okay?" My response was, "Yes, you will be fine. But I may have to take you to the OR in a minute if your bleeding continues this way."

Finally, Michelle's tired uterus contracted and stopped her bleeding. Being young and healthy was a huge advantage for her. Despite the fact that she lost a large amount of blood—about two liters—she remained stable throughout the dramatic time as her body was able to compensate. After it was all over, she showed signs of anemia, so she did require a transfusion of blood, but that too went smoothly. Just a few days later, Michelle left the hospital with a beautiful infant son in her arms.

Over the years, we've moved away from transfusing moms unless absolutely necessary. Many factors, including maternal health, will influence the need for transfusion. Because Michelle felt quite dizzy, we knew that she would struggle with her anemia at home trying to care for and breastfeed a newborn. The blood transfusion was just what her body needed to help in its recovery from her dramatic birth experience.

—Alane ◀ ◀ ◀

Risk Factors

The risk factors for postpartum hemorrhage are:

- Uterine atony,
- Lacerations of the vagina or cervix,
- Abnormal placentas,
- Severe preeclampsia,
- Blood clotting disorders.

Uterine atony is the most common reason for excessive bleeding. Normally, after the baby and the placenta have been delivered, the uterus contracts to slow down and stop the uterine bleeding, called involution. Atony means the uterus resists contracting, stays soft, and continues to bleed. At term, an enormous amount of blood flows through your uterus every minute, so it does not take long to lose blood to the point where you become anemic. Remember, also, that your uterus has been distended for months, making room for a term infant, placenta, and amniotic fluid. A term uterus that was carrying your seven-pound baby must contract to half its size within minutes. The following conditions put you at risk for having uterine atony:

- Any condition that distends your uterus more than the usual, such as twins, a very large baby, or polyhydramnios (excessive amounts of amniotic fluid)
- Your uterus working to the point where it is totally overtaxed and exhausted and is unable to contract well anymore because the muscles are so fatigued
- Long inductions, which lead to an overtired uterus
- Developing an infection in the uterus during your labor

These are simply risk factors, and having any of these conditions does not necessarily mean you'll have uterine atony. A mother's body is resilient; you'd be surprised by what it's able to handle.

Lacerations: Lacerations are spontaneous tears in your vagina or on your cervix that result from the baby coming through the birth canal. Depending on their location and extent, some lacerations can bleed profusely after delivery. In addition, episiotomies (a cut in the perineum made by your doctor) can also be associated with bleeding.

Abnormal placentas: The uterine blood vessels where your placenta implants are large with life-giving blood coursing through them. After the delivery of the placenta, these vessels are supposed to constrict to stop the blood flow. In abnormal placentas, such as placenta previa or accreta, the vessels may have a harder time clamping down, causing you to bleed excessively. In addition, if your placenta does not separate from the wall of the uterus completely and pieces of it are left behind, the uterus may continue to bleed.

Certain medical conditions: Some of these conditions are severe preeclampsia or blood clotting disorders.

Management

If your doctor determines that you are bleeding excessively, you will be given an IV with fluids to help replace what your body has lost and maintain your blood pressure. The medical team will massage your uterus to help it to contract, identify any tears that need to be repaired, and examine the placenta to be sure no small fragments have been left behind.

If fundal massage is not effective, medication to help your uterus contract may be given through the IV, as an injection in your arm or thigh, or as a rectal suppository. The blood bank will be notified in case you need a blood transfusion. If all fails, your doctor may need to take you to surgery to stop the bleeding. In some cases, the large blood vessels that feed your uterus need to be tied off or, in more serious scenarios, your uterus may be removed. Remember that your doctor and nurses have been well trained for this complication, and you have to trust that they are making the right decisions for you.

You will be evaluated for anemia through a blood test. We can determine how well your body is adjusting to the anemia by measuring your vital signs and urine output. You may be able to forego a transfusion if you are healthy, your vital signs are stable, you can walk around without dizziness, and we can see that you're able to handle your baby well.

Stillbirths

Stillbirth, any fetal death that occurs after twenty weeks of pregnancy, occurs in one out of two hundred pregnancies. Experiencing a still-birth is one of the most tragic events a woman may ever go through in her life. Nothing can describe the devastation of a mother who no longer feels her baby moving inside her.

Causes

The causes for stillbirth follow, along with their incidence:

- Birth defects and chromosomal abnormalities: 30 percent
- Umbilical cord accidents (not simply the cord around the fetal neck but knots in the cord, problems with the umbilical cord placement, or blood clots within the cord): 15 percent
- Problems related to the placenta, such as abruption as a result of abdominal trauma: 10 to 20 percent.
- Maternal disease, such as high blood pressure, diabetes, and kidney disease: 10 percent
- Infections such as parvovirus, cytomegalovirus (CMV), or Listeria: 5 percent
- Unknown causes: 25–35 percent

As the last statistic shows, we don't always know what causes a still-birth. In 25 to 35 percent of cases, no reason is ever found, leaving the parents wondering what went wrong and fearful of trying again.

Management

When a stillbirth is discovered, the baby must be delivered. Some women will opt for an induction, but others do not want to go through a lengthy labor and may choose a cesarean. After delivery, an autopsy can be performed to look for any birth defects or chromosomal ab-normalities.

In subsequent pregnancies, women often feel anxious and scared, especially if the reason for the stillbirth was not identified. These pregnancies will be monitored more closely, often with frequent ul-trasound exams and nonstress tests to ensure that the fetus is grow-ing well and receiving all the oxygen it needs.

Prevention

If there are preexisting maternal conditions, such as hypertension or diabetes, that could have caused the stillbirth, excellent control of these conditions may prevent a future demise. In a woman with a known history of stillbirth, antepartum testing is begun one week prior to the time at which the stillbirth occurred or at 34 weeks, whichever comes first. Early delivery can be at 37 weeks with documentation of fetal lung maturity by an amniocentesis.

▶ ▶ ▶ THE COURAGE TO TRY AGAIN

Last spring, my husband and I sat together in the school auditorium, beaming with pride at our son Matthew's performance in his annual end-of-year concert. From my seat on the aisle, I could clearly see Arianna, Matthew's warm-hearted music teacher, standing in the wings, making sure all the children were remembering their lyrics. Arianna had the belly of a woman almost ready to deliver, and I remember how happy and excited I was for her. When she returned to school in the fall, I mused, she would be a new mommy, with a new adventure in life just beginning for her.

Matthew's summer came and went. The new fall year started. Matt was busy with his new schedule, and one day he said, "Mom, Mrs. Hillman lost her baby."

I said, "What are you talking about, Matt? What happened to her baby?"

"I'm not sure Mom," Matt replied.

My heart sank.

Not long afterward, I met Arianna for coffee to ask her what went wrong. She had gone two days past her due date, and at a regular check-up, she was told that her baby had demised. She was beyond devastated. I can't imagine what it must feel like to go through forty-plus weeks of carrying a child, only to lose him so unexpectedly. I'm not sure that I could have handled the pain and sadness. But Arianna looked strong. She wanted answers to why and how something like this could have happened to her and her beautiful son. Her doctors ran all sorts of tests, but as is sometimes the case, she was told that they could not find a cause. Everything had appeared to be perfect.

Arianna had enough courage to try again. She asked if I wouldn't mind taking care of her. I felt it was such an honor that she asked me that I broke my rule of not having close friends or family members as patients.

Arianna and her husband, Dennis, conceived easily. During most of her pre-natal visits, I could sense her uncertainty. To help ease her anxiety, I had her come in to see me more often than most patients. Finally, sometime in the second through early third trimester, she started looking a little more comfortable and confident.

Months passed, and suddenly it was that time of year again—Matthew's spring concert. My husband and I sat in the same spot in the audience, and there was Arianna, pregnant again, sitting on a chair with a smile on her face, watching over the performing children. The pregnancy was going smoothly, but as we approached thirty-five weeks, she began to panic. Her first pregnancy had been fine on the surface as well. I saw her practically every day during her last weeks, to reassure her that her daughter was doing fine. She told me, "My son was with me at all times in my belly, and I still could not protect him. I want my daughter out as soon as you think she's ready." At around thirty-six weeks, her amniotic fluid began to decrease. Because she had a history of a myomectomy (fibroid tumor removal surgery) and had delivered her first son by cesarean, she was going to deliver by cesarean this time too.

I remember seeing her on the big day. Most moms look nervous on their scheduled cesarean day because, after all, it is surgery. Arianna, on the other hand, looked more relaxed and relieved than I had ever seen her.

She delivered a beautiful baby daughter that day. Arianna and Dennis could not have been happier. Little Lily was a bit premature, so she had to be in the NICU for a short while, but Arianna didn't care. She was just happy to be able to hold Lily, alive and healthy, in her arms at last.

—Alane ◀ ◀ ◀

Intrauterine Growth Restriction

Intrauterine growth restriction (IUGR) describes a baby that is small for its gestational age (see Figure 9-5). If the fetal size is less than the tenth percentile (that is, smaller than 90 percent of all fetuses in its age group), it is diagnosed with IUGR. At term, this means the baby weighs less than twenty-five hundred grams, or five and a half pounds.

Complications for growth-restricted infants are similar to those for preemies. They may have a harder time maintaining their body temperature (hypothermia) and controlling their blood sugars

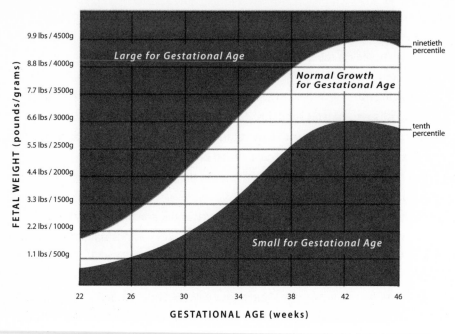

Figure 9-5: Normal Fetal Weight Chart

(hypoglycemia). They may also be prone to cerebral palsy and developmental delays later in life.

Risk Factors

- Physically small moms
- Poor nutrition
- Lifestyle factors (alcohol, smoking, drugs)
- Infections, such as rubella, hepatitis A or B, Listeria, syphilis, toxoplasmosis, CMV
- Birth defects
- Chromosomal abnormalities
- Bone and cartilage disorders, such as dwarfism
- Preeclampsia
- Medical conditions: kidney disease, diabetes, chronic hypertension, asthma, sickle-cell disease, blood clotting disorders, and systemic lupus erythematosis (SLE)
- Placental and umbilical cord abnormalities

- Multiple gestation (twins, triplets, and so on)
- Living at high altitudes

Prevention

Prevention of IUGR focuses on controlling any medical conditions that may cause it, such as hypertension and diabetes. In addition, having good nutrition and eliminating dangerous habits such as cigarette smoking and drug use can decrease its incidence.

Diagnosis

IUGR can be detected during your prenatal care visits. At each visit after twenty weeks, your doctor will measure your fundal height (see Chapter 4, page 138) to assess the growth of your baby. If the fundal height does not correspond to the gestational age, an ultrasound will be performed to estimate the baby's size and weight. Ultrasound measurements of your baby are usually more accurate than fundal height measurements. If the baby's weight is less than the tenth percentile, the baby is growth restricted.

In addition, during the ultrasound, we can check the *umbilical artery velocimetry*, which measures the flow of blood through the umbilical artery. In severe cases of IUGR, there may be great resistance in the placenta, decreasing the blood flow. As a result, the baby is not getting enough nutrition or oxygenation and is at a very high risk for growth issues and even stillbirth.

Management

Early detection of IUGR by regularly measuring the fundal height is critical. After IUGR is diagnosed, the patient may be instructed to decrease her physical activities and increase caloric intake to provide more nutrition to the growing fetus. In addition, we monitor the fetus by performing a biophysical profile, measuring umbilical artery velocimetry, and every two to three weeks assessing the growth of the fetus by ultrasound.

The goal is to allow the baby to grow inside the mom as long as possible, until its lungs are mature. However, if the baby stops growing or shows signs of distress, delivery is recommended.

Macrosomia

Macrosomia describes the other end of the spectrum—an excessively large baby. The average birth weight of a baby born in the United States is thirty-three hundred grams, or seven and one-third pounds. Although there's disagreement among doctors about exactly how big is too big, most consider a baby weighing more than four thousand to forty-five hundred grams (eight and three-quarters to ten pounds) to be very large. The definition of macrosomia is when the baby hits forty-five hundred grams, or ten pounds.

The National Center for Health Statistics reports the incidence of macrosomia as 1½ percent of all pregnancies.

Risk Factors

Risk factors for macrosomia include:

- Uncontrolled pregestational or gestational diabetes
- Maternal obesity
- Excessive weight gain during pregnancy
- Prior history of macrosomia
- Multiparity
- Post-term pregnancy
- Male fetus
- Hispanic ethnicity

Prevention

Prevention of macrosomia is largely dependent on the risk factors. For diabetic moms, tight control of sugar levels before conception and while pregnant may prevent excessive growth of the baby. For obese patients and patients with excessive weight gain during the pregnancy, we recommend watching your diet and regular exercise regimen.

Diagnosis

We can estimate your baby's weight near term in two ways: ultrasound and Leopold's maneuvers. With an ultrasound, we measure the baby's head, belly, and thigh bone to calculate an estimate of your baby's weight. In *Leopold's maneuvers* (see Figure 9-6), we use our

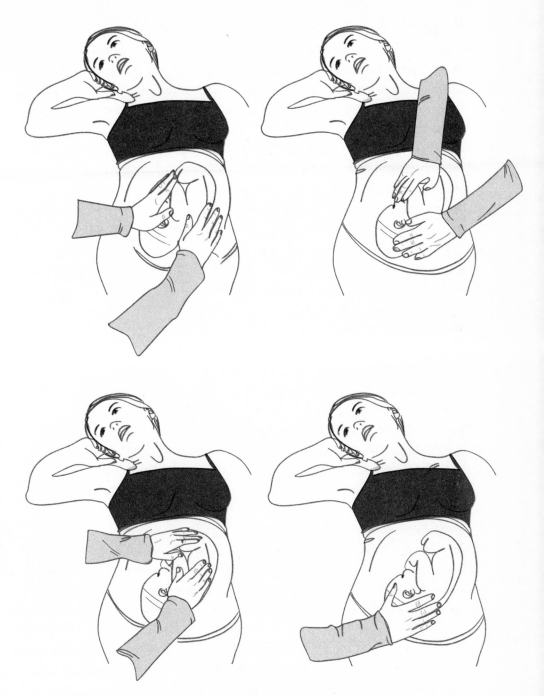

Figure 9-6: Leopold's Maneuvers

hands on your abdomen to feel your baby and estimate its size. Unfortunately, both methods have a margin of error of 10 percent. In addition, after thirty-eight weeks, fundal height measurements lose their accuracy because the baby starts its descent into the birth canal. Macrosomia can be truly diagnosed only after the birth of your baby, when we can measure him on the outside.

Management

Studies have shown that inducing labor in nondiabetic women for suspected macrosomia did not reduce the rate of birth injury or cesarean delivery. The current guidelines are to offer an elective cesarean delivery to nondiabetic mothers with a fetus estimated to be more than forty-five hundred to five thousand grams (ten to eleven pounds) and to diabetic mothers with a fetus of four thousand to forty-five hundred grams (eight and three-quarters to ten pounds).

Complications

Birth injuries from shoulder dystocia are the most common complications for a macrosomic baby during a vaginal delivery. *Shoulder dystocia* is an obstetric emergency where the baby's head has delivered but the shoulders are stuck behind the mother's pubic bone, causing injury to both the mother and the baby. Macrosomic babies often have their fat distributed around their shoulders and trunks. Although the mother's pelvis may be large enough to allow the delivery of the baby's head, the wider part of the baby—the shoulder area—gets stuck behind the mom's pubic bone. To facilitate delivery, your doctor will attempt different maneuvers to dislodge the stuck shoulder. In addition, you may require an episiotomy to enlarge the vaginal outlet. Consequences of shoulder dystocia for the newborn are a broken collarbone or arm, nerve damage within the arm, or brain damage from decreased oxygen supply.

As a result of more difficult births, macrosomic babies tend to have lower Apgar scores and are more likely to be admitted to the NICU. Macrosomic babies are at higher risk of obesity later in life.

Complications for the mother include increased risk of cesarean delivery, postpartum hemorrhage, and vaginal lacerations.

▶ ▶ ▶ **ATTACK OF THE GIANT BABIES**

Our patient Dominque, a six-foot, statuesque woman, and her husband Wayne, who stood about five inches taller than his wife, always turned heads when they walked into a room. Bubbling with enthusiasm and always ready with a joke to lighten the moment, Dominque had delivered her first daughter, Hailie, with us three years earlier; a beautiful baby girl who weighed eight pounds, six ounces at birth. Dominque pushed Hailie into the world naturally, without pain medication and without difficulty.

Dominque's second pregnancy moved along smoothly, but at around thirty-six weeks, her belly was measuring bigger than average by the standard Leopold's maneuver and fundal height measurements. To confirm our suspicion, our perinatologist performed an ultrasound, and estimated the current fetal weight was more than eight pounds. Based on this prediction, if Dominque carried to term, her baby would weigh more than nine pounds.

We spoke frankly with Dominque, counseling her that a vaginal birth with a baby this large carried a risk of shoulder dystocia. At thirty-nine weeks, Dominque's blood pressure was elevated (consistent with mild preeclampsia), so she agreed to undergo labor induction. She felt confident that she would be able to deliver a large baby because she had delivered so easily the first time. Her induction progressed quickly until, despite all our medical efforts, the cervix would not open beyond nine centimeters. Dominque agreed to proceed with a cesarean, where, to her surprise and ours, she delivered an eleven-pound, twelve-ounce boy, Logan. Dominque's son was the size of most three-month-olds! It seemed that her body knew exactly what to do to avoid a dangerous birth—in this case, to stop dilating mom's cervix.   ◀ ◀ ◀

Post-Term Delivery

"What happens if I go past my due date?" As the magical date approaches, this question is one of the most common discussions we have with our patients. An average pregnancy lasts 280 days, from the first day of the last menstrual period. However, the due date is only an estimate of when your baby will be born:

- 80 percent are born at full term, between thirty-seven to forty-two weeks

- 10 percent are premature
- 10 percent are post-dates, after forty-two weeks

A woman may go past her due date for a variety of reasons. If the original due date was calculated incorrectly—especially if it was based only on the menstrual cycle and not confirmed by an ultrasound—the pregnancy may seem to continue past forty-two weeks. For example, if a woman ovulated and conceived later than the predicted time, her due date may have been set too early. This issue can be avoided with the more widespread use of first trimester ultrasounds. In other cases, an abnormality in the fetus or low levels of placental hormones could allow the pregnancy to progress past the forty-two-week mark.

In most cases, however, we don't know exactly why a certain baby decides not to come out on time. It may simply be that every pregnancy is different and every woman's body is different. Note that if your first baby was born post-dates, you have a 50 percent chance of being late with the second baby as well.

Management

So what will happen if you are approaching forty-two weeks? We check that the environment in the uterus is still safe and that the baby is getting enough oxygen by performing the modified biophysical profile (described at the beginning of the chapter). If these tests are normal, we feel confident that we can continue to wait for labor to come spontaneously. If the test shows that the baby is compromised in any way, however, we will recommend delivery.

Stripping the membranes can decrease the chance of getting to forty-two weeks. (see Chapter 6, page 252, for details). During the cervical exam, we try to separate the amniotic bag away from the cervix with our fingers. This releases prostaglandins from the cervix, which can initiate part of the chain of events that causes labor or, at least, can ripen the mom's cervix a little more. Studies have shown that this procedure can shorten the length of a post-term pregnancy by an average of four days.

Ultimately, if a mom passes the forty-two-week mark and still shows no signs of delivering, labor induction may be our only option.

Complications

Ideally, we would like most of our patients to deliver by the forty-second week. The placenta acts as a filter, such as the filter in your coffee machine. The more you use it, the less efficient it becomes at making your tasty morning cup. As the placenta ages, it also becomes less efficient at its most important job, providing oxygen and nutrition to your baby. As a result, perinatal mortality (stillbirths and early neonatal deaths) increases, as follows:

0.4 per 1,000 births at thirty-seven weeks

2.5 per 1,000 births at forty weeks

5.5 per 1,000 births at forty-two weeks

11.5 per 1,000 births at forty-three weeks

15 per 1,000 births at forty-four weeks[5]

The aging placenta can also affect the baby's ability to tolerate labor. Contractions squeeze the blood vessels throughout the uterus and placenta, resulting in less blood flow to the baby. In addition to this normal phenomenon, if the placenta is also not functioning optimally because it is older, fetal distress can occur and sometimes a cesarean delivery is required.

Another consequence of the post-date pregnancy is the increasing size of the baby. From thirty-seven to forty-two weeks, the baby continues to grow, but at a slightly slower pace than earlier in the pregnancy, gaining about one-third pound per week. Depending on how long the pregnancy lasts, the baby can get quite large, increasing the risk of shoulder dystocia (a baby stuck during a vaginal delivery) and of vaginal tears.

Meconium passage is another risk when you go past the due date. Meconium is the first stool of the baby. It usually comes out after the baby is born, but in about 10 to 15 percent of pregnancies, the baby passes the meconium while still in the uterus. From the outside, we cannot tell if meconium has passed. It is diagnosed by seeing the green color of the meconium-stained amniotic fluid after the water has broken. In 5 percent of these cases, the baby will breathe the meconium into its lungs, causing pneumonia, also known as *meconium aspiration syndrome.* The risk of meconium aspiration syndrome is three times higher in post-date pregnancies than in babies delivered at term.

▶ ▶ ▶ IT'S A LONG STORY

Sandra, an imaginative writer, had been a patient of mine for four years. I first met her when she was pregnant with her daughter, Violet. That pregnancy was wonderful, except that it seemed as if it would never end. Sandra strongly desired an unmedicated, natural birth and went to great lengths to prepare herself for the process. Her pregnancy continued all the way to forty-two weeks, but ultimately she had to have her labor induced after we discovered her amniotic fluid was low. Although she was still able to have a vaginal delivery, the process of induction was long and arduous, lasting nearly thirty-six hours. Sandra never would have scripted this birth scenario for herself.

Two years later, Sandra found herself pregnant again, with a little boy. Like the first time, she had a textbook-perfect pregnancy but her due date came and went with no signs of labor. This time, Sandra took matters into her own hands, trying everything she could to jump-start the process. She had sex, went on long walks, ate spicy salad dressing, and used evening primrose oil. She went to an acupuncturist who even gave her free sessions because she had been there so many times without success.

Finally, after forty-two weeks and two days—a full 296 days of pregnancy—Sandra's contractions began. Because her first labor had lasted so long, Sandra and her husband, Andrew, decided to relax at home for a while before heading to the hospital. Unlike the first time, however, the contractions quickly became strong. They rushed to the hospital, but before Sandra could get out of the car, she could feel the baby coming. She delivered a nine-pound six-ounce baby boy in the parking lot without any problems. Although she was stunned, ultimately she was able to experience the unmedicated natural birth that had been her first draft. Her son, Robert, is a testament to the fact that the good things in life are worth waiting for.

—Allison ◀ ◀ ◀

▶ ▶ ▶ WHY HIGH RISK IS LESS RISKY THAN EVER BEFORE

I have been blessed to spend my career as a perinatologist, a subspecialty of obstetrics that focuses on taking care of complicated or high-risk pregnancies. Although taking care of a woman and her unborn child is a huge responsibility, the gratification this work brings is enormous.

It has been my experience that patients and their families undergoing a complicated pregnancy find sources of courage, unity, and love for each other that they never experienced before. Although much anxiety is associated with any pregnancy that develops a complication, we are fortunate that we now have the means to help the great majority of patients have a successful outcome. I cannot imagine a more fulfilling way to spend my life than to help these courageous mothers maintain their own health and give birth to a thriving, healthy baby.

—Dr. Cliff Bochner ◀ ◀ ◀

We realize we've just taken you through a litany of serious issues related to pregnancy. We're not trying to scare you; our intention is exactly the opposite. We want to arm you, educate you, and inform you with facts so that you will feel more confident and empowered should any of these complications happen to you. Modern obstetric medicine has come a very long way and is still growing in leaps and bounds. Our goal is to keep you and your baby healthy.

chapter ten

THINGS YOU NEVER EXPECT WHEN YOU'RE EXPECTING: COPING WITH CURVEBALLS

Pregnancy: The Forty-Week Emotional Roller Coaster

The forty-week interval that defines pregnancy is a whirlwind of contradictory feelings and emotions: excitement, joy, apprehension, anticipation, confusion, fear, and delight. But here's what they don't tell you . . .

Care during pregnancy involves much more than blood tests and ultrasounds, eating healthy, and exercising. Prenatal care also goes beyond the physiology of your developing fetus and details of your labor curve. In addition, you'll need emotional support. This book is primarily a guide to the physical and medical aspects of pregnancy. But getting pregnant can unleash a flood of feelings and potential psychological concerns for just about every woman, her partner, and often the rest of her family. As joyful as pregnancy may be much of the time, it puts a new stress on a woman's body, mind, and emotions and can amplify already existing stressors in her life as well.

As obstetricians, for every hour of medical analysis, we sometimes spend just as much time helping a patient overcome her fears and anxieties, or assisting her with the unexpected emotional pressures of being with child. We're not trained therapists but we've certainly heard, seen, or dealt with just about every personal issue that can arise for our pregnant patients. We want to share some of the most common experiences with you here, to help you prepare for what can often be an emotional roller-coaster ride.

Throughout our years of practice, we've tried to make our office a safe, friendly place where women can feel free to talk about their personal issues during their prenatal visits if they need to. Every patient has her own story about what is going on in her life—maybe she has a difficult boss, a seemingly unsupportive spouse, or a jealous sister . . . or all three. Others are dealing with more serious issues, such as illness, divorce, or aging parents. Often, they bring these burdens with them when they come to their appointments. Sometimes the only place they can open up is in the OB-GYN office.

You should know that your doctor or midwife is there not only to make sure you deliver your baby safely but also to support you emotionally as a new chapter in your life begins. If your emotional issues become so overwhelming and complicated that they go beyond their level of expertise, practitioners can refer you to a therapist, psychiatrist, or another specialist with experience in these situations.

▶ ▶ ▶ NO BUBBLE-WRAP REQUIRED

Abigail, a thirty-five-year-old interior designer, was overjoyed when she found herself pregnant for the first time. In the year before her pregnancy, she had come to me for preconceptional counseling. Even before she and her husband, Ryan, started trying to conceive, she was charting her menstrual cycles for months. In that first session, I also learned she had already started taking prenatal vitamins and had even combed through her family tree for any evidence of genetic diseases. Abigail was a planner.

Abigail and Ryan conceived on their third try, and came to my office for their first OB visit. Everything checked out fine—she was six weeks pregnant, and the baby was growing well with a strong heartbeat. After receiving their clean bill of health and making a two-week follow-up appointment, the couple left the exam room with joy in their eyes and big grins on their faces.

When they came in for their eight-week check-up, however, it seemed that Abigail was under a dark cloud. She plopped down in a chair, pulled a dog-eared notebook out of her purse, and began reading off a list of questions and concerns: She had eaten cheese and crackers at an office party before she knew she was pregnant; her indoor cat had been sitting in her lap; she woke up in the middle of the night to find herself sleeping flat on her back. The list went on and on, and as Abigail continued to read, I could see her becoming increasingly distraught. She was terrified that by her everyday actions, she had somehow caused some terrible harm to her baby.

As I calmly went through Abigail's list item by item, addressing each concern, Ryan spoke up. He confessed that Abigail had purchased four pregnancy books in the last two weeks and had been online nonstop, finding site after site chronicling pregnancy horror stories and disasters. Abigail had hoped pregnancy would be one of the most joyful times in her life, but instead it was evoking incredible anxiety. "I feel like nothing is safe anymore," she told me. "I wish I could just be in a bubble for the next nine months, to avoid all the dangers around me."

I was happy to see that Abigail wanted to be informed and make sure the pregnancy was a healthy one. But she also needed to limit how much time she was spending stressing over minor details. I advised her to try to enjoy her life day by day and embrace her pregnancy as just another part of it. I reassured her that most pregnancies *do* progress in a perfectly normal, healthy way. By the time she and Ryan left the office that day, she finally agreed that the bubble wrap would not be necessary.

—Allison ◀ ◀ ◀

The Department of Misinformation

myth: The color change resulting from mixing Drano with a pregnant woman's urine can tell her the sex of her unborn child.

FACT: Many swear by the Drano test—after all, it has a 50/50 chance of being right! However, absolutely no science is behind this test.

One of the most persistent causes of anxiety for our patients is the legion of pregnancy-related myths we have been working to dispel throughout this book. Women are bombarded with half-truths, propaganda, and personal opinions from the moment they find out that they are pregnant. They are afraid that anything they eat, touch, or breathe will cause harm to their unborn child. Hot dogs, cheese, a turkey sandwich, lifting the laundry basket, a fresh coat of paint in the nursery, acrylic nails—the list of so-called dangers goes on and on. Where does this misinformation come from? Family, friends, total strangers, and, of course, the Internet are all dispensers of strange recommendations, crazy myths, and outright falsehoods when it comes to pregnancy.

Some women who have had babies themselves automatically think that the significant act of surviving their own pregnancy qualifies them as experts, ready to dish out free advice to anyone else going through it. Others, both men and women who haven't even had kids themselves, are all too willing to proclaim their opinions as medical fact. And the vast majority of unofficial experts take secondhand experiences and assume that is how it is for everybody who is having a baby.

Too Much Information

As the birth day approaches, some patients start to feel fearful and become obsessed with everything that could possibly go wrong. The more these moms educate themselves by surfing the net and reading every worst-case scenario that the Web can serve up, the more terrified they often become. There really is such a thing as too much information, especially when it comes from an uninformed source or hasn't been filtered through the perspective of a professional. We find ourselves having to clarify a lot of this misinformation to keep our moms calmer and more balanced.

Type the word *pregnancy* into a search engine and be prepared to take what you read with a grain of salt. As wonderful as the Internet is as a tool for educating and finding information on a variety of subjects, it can also be a place where women can hear some frightening things that—even if true—may not apply to their situation. For example, if you look up *cramping during pregnancy* online, you might find a Web site that leads you to believe you are having a miscarriage, that something's terribly wrong with your pregnancy, or that you've damaged your baby by lifting a heavy item onto the top shelf of the closet.

In truth, it's hard for women to know whether the warning they are reading or the fact someone is claiming applies to them and their unique, individual situation. When in doubt, call your doctor.

Unsolicited Advice

Our patients tell us again and again that after they are visibly pregnant, they suddenly become public property overnight. Not only does everyone—including complete strangers—feel the need to touch your growing belly without permission, they also can't wait to share a litany of tips, suggestions, and unsolicited advice. You will also be likely to hear everyone else's childbirth story in greater detail than you'd ever want to know. Like a minor celebrity besieged by advice-dispensing paparazzi, just walking around with a pregnant belly can make you a target for a well-meaning strangers' remarks, warnings, or even lectures. You'll get stern admonitions to stop eating what you're eating or be handed the weekly schedule to a person's favorite yoga class.

Our patients are often barraged with worrisome statements like "Is something wrong? You're awfully small to be so far along," or "Oh my god, I've never seen anyone so huge." If patients get enough of these unsolicited remarks, they're often concerned by the next time they come in for an appointment. "Why are so many people asking me if I'm having twins?" they'll ask with frustration. We almost always find ourselves telling them, "Don't worry, you're normal." It's natural for a woman to be a little self-conscious when she's pregnant, but random comments and criticisms from loved ones and strangers don't help.

We recommend that you take these comments lightly. Most likely, people aren't trying to scare you. They may simply be trying to make conversation and acknowledge your obviously pregnant state. Or they may want to bond with you through the universal pregnancy experience. Bring up any fears you may have with your doctor so you can be reassured that your baby is perfectly fine.

▶ ▶ ▶ THE BEAUTY DRAIN

Whenever I think I've heard it all from my pregnant patients, one of them brings me a new anecdote that leaves me shaking my head with amazement.

When my patient Sabrina was about thirty weeks pregnant with her third child, she was picking up her dog from the local groomers when a woman approached her and inquired whether she was having a boy or girl. Sabrina responded politely that she didn't know the sex of her baby yet, and that she was waiting to be surprised.

Then the woman shocked her.

"You must be having a girl because all the beauty has gone out of your face."

Sabrina was stunned. This was a comment from a total stranger who didn't even know what Sabrina looked like before she was pregnant!

Sabrina left the dog groomers trying to choke back a wall of tears. A lovely young woman, she was already feeling self-conscious about how her appearance had changed with her pregnancy. Like most moms-to-be, she had gained some weight and felt out of shape. She felt even more discomfort and swelling than the first two times around. The last thing she needed to hear was a thoughtless, mean comment.

Ironically, it turned out that Sabrina did deliver a beautiful, healthy girl. She came in and asked me, "Did I look horrible when I was pregnant?"

I reassured her that she always looked beautiful—and still does!

—Allison ◀ ◀ ◀

Bonding with Your Unborn Child

myth: If you have a cesarean, you won't be able to bond with your baby.

FACT: No matter which way your baby enters the world, your maternal instinct will take over and you will fall in love with your child.

For many women, the instant the urine pregnancy test turns positive, a warm sensation begins to grow within them. They are truly overjoyed and excited and are already falling in love.

But what if you *don't* feel that way? What if you confess you are not a baby person? Despite doing everything you could to get pregnant, you are now faced with a feeling of anxiety, wondering if you will be a good mother, and doubtful that when the time comes, you'll be able to unconditionally love your child the way everyone else seems to love theirs.

In our practice, we have met mothers who have felt disconnected from their pregnancies and are scared that this feeling will never change, even after they deliver. Maternal bonding is an instinct in the animal kingdom that ensures survival of the species. In many animals, this instinct is related to the hormone oxytocin. Similarly, in primates and in humans, higher levels of oxytocin in the first trimester of pregnancy lead to more nurturing behaviors after birth.

We want to assure you that feeling detached during pregnancy is common. It doesn't mean something is wrong with you or that you are not going to be a good mother. Rather, the maternal instinct develops differently for everyone. The bonding experience happens gradually over time and can change from week to week. Although it may take days, weeks, or even months, eventually you will fall in love with your baby. Be patient during this time. Don't let anyone else's experience define what is normal. Your process of forming that deep, loving connection between mother and baby will be unique to you and your little one.

Relationship Issues

myth: Having a baby with your partner can strengthen and possibly save your shaky relationship.

FACT: Sadly, in our experience, a pregnancy more likely adds additional stress to an already troubled partnership. It is important to take an honest look at the state of your relationship before conceiving.

▶ ▶ ▶ COLD FEET

Whitney and Seth had been dating for two years. Whitney, thirty-six, was the oldest of three sisters and two brothers, yet she was the only one in her large, old-fashioned family who had yet to get married and have children. She and Seth were in love, and she was ready to move on to the next phase of their relationship, which for her meant a wedding, a home, and a family of her own. For an entire year, they had gone back and forth about this topic. Seth was hesitant because he had recently been divorced and, at this point, wasn't sure he was ready to make another lifetime commitment. They had broken up and reconciled twice in only a few months. During one of their breaks, Whitney decided to stop her birth control, not knowing what the future would hold.

Then, next thing she knew, Whitney found herself pregnant. Despite her fears, she was hopeful that this would be the extra push that Seth needed to solidify their relationship and finally make the commitment she desired. She knew he loved her and believed this news would inspire him to take the plunge into becoming a husband and father.

Unfortunately, Seth didn't see things the same way. He told Whitney that he cared for her deeply but truly didn't feel ready to make the next move. He promised to stand by her during the pregnancy and seek the advice of a counselor.

Although the pregnancy was perfect, their relationship was not. Anger and resentment festered between them and the tension was palpable during every office visit. Whitney felt disappointed and let down by Seth's lack of enthusiasm about what she had hoped would be the happiest time in their relationship. She gave birth to a beautiful son but found herself going home from the hospital on her own. Although Seth continued to lend his support, the pregnancy did not transform them into the happy family of Whitney's dreams.

We aren't psychologists. We aren't couples' counselors. We don't have therapy licenses claiming that we can help our patients work out the kinks in their personal relationships. At the same time, our job as obstetricians means intense involvement in the most intimate areas of our patients' lives, so we often end up playing the therapist role at moments of high crisis. At the very least, we try to listen to our patients, act as outside observers, and recommend professional help in this area if necessary. In the thousands of patients all three of us have come to know over the years, we have recognized some troubling patterns.

It's always a pleasure to see the partners supporting our patients by being part of the prenatal care. But sometimes a woman will come to her visits alone and make no reference to any partner or husband. On other occasions, we'll have a couple who are fraught with tension as the man sends signals with his attitude and body language that he is either totally terrified or doesn't want to be there.

These visits are red-flag moments for us because we have seen them so many times before. On such occasions, we may ask the woman, "Is your partner supportive of this pregnancy?" or "Will your partner be involved in raising the baby?" Some adult women are truly excited about embarking on the journey of raising a baby on their own. But in our experience, being pregnant all by yourself can be scary, and if you have a partner who isn't wholly supportive going in, he or she may not hang in with you for the duration.

We've seen a significant number of patients who've confided to us that they were counting on their pregnancy to solidify their relationship with their partner. Many admit that their relationship isn't currently exclusive or established, but they are hoping that this pregnancy will make the relationship permanent. Others hope that having a baby will correct a problem in a marriage, or convince a partner who is on the fence to stay. Society paints such a relentlessly glowing picture of the concept of childbirth and childrearing, but having children is far more likely to put a strain on a relationship, not make it easier. Caring for children is hard work—especially for the first few years—and it takes a strong partnership or a strong support system to pull it off well.

Even with comfortably married couples, a seismic shift can occur. You make a commitment when you marry somebody, but you make a different and deeper level of commitment when you choose to have children with that person. A couple without children can get divorced, walk away, and never deal with each other again. But if you get divorced when kids are in the picture, your ex will probably be part of your and your children's lives for decades to come.

We find it surprising to see how many married people get pregnant accidentally. Married couples often have unprotected sex, even though they have no intention of having children or adding to their already established families. Accidental pregnancy can be a blessing in disguise or it can put an unexpected strain on a relationship.

If you have the luxury of being able to choose whether or not you will get pregnant, use that time to take an honest look at the state of your relationship and your circumstances and figure those into the equation. After you bring a baby into the world, it's not all about you anymore.

Having a Baby on Your Own

▶ ▶ ▶ FINDING A NEW DREAM

Our patient Pamela, a thirty-five-year-old attorney, and Sean, also an attorney, had been married for eleven years. They already had a beautiful three-year-old daughter, who had been born two months prematurely after preterm labor. Together, they made the decision to have a second child to complete their family, especially because they wanted their daughter to have a sibling.

Around twenty-nine weeks, while paying some bills, Pamela came across an unusual charge on the credit card. It was for a local hotel she had never been to. She began to look at the rest of the bill and the phone bills, noting hundreds of calls and text messages to one number. Her heart sank as she realized the obvious: Her husband was having an affair. Pamela called her husband, confronting him about her suspicions. Instead of denying it, he confessed that he was not in love with her anymore and had met his soul mate.

For weeks, Pamela could do nothing but lie in bed, devastated by the news that she would now be a single mother. She begged Sean for another chance, to try counseling before throwing in the towel. She asked him why this happened now, when she was pregnant. He responded that he felt so trapped by the idea of another baby coming into their family that he realized he needed his freedom. When Pamela got pregnant the second time, he said he felt like the jail cell was closing in on him.

Pamela gave birth to her second daughter at thirty-five weeks. She, too, was a preemie, but she was strong and able to go home with her. For Pamela, her birth was the saddest day of her life. While hearing the scores of congratulations, all she could think about was the loss of her marriage and the uphill battle before her, raising two kids on her own. This was not the life she wished for herself. She wanted to have children to be a family, to raise them together with her husband. Now that dream was shattered.

For the first few months after her daughter's birth, Pamela went through her daily routine in a haze, feeling numb. She wasn't sleeping or eating well. At work, she was unfocused and forgetful. But her spirit wasn't dead, and with time, the fog began to clear. She made a decision to be an example for her daughters of a strong, resilient woman. And eventually, her heart followed her actions. She and her two girls started over with a new dream that may prove to be even better than the first.

◀ ◀ ◀

Many times we've been called in to support our patients after a husband or a partner has left them alone, three-quarters of the way through their pregnancies. They're heartbroken, devastated, and terrified. They had never dreamed of being alone and pregnant, let alone facing the possibility of raising a child by themselves.

In taking care of thousands of women over the years, we have learned how strong they are! A parade of unsung heroines walk in and out of our offices every day. They may be with or without partners, struggling through job loss and financial ruin, caring for a family member who's dying, dealing with problem pregnancies that may result in a sick baby or a baby with a birth defect, but whatever obstacles life throws in their way, they never fail to show daily how resilient women can be.

◗ ◗ ◗ SOMETIMES, THINGS DO WORK OUT

Maria is a young, beautiful woman from a modest family background with a healthy four-year-old boy from a previous marriage. Her partner, Lee, is a handsome, successful man with no children from a well-to-do, class-conscious family. They fell in love, and Maria got pregnant. They were overjoyed at having a baby together. Maria's family embraced Lee into their circle, but Lee's father had always disapproved of Lee's relationship with Maria. She confided to me that she was not certain Lee would be there for her because his parents, especially his father, were pressuring him to move on with his life. Lee felt torn between being a supportive partner to Maria and making his father happy.

When Lee came to Maria's OB appointments, he asked thoughtful questions and seemed genuinely interested and concerned about the baby's well-being and the entire birth process. When the big day finally arrived, Lee stood firmly by Maria's side throughout her labor, and you could see the love in his eyes when their baby girl made her way into the world. Maria also had an army of extended family and friends who were right there to show their support for the birth of her child.

Although Lee's father never came around to accepting Maria, her son, or even Lee and Maria's new baby, the beautiful birth experience that Lee shared with Maria and her family convinced him to commit himself wholeheartedly to the relationship. During her postpartum visit, Maria looked wonderful and was pleased to inform me that they were all planning on moving in together as a family.

We're happy to report that sometimes it really does work out.

—Alane ◀ ◀ ◀

Coping with Pregnancy: The Gender Gap

▶ ▶ ▶ DON'T FORGET YOUR PARTNER!

We know that for a new mother, the hours fly by at double time. The next thing you know, your baby is twelve months old and you realize that every ounce of your energy has been going toward your baby. But do not forget your partner in all this. He or she may not do things exactly the way you would do them— the bottle may not be clean enough, the diapers may be too loose, and your baby may end up with mismatched socks—but your partner is doing his or her best. As long as your baby is healthy and happy, it's okay to let someone else do it their way sometimes. Please remember to take your partner's feelings into consideration during this hectic time in your life. Your significant other needs your love and attention just as much as your baby does.

—Alane ◀ ◀ ◀

When some women see that second line turn blue on their plastic pregnancy test stick, they immediately wonder whether it's a boy or a girl, imagine future Christmases, or plan their grown child's wedding. We see how instantly connected our patients become to the life that is starting to grow inside them. Because men don't experience the physical symptoms and changes of pregnancy firsthand, they may view a new pregnancy differently.

We are not saying that only the pregnant woman is attached to the embryo growing inside her. A lot of dads embrace pregnancy and are excited about being full-time participants in the process. More and more couples who come to us have a male partner who is very much a part of the planning of the pregnancy and shares a deep, emotional investment in the outcome. However, that doesn't mean men always understand or know exactly how to cope with what their partner is going through.

All women deserve support to help them deal with the physical and emotional aspects of pregnancy, particularly when someone is having their first pregnancy and things go wrong. Maybe the woman had an anembryonic gestation, where the baby never developed. Or a fetal heartbeat seen at one visit is gone at the next. Remember, the chance of a miscarriage is one in five. These types of devastating events can put a strain on just about any relationship.

We've heard some men say, "Honey, try not to worry about it. It wasn't quite a baby yet." They are trying to make their partner feel better, but that statement often just emphasizes and increases the emotional distance between mother- and father-to-be. In many women's minds, just because there wasn't an actual baby doesn't matter; it still feels as if she lost a real baby. "But it was a baby to me," the woman will reply. Partners don't say these things maliciously, but they can unintentionally cause hurt. Often, the guy wants to do the right thing but doesn't know exactly what he's supposed to do or say. He may be just as sad as she is but can never know exactly what it feels like because he's not the one who was pregnant.

Many women have high expectations of their partners and definite ideas about how they should behave and the kind of emotional support they should provide during all aspects of the pregnancy. Sometimes, these expectations are fair and realistic, but other times, they are not. We've seen many a well-meaning partner try his best to provide the strength and comfort a woman needs, but he just can't live up to his partner's unrealistic standards. In these situations, we may counsel the husband or partner about specific ways he might be more supportive. If nothing else, we try to make sure that the couple is engaging in open and honest communication about what's going on. Sometimes we find ourselves defending the partners. We don't want the relationship to go awry because our patient came into the pregnancy with unrealistically high expectations of how comforting and understanding her partner should behave at all times.

We believe it's a good idea for couples who are facing extreme emotional challenges to seek the advice of a professional therapist. Those who do invariably tell us it was a great help in getting them through the experience together, while keeping their relationship strong.

▶ ▶ ▶ THE LINGERING WOUND

On the very first day we began filming our series, *Deliver Me,* one of my favorite moms-to-be came in for her five-month check-up, complaining of a strange discharge. During her vaginal exam, I could see that her amniotic sac was coming out the cervix and she was over two centimeters dilated. My heart fell—I knew instantly that her pregnancy was doomed and she was going to lose her first baby. I sent her to the hospital, and then the cameras caught me in the hallway. She was not a patient on our show, but the crew knew something serious was happening and wanted to catch my reaction on film. I told them that one of my favorite patients was about to lose her twenty-two-week baby and I could do nothing. I then began to cry, explaining that I was now blessed with a beautiful son but had also lost a pregnancy years before. Through my tears, I tried to convey how much I had been affected by my loss and how it gave me empathy for my patients in a similar situation.

Many months later, that first show aired on television. I was getting out of my car in the doctor's parking lot the next morning when Michael, a fellow physician, approached me. He said, "I watched *Deliver Me* with my wife last night, and when you got to the story about the patient losing her baby and you having your miscarriage, my wife also started crying. We lost a baby more than thirteen years ago and have two grown boys now. Until that moment, I had no idea how much it still affected her."

—Yvonne ◀ ◀ ◀

The Difficulties with Infertility

Infertility, especially the in vitro fertilization process, can take a toll on relationships. We've worked with couples who've endured months or years of fertility treatments without getting pregnant, draining both their patience and their finances as they struggled to conceive a baby. Then one day, one or both decides that he or she just can't do it anymore. They decide to take a break for a few months or give up on the idea of parenthood altogether. If both partners agree that this hiatus is needed, it can be a breath of fresh air. Maybe it's time to pursue a new route, such as adoption. But if one wants to take a break and the other wants to continue full steam ahead, a rift can develop. The stress, anger, and frustration test their relationship. Most couples are strong enough to weather this storm, but others can be pulled apart by it.

We strongly recommend that anyone who feels that the path to pregnancy is eroding their relationship should seek counseling from a family therapist. These sessions can help to refocus on what brought you together as a couple in the first place.

Single Motherhood

▶ ▶ ▶ CHOOSING TO GO IT ALONE

One of my patients has an astonishing story. Chloe, a bright, adventurous location manager for feature films, was in her mid- forties and had always wanted to have a baby. She had many long-term relationships during her life, but never found the perfect guy to start a family with. After much reflection about motherhood, she decided to find out how she could pursue this on her own. Considering the option of donor sperm from a sperm bank, Chloe had a consultation with a fertility specialist and learned that she would need donor eggs in addition to donor sperm because of her advanced age. She reconsidered going through IVF and finally reconciled herself to the idea that being a mom was not in the cards for her.

Not long after that, she met Chase on a blind date. They instantly hit it off and started seeing each other regularly. Chloe confided to Chase her disappointment about her meeting with the fertility doctor. Chase assured her that parenthood is not for everyone and that she could have a wonderful life, even without children. Then unpredictably, after dating for two months, Chloe suddenly found herself pregnant.

When they came in to see me, I confirmed the pregnancy and could see that both of them were still in a state of shock. The couple had not been using any birth control because Chloe had believed that she couldn't have a baby because of her age. She was happy but also frightened about the effect this would have on her new relationship. She realized that she barely even knew this guy—they had been dating for only a few months.

Chloe's boyfriend was terrified, too. He wondered if they would even be together to raise the baby and suggested that she consider terminating the pregnancy. Chloe, however, couldn't help but remember how much she had wanted to be a mother, and the lengths to which she'd been willing to go to

have a baby on her own. She decided to continue the pregnancy and not involve her partner. She delivered her healthy daughter, Brittany, at thirty-nine
weeks. With her characteristic courage, she happily embarked on her new journey into motherhood.

—Allison ◀ ◀ ◀

These days, we've found more and more women deciding to keep
and raise babies on their own, without a partner. Some patients are
quite young, even still in their twenties, and feel they are ready, willing, and strong enough to take on the responsibilities of being a single parent. Others are older, more successful women who can
financially sustain themselves, hire child care support, or have the
support of their families. These resources or support systems allow
them to have a baby without a partner.

Other single women who unexpectedly find themselves pregnant—including many who aren't financially well off—may simply
decide that this may be their only opportunity to experience motherhood. They choose to continue a pregnancy by themselves and often
come in to see us with their own mothers by their side for support.

A new baby is a nonstop "needs" machine, and taking care of that
child by yourself can be an overwhelming prospect. In the early days,
sometimes you just need to have someone who can watch the baby so
you can shower or go out for more diapers. You need an external support network in place. Our patients often have a helpful mother, sibling, or close friend to assist them. Ask for help. The saying is true:
Raising a child in this complicated modern world truly does take a
village.

When we think of a single mother, we envision a woman who is
packing a diaper bag, loading the stroller into the car, driving her
child to day care, and trying to get to work on time to concentrate on
the "other" job at hand. She has the usual stresses of life and dozens
of tasks to juggle. How do I do the laundry? When do I pick up the dry
cleaning? What happens if the baby is sick and can't go to day care?
When will I clean the house? What will I do for meals? As her children get older, the questions become more complex. Will I be able to

help them with their homework after a long day at work? How will I manage to pick up my kids from their afterschool activities on time? How do I get them to the doctor?

Single motherhood is easier if you can afford to have help around you all the time. We had one single mom who mapped out her pregnancy years in advance by doing some serious financial planning and money managing. When she gave birth, she was financially prepared to be off work for two years to be a mom full time. Her careful long-term planning paid off and she loves it.

▶ ▶ ▶ GETTING THROUGH HARD TIMES

I recently ran into one of my son's teachers, Leila, who was a single mother for quite a while before recently getting remarried. She is a delightful woman—smart, hard working, and always optimistic. She told me about one memorable incident when her son was a newborn. She was at a fast-food restaurant with her infant son. It was the first time she had ventured out on her own since her delivery. When her order arrived at the pick-up counter, she realized that she had not planned on how she would carry the food, with her son in one arm and a diaper bag and bottle in the other. For some reason, at that moment, she felt very alone, helpless, and overwhelmed and just started crying.

Figuring out how to manage all the routine needs of a baby plus all life's regular chores can be a tough road—with or without a partner. Still, in time, Leila more than managed well. That little infant in the burger joint is a strapping, well-adjusted seventeen-year-old today. Leila is happily remarried with a supportive partner. I loved hearing Leila tell me her story. Despite her struggles as a single parent, her positive, upbeat attitude and sense of humor got her through it all.

When faced with challenges, we may break down for a moment, but we also know that the best way to get through a crisis is to get right back up and keep moving.

—Alane

Kids and Their New Siblings

When a new baby joins a family, reactions differ, especially from the children who are already there. Some kids are excited to have a sibling, but others may be too young to even understand the concept. Still others start off suspicious or resentful. Kids display a wide spectrum of emotions when a new brother or sister arrives.

▶ ▶ ▶ WHERE'S MY BROTHER?

I was taking care of an energetic third-time mom named Kendra. She had two charming boys—Tyler was five and Caleb was three. The boys excitedly accompanied their mom to every prenatal appointment, and at about twenty weeks, everybody was thrilled to learn that there would soon be a third brother joining the family. At each visit, the boys would chatter on and on about their new brother, where he was going to sleep, what games they would play with him, and whether he would prefer Batman over Spiderman.

The day finally arrived when Kendra gave birth to beautiful seven-and-a-half-pound Austin, with her other two boys waiting anxiously in the hallway. Cautiously, they entered the room to meet the new addition to their family—and three-year-old Caleb's face fell with disappointment.

Caleb looked around the room, confused, and then blurted out, "Mom, that's not a brother. That's a baby!"

Kendra laughed as she realized that to Caleb, a new brother was a boy like his brother Tyler. It never occurred to him that his new brother would be a baby!

—Allison ◀ ◀ ◀

The process of introducing a baby into a family begins with the other children first discovering that their mother is pregnant, and continues through the first months after the baby arrives home. Parents might find that they have to deal with jealousy. If they have a two-year-old toddler, he or she might not be able to comprehend exactly what is going on and might erupt into unexplained temper tantrums. Sometimes, these outbursts seem to come out of the blue, but they generally happen because the child senses that their mother can't provide the same level of attention that he or she is used to getting. The important process of smoothing things out with her other children can be another unexpected strain on an already stressed new mom.

We like to offer our patients support in heading off these situations. Many approaches are available. We encourage our moms to bring their children to the prenatal visits with them and let them see the ultrasound of the growing baby in her tummy. The goal is to integrate the children, particularly older siblings, into the entire process. When children feel included, they don't feel as threatened by the changes happening around them.

▶ ▶ ▶ BROTHERLY LOVE

It took my husband and me a long time to conceive a second child. After years of trying, my impatient son Ryan was getting older and anxious for a sibling. Every year, he would list "Baby brother or sister" as the number one item on his Christmas list.

I ultimately went through in vitro fertilization to have a baby. Ryan would come to my ultrasounds with the perinatologist, and everyone would ask Ryan what he wanted, a boy or a girl. He would say, "I don't care, I will be happy with either one." When we discovered that the baby was a girl, he never wavered; he stuck to his guns and said it didn't matter that the baby was a girl. Ryan walked me to the OR when I went to have my cesarean delivery with Kylie, and he was the first person I saw in my recovery room. The first time he laid eyes on Kylie and was able to hold her, he was glowing.

After we were home, however, the days and nights of constant caring for the newborn soon lost their luster. Ryan realized his own needs were not being attended to as quickly as before. He saw that his mommy was spending most of her time with the baby and not with him. After several months, Ryan began to say, "I wish I had a brother instead of a sister."

Our own family story illustrates how even the most supportive sibling can lose his enthusiasm when the reality of life with a newborn sets in. Thankfully, my wonderful husband stepped up to the plate, keeping Ryan busy with sports and other activities, and their bond grew even stronger in the process. Kylie eventually grew and was soon able to show her affection for her big brother. He was the first one she kissed—and many times, he's the only one she will kiss.

—Yvonne ◀ ◀ ◀

Another solution is for parents to have a gift to give to the other children from the new baby, as a housewarming surprise when the baby comes home. Other moms and dads will sit down with their kids and explain that the role of big brother and big sister is one of the most important jobs in the world. Whatever method the parents choose, we want to offer them whatever support they might need from our end.

▶ ▶ ▶ MATTHEW'S TRANSFORMER TRUCK

As I approached my due date with my second son, Max, I recalled all the stories I'd heard from friends and patients about adjustment problems they'd had with a second child. I began to fret about how I would introduce our four-year-old, Matthew, to his new little brother. I turned to Carmen, one of my favorite doulas, for some expert advice.

Carmen counseled me to always keep Matthew involved in the pregnancy and birth, and to never make him feel left out or replaced. She recommended that I install the baby's car seat in the car before Max's arrival, so that Matthew would have a chance to adjust to dealing with the changes that were coming. When Matthew walked into the postpartum room for the first time, she suggested that I not hold the baby in my arms but rather have baby Max in his crib next to me. Then, after Matthew was introduced to the baby, we could hold and touch the baby together.

Carmen also suggested that when family and friends come to visit, they be advised to always address Matthew first, asking, "Can you introduce me to your new baby brother Max?" When a new baby is born, everyone wants to go to the baby, who has no idea what's going on. The older sibling does, however, and can sense that attention is now being taken away from him or her.

I also got a gift, a Transformer toy truck for Matthew. It was wrapped and given to Matthew as a gift from his little brother, Max. Matthew was ecstatic. To my surprise, when we saw the truck reappear several years later, Matthew exclaimed, "Look mom, there's the truck Max gave me when he was born!" My two boys have their moments, believe me, but Carmen's pearls of wisdom helped our family make a healthy transition from three to four.

—Alane ◀ ◀ ◀

We have written about how your firstborn will adjust to the second child, but we haven't forgotten about you. Many patients wonder how they will adjust as moms to having a second child. You may wonder, "How could I possibly love another child as much as I love this first one?" You will be surprised by how much love you have to give. Or you'll ask yourself, "How will I have time to pay attention to both?" We still grapple with these issues now, as moms and as career women. The juggling is the biggest challenge we face every day. However, our children learn to be loving and tolerant. They discover how to deal with disagreements, how to share, and how to voice their wants and needs. They learn these important life lessons not only from their mom and dads but also from their siblings.

Parents, In-Laws, and Other Interested Parties

Extended families are an important part of many of our deliveries. As doctors, we walk a fine line between making sure the families are happy and advocating for our patients. Our job is about being there for the mother, so if a family issue is causing stress for our patient, we try to help her avoid that stress if possible.

It's always an adventure for us to walk into a labor and delivery room, wondering who's going to be along with us for the ride. Most of the time, we see the partner and maybe one other support person, such as a doula, mom, sister, or best friend. Sometimes, we find ourselves entering what feels like a big party, with both sets of parents, a passel of siblings, friends, and sometimes even office mates. Seeing the amount of support and bonding that the arrival of a new life can bring is nice, but sometimes our patients may be overwhelmed by the number of bodies in the room. However, if you are okay with having lots of support, of course we're going to welcome it. If you start to feel that the festival atmosphere is causing you stress, let us know and we can assist you in paring things to make you more comfortable. We are all for family support, but our first and foremost concern is mom.

Many of our patients have mothers who want to be involved in the pregnancy from beginning to end. Thankfully, often a mother is a great help and support. In the majority of cases we've seen, the soon-to-be grandmas and even our patients' mothers-in-law offer comfort and cheerleading in the delivery room.

Some mother-daughter relationships or in-law relationships, however, are fraught with tension. We've seen some mothers or mothers-in-law act controlling. These women want to help; perhaps they genuinely believe that they really do have all the answers, because they had a baby themselves. Many of our patients become even more anxious and stressed when their own moms or mothers-in-law insist on being in the picture.

Unfortunately, sometimes grandmas-to-be can cause more conflict than goodwill, especially at the time of the actual delivery. Perhaps they are afraid for their child or don't trust the doctors. Or maybe an unhealthy dynamic exists between the mother and the daughter that prevents the daughter from relaxing. For example, we've seen a grandma-to-be refuse to allow her daughter to get an epidural because she herself didn't have one. In these cases, the pregnant woman will actually send her own mom home or request that she wait in the waiting area because she's adding more stress to the situation. In other cases, a mother-in-law is being a liability. The birth day will be a stressful day in any case. If anyone in the room is making it more so, we think it's better that he or she go home or spend some time somewhere outside the labor and delivery room.

Patients with divorced parents can also present a challenge. Imagine a grandfather-to-be and grandmother-to-be, both waiting expectantly for their new grandchild, neither having spoken a civil word to the other in ten years. These kinds of volatile family dynamics don't make a soon-to-be-mom's job—or ours—any easier. On the positive side, we've seen many wonderful occasions in which a new baby served to bring a fractured family together.

If you are experiencing discomfort with your mom or mother-in-law in the room, ask your doctor or nurse to step in. We can say, "As Susan's doctor, I think it's best that only her husband be in the room with her." It's important for mothers, fathers, and others to realize that every pregnancy is different and every labor is different. Just because it went a certain way for you doesn't mean it's going to be the same for your daughter.

Having a Sick Baby or Special Needs Child

▶ ▶ ▶ A LIFE-CHANGING DELIVERY DAY

I have had several first-time parents who decided not to do genetic screening tests because they knew that they would continue the pregnancy no matter what. Pamela was a thirty-year-old literary agent and her husband, Bradley, was an advertising executive. Their pregnancy was perfect. Pamela had an ultrasound at twenty weeks, and they learned they were having a baby boy.

Pamela was less nervous about her baby than she was about the family dynamics that would be at play during the birth. Her mom and dad had a bitter divorce and were both remarried. They had not spoken in more than ten years and had a nightmarish encounter at Pamela's wedding. For the delivery, they both insisted on coming into town and being there when the baby was born. Because Pamela had experienced the uncomfortable tension between them for most of her life, she was stressed about the potential fireworks.

During labor, both grandparents were present with their new spouses—keeping on opposite sides of the room. Serious tension was in the air. Pamela pushed for about two hours until she finally delivered her little boy, Troy. When he was born, just Pamela and Bradley were in the room. Because of the length of time the mom had pushed, the baby's face was swollen, making his features hard to distinguish. Still, when I handed the baby to the nurse, I immediately noticed something different. I tried to tell myself that the lighting in the room made me see an unusual shadow and abnormal swelling in the baby's face.

As soon as mom was cleaned up, all the new grandparents came into the room. They passed the baby around—still keeping to their own sides of the room—and oohed and aahed about how beautiful he was and how happy they were to be grandparents.

Every time I glanced at the baby, I was more convinced that he had Down syndrome. I asked another experienced obstetric nurse to look at the baby to confirm my suspicions, which she did. Finally, I heard one of the grandmothers say "look how cute—he's sticking out his tongue." I knew the diagnosis was correct at that moment. Down's babies often stick out their tongues because they are larger than normal.

I went outside and sat down at the nurses' station to figure out how I was going to break the news to this family, who seemed to be tolerating each other for the first time in years. I went back in the room and sat down on the bed with Pamela. The baby was still making the rounds with the grandparents. I quietly told her that there was something different about the baby's features—that I thought he may have Down's. Pamela looked at me like I was crazy. She told her family to be quiet and pass her the baby. She looked into his face and saw it. She quietly started to cry.

Her parents came to her side—and now saw what she saw. Some cried; some were quiet. But most importantly, the air had changed. They weren't fighting. The tension was gone. They all agreed to do whatever it took to take care of their special baby boy. In his first moments of life, baby Troy had already brought a long-divided family together.

A follow-up: Not only did Troy repair the dynamics of his grandparents' relationships, he also profoundly changed his mother's quality of life as well. After Troy was born, Pamela quit her job at the literary agency and joined the board of the Special Olympics. She said she had been looking for a reason to get out of the rat race and was now so grateful that her life could be devoted to something more meaningful.

The entire family is now united and happy, and Troy has the best possible extended network of parents and grandparents to help raise him.

—Allison ◀ ◀ ◀

When asked whether they desire a boy or a girl, nearly every set of newly pregnant parents tells us, "We don't really care. We just want a healthy baby." This is the universal wish of every mom and dad. Happily, only a very small percentage of babies are born with birth defects or with some sort of an illness or chromosomal abnormality, such as Down syndrome. But despite the fact that the majority of babies are born healthy, some babies will inevitably come into the world with an illness, a birth defect, or a condition that requires short- or long-term medical care. Even if a mother lives in a bubble during her pregnancy, breathing filtered air, eating only organic foods, with a personal yoga teacher guiding her every movement, in some cases, we cannot prevent a child from being born with special needs.

We have a helpless feeling when we deliver a baby that we know will require lots of medical care, but we are consistently impressed with how the parents of these babies rise to the occasion. Under these trying circumstances, we have seen so many ordinary moms and dads gather their strength, faith, and the circle of support around them and become almost heroic. We are always amazed at the amount of inner strength moms will muster for their children, even under the most devastating circumstances.

Discovering that your child has a serious medical condition, either during pregnancy or after birth, can be overwhelming. If you find yourself in this situation, educate yourself and your family about the latest medical advances. Make sure to reach out for help—seek family support services and a team of medical specialists to assist you. Most important of all, remember that you can never give your baby too much love.

▶ ▶ ▶ MY CHILD NEEDS ME

Camille is a physician by training, an amazing woman who gave up her career to raise her children. She comes from a long line of doctors, as does her husband and his family. I am so grateful to her for sharing her story with us here. No matter how many times I read this, I feel a surge of emotion. Camille captures the essence of what it means to be a mother:

"Two and a half hours from my first contraction, our daughter is born. She comes with a fierce determination, and we are so full of joy to see her beautiful face. My husband and I can't wait to introduce her to her five-year-old big brother.

"The next morning, our family practice doctor comes in to do a well-baby check. I see her face change. She is no longer playing with the baby but has gone into examination mode. And the first tears of many start to come. I ask her to tell me straight on what she is seeing.

"She says, 'I think your daughter may have trisomy 21.'

"When I see my husband, he says, 'There is no way that she has anything wrong with her. Just look at her face.' He is right; I do not see the characteristic facial features present in children with Down syndrome.

"The day is full of doctors and nurses who are now talking in quiet tones and explaining that our daughter must undergo testing, the first of which is a blood draw to do chromosomal testing. This test will give us a definitive answer in ten to twelve days. If they are not sure, surely there is reason to hope.

"Our hope dangles by a thread until our daughter gets so sick that they have to take her to the NICU and hook her up to machines that will keep her alive. We held out that hope right up until the moment that her neonatologist takes us aside and says she is certain that our daughter has Down syndrome.

"For a moment, I feel a rush of pure, unadulterated hate for the woman who gives me this news. And then she tells me that our daughter needs us.

"Our daughter *needs* us.

"Those four simple words change our lives in an instant. They kill our self-pity and turn our attention to our daughter. She didn't ask this to happen to her. She is relying on us to love, nourish, and raise her, and help her reach her full potential. Now the new question becomes, 'Will we be enough for her?'

"I would like to report that everything has been a smooth ride from that moment on, but the truth is, we have experienced many more tears and sleepless nights. We have faced challenges with her health, her school, and her community. But the more important truth is this: My daughter taught me to draw on reserves of strength I did not know I had.

"She turned seven yesterday. She is in first grade with her peers and gets support in areas where she needs it. She is bubbly, sweet, strong, kind—and even a little bit mischievous. And she is determined to accomplish the things she desires.

"Her gift to us is her enduring sense of herself. She knows who she is and she is content, happy, and loved. We can only strive to be the best we can be for her. Our daughter needs us, and she deserves no less."

—Alane ◀ ◀ ◀

Work-Related Issues

When it comes to workplace issues, we've seen a variety of scenarios. Some women have nurturing bosses or work in a supportive atmosphere with coworkers who are willing to fill in as needed. Each time one of the three of us had a baby, we could rest easily, knowing our professional partners, colleagues, and staff were standing by to support us in any area where we needed help.

Unfortunately, some of our patients face the opposite. These patients tell us that their work lives are miserable. Their bosses don't want to change their duties or don't understand why they're tired and can't push themselves to work the hours they used to. We've even had patients who needed to start antidepressants due to work-related issues. Some professional environments still discourage pregnant women from leaving in the middle of the day to go to their prenatal appointments. The boss gets upset and the mom-to-be gets stressed out, which is the last thing she needs.

In some situations, a pregnant woman is discriminated against by her boss or coworkers. Maybe they won't let her take a full lunch break, or they won't let her sit down or use the bathroom as frequently as she needs to. We often counsel patients to open up and discuss their feelings and difficulties with their bosses or colleagues. It may take courage, but many women are pleasantly surprised at the results when they address concerns face to face.

If you are going through significant workplace problems, talk to your obstetrician or midwife. We may be able to send a letter to your employer with a list of restrictions such as the following:

> No lifting of more than twenty-five pounds.
> Take time for more frequent bathroom breaks.
> If you sit or stand for long periods, change your position every two hours.

In addition, you can discuss your concerns with a member of your company's human resources department, who may be able to make your job environment more manageable.

Because every employment situation and every pregnancy is different, you need to decide what's best for you. Certain things about pregnancy are truly beyond your control—or your doctor's. Although you may want to keep your pregnancy private until you know that everything is all right, it may be helpful for management to know why you are going to the bathroom every hour or why you keep vomiting into your trash can.

For moms who have jobs where they need to sit or stand most of the day, our recommendation is similar to the one we give women who go on long airplane trips. If you sit or stand for a long time, you increase the risk of developing blood clots. We advise pregnant patients to change their positions roughly every two hours, for a few minutes duration each time. If they're standing, they need to sit down for a few minutes every hour. This is particularly true for jobs such as cashier or counter clerk, where women stand in one place for most of the day. In addition, consider wearing support stocking if you are on your feet all day.

Our Final Words to You

Pregnancy, labor, delivery, and the aftermath can be overwhelming. As moms, each one of us has been through it twice, and found it both the hardest and best thing we've ever accomplished: harder than the intensive study of med school, the pressures of internship, and even the impossible hours of residency. But the rewards are indescribable. The miracle of life and the transformation from person into parent can't truly be understood until someone has gone through it herself. You are forever changed when you become a mom. The road can be rough and rocky, but the destination is always worth it.

What we'd like you to take away from this book is a sense of comfort and security. Pregnancy and raising a baby afterward can be a joyful journey if you follow the right guidelines, connect with a good support system, and find the right doctor or midwife to entrust with your questions, concerns, and fears. Even if you are high risk, with the proper care you can have the outcome you desire: a healthy you and a healthy baby.

We knew that writing this book together would be a challenging experience, but it didn't occur to us that it would be an emotional one as well. When writing something about our personal experiences or relaying one of our patient's stories, we often found our eyes welling up with tears as we typed. Once again, we are reminded of how fortunate we are to be able to do this job. We love what we do. Our jobs are personal on so many levels, especially because we've been on both sides—as doctors and as patients, moms, and women. We'd like to think that we get it, or at least, we try hard to. Aside from the hectic, unpredictable schedule, we can't imagine a better job.

chapter eleven

FREQUENTLY ASKED QUESTIONS AND FREQUENTLY REPEATED MYTHS

ONE OF THE GREAT THINGS about being in practice together is having the opportunity to compare notes. Over the last fifteen years, we've noticed a number of questions and concerns that we hear repeatedly from our pregnant patients, sometimes several times a week. We also hear a lot of misleading pseudo-information and myths echoed repeatedly. We've compiled a list of these questions and myths that are clearly on the minds of pregnant moms. Most of the items in this section are covered in greater depth elsewhere in the book.

Getting Pregnant

Do birth control pills cause birth defects?
No studies link birth control use to birth defects, even if a woman is taking birth control pills before she discovers she is pregnant.

Must my system be cleansed of birth control hormones before I conceive?

You do not need to wait after you stop the pill before you conceive. As soon as you take your placebo pills, the pill is out of your system and you can get pregnant that next cycle. (See Chapter 1, page 33.)

Can you get pregnant while breastfeeding?

When you are breastfeeding exclusively, at least eight times a day, it is hard but not impossible to get pregnant. The hormonal changes associated with nursing—specifically, the production of a hormone called prolactin—prevent ovulation. But as soon as you start to breastfeed less, your prolactin levels drop and you might start to ovulate again. We always recommend that people use a contraceptive method during this time. (See Chapter 7, page 296.)

Is it harder to get pregnant after a miscarriage?

One long-standing myth is that if you have a miscarriage, you should wait for six months or a year to conceive again. After you have had a

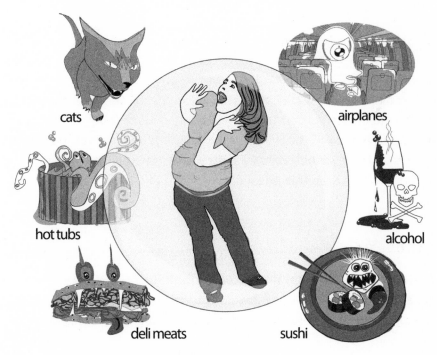

cats

airplanes

hot tubs

alcohol

deli meats

sushi

Figure 11-1: Scary Myths

normal menstrual cycle, the uterus has healed and can accept a new pregnancy. No medical reason exists for waiting, but some women may not be emotionally ready to try again and may benefit from a short break. (See Chapter 8, page 362.)

If you've had a cesarean delivery, when can you get pregnant again?

If you've had a cesarean and want a vaginal birth with your next baby, you may want to space the pregnancies so the babies are at least eighteen months apart. The risk of uterine rupture during VBAC is three times higher if the previous cesarean was less than eighteen months ago.[1] If you are planning a repeat cesarean, however you do not need to wait to get pregnant. As soon as you feel well enough, you can start trying again.

I was told I have a tipped or tilted uterus and will not be able to get pregnant. Is that true?

The position of your uterus has nothing to do with fertility or your ability to conceive. (See Chapter 8, page 350.)

Pregnancy Symptoms

When can I find out if I'm having a boy or girl?

You can discover the gender of your baby at around twenty weeks by ultrasound and slightly earlier if you do genetic testing. (See Chapter 4, page 153.) How you carry the baby, how you feel, what kind of food you are craving, or how fast the baby's heart rate is will not give you a definitive answer to this question.

How much should I weigh during pregnancy?

In a perfect world, a mom-to-be will start her pregnancy near her ideal body weight. Maternal obesity is linked to many pregnancy and birth complications and may effect her child long term. An average-weight woman should gain twenty-five to thirty-five pounds during the forty weeks. This weight gain can be accomplished by adding 300 extra calories per day. (See Chapter 2, page 56.)

I'm pregnant but I'm not feeling sick. Is this normal?

Usually during the first trimester, people ask us if it is normal to feel normal. The answer is yes—feeling okay doesn't mean anything is wrong. Some women just get lucky and have few or no pregnancy symptoms. However, if you have severe symptoms that disappear suddenly, something could be wrong with the pregnancy. If your doctor gives you a clean bill of health, we tell our moms that it can be normal not to feel anything. (See Chapter 3, page 114.)

How long does morning sickness last?

At the twelve-week mark, most women's symptoms of nausea will improve. Nausea is linked to hCG levels, which peak at ten weeks and then decline. (See Chapter 3, page 106.)

Can the baby move too much?

No, your baby cannot move too much. Often, women become concerned when the baby begins moving all of a sudden, as if he or she is in pain or distress, is having a seizure, or is struggling to get out. An active baby just means the baby is getting the necessary oxygen and nutrition. With some moms, extra movement might be a response to being cramped in a very small space and needing to shift position to move an elbow or a knee. Also, babies develop hiccups in the last trimester, which can also feel like frequent, regular, rhythmic movements. All these patterns of movement are normal. (See Chapter 5, page 174.)

If my husband or I were big babies, does that mean I will have a big baby?

Whether or not you will have a big baby depends on many factors. Yes, part of it is genetics, but not necessarily related to how much you weighed when you were born. However, if you or your husband are tall adults, you may have a larger baby. Following are other factors that are just as important:

- How much weight have you gained during the pregnancy? A weight gain of more than thirty-five pounds is associated with larger babies.

- Do you have diabetes? Both pregestational and gestational diabetes have the potential to raise your blood sugar. In turn, the baby's blood sugar is higher so the baby will grow larger in uncontrolled diabetes.
- Will you deliver before or after the due date? A longer time pregnant means the baby can grow larger.
- Is this your first baby? Second and third babies tend to be larger than the first. The uterus becomes more efficient with a better blood supply if you've been pregnant before.
- Are you having a boy or girl? In general, boys are larger at birth than girls.

How do you know the baby is okay on the inside by checking it on the outside?

We can evaluate your baby in several ways. By the end of the second trimester, the simplest way is to observe the baby's movements. We teach our patients how to assess the movements by fetal kick counts (see page 174). We follow fetal growth with fundal height measurements. In high-risk pregnancies and during labor, your baby will be monitored by a non-stress test, or NST (see page 373) to make sure he is getting all the nutrients and oxygen on the inside.

Why do I get dizzy?

During pregnancy, your blood vessels are more dilated so more blood is in your legs and less flows to your brain, causing dizziness, lightheadedness, or even fainting. These symptoms are normal. If changing positions quickly exacerbates dizziness, get up slowly when moving from a lying down or sitting position to a standing position. Also make sure that you are well hydrated, your blood sugar isn't low, and you are not becoming anemic. Your doctor should check you if you have severe or persistent dizziness. (See Chapter 3, page 109.)

What are these painful hot areas on my belly?

As the uterus and the belly start growing, some women can get painful, burning, or tingling areas on their skin, usually on their belly.

This condition is a neuropathy, in which a nerve is being pinched or stretched by the growing uterus. The painful area usually persists a few weeks, until the baby grows and moves off the nerve. (See Chapter 5, page 180.)

Why do my hands get numb?

In the late second or third trimester, extra fluid in a woman's body compresses the nerves in her hands and arms and can cause a carpal tunnel–like reaction. This form of neuropathy can be worse in women who have jobs that require a lot of repetitive hand motion, such as typing on a keyboard. One way to alleviate this condition is to wear hand splints at night, which keep the wrist straight and allow excess fluid to drain out of the joints. These symptoms usually go away when the extra fluid in the body is excreted postpartum. (See Chapter 5, page 180.)

Is it okay to sleep on my back?

A persistent pregnancy myth that scares many women is that they will harm their babies if they sleep on their backs. A major blood vessel (vena cava) runs along the right side of your vertebral column (your backbone), and as the baby gets bigger and your uterus expands, the combined weight can compress that vessel. Theoretically, it could inhibit blood flow back to the heart and then back to the uterus. But this shouldn't be a problem if your baby is small (even at thirty weeks, the baby weighs only about three pounds).

We have never seen a baby hurt by a mother sleeping on her back. We tell our moms that if they wake up in the middle of the night and are on their backs, don't panic. Just turn over on your side, preferably the *left* side because the vena cava runs along the right side. A long body pillow or a regular pillow can help angle your body in that direction. Toward the end of the pregnancy, as the baby gets larger and the weight of the baby and uterus become greater, laying flat often may make you a bit nauseous or will cause you some difficulty with breathing. Your body is giving its own direction to you, telling you to turn over on your side.

Foods and Medications

How much caffeine can I have?

You don't need to eliminate caffeine, but limit yourself to two hundred milligrams a day, which is approximately one cup of coffee. Caffeine increases your heart rate. When you're pregnant, you already have a higher heart rate than normal, so adding caffeine can cause palpitations (a racing heart). One study indicated higher miscarriage rates in women consuming a lot of caffeine, but that study is still being debated.[2] And caffeine does not cause birth defects. (See Chapter 2, page 75.)

Can I eat deli meats?

Bacteria called Listeria can be potentially harmful to a developing fetus, resulting in miscarriage and stillbirth. If deli meats are heated to 160 degrees, which kills any Listeria infection, they are considered safe. Listeria infections are extremely rare, with about three cases per million people each year in the United States. (See Chapter 2, page 73.)

What types of cheese should I avoid?

You should avoid unpasteurized and soft cheeses such brie, feta, blue cheese, and Mexican cheese because of potential Listeria contamination. These cheeses are okay if they are made with pasteurized milk or are cooked. (See Chapter 2, page 72.)

Is it safe to eat hot dogs?

You may eat hot dogs as long as they are cooked to over 160 degrees. The fear about eating hot dogs concerns bacterial contamination, such as Listeria, and nitrate concentrations. If the hot dog is cooked, the bacteria will be killed. In addition, no studies in humans show that nitrates in hot dogs are associated with any birth defects. (See Chapter 2, page 73.)

Can I safely eat sushi?

You can eat sushi if you follow several precautions. First, avoid fish high in mercury: shark, tilefish, swordfish, and mackerel. Limit your intake of albacore (white) tuna to one six-ounce servings per week. Raw fish, like any other uncooked food (including meats, fruits and vegetables), can carry bacteria and parasites. Sushi in the United States is flash frozen to kill parasites. Bacterial infections such as Listeria can occur but the incidence is extremely low (three people per million). According to the Center for Evidence Based Medicine, "there is no conclusive evidence in published literature that eating sushi in pregnancy has an adverse effect on the pregnancy." (See Chapter 2, page 74.)

Can I eat honey while I'm pregnant?

One interesting myth states that babies can't digest honey, so the mother shouldn't eat it. Please remember, your unborn baby isn't digesting anything. You are. The fetus is simply receiving the nutrients from what you've already eaten, filtered through the placenta. So you can put honey in your tea without fearing that it will harm your unborn baby.

Do I need to stop drinking alcohol?

According to the American College of Obstetrics and Gynecology, no amount of alcohol has been proven safe during pregnancy. However, recent data from a study published in the *Journal of Epidemiology and Community Health* suggests that moderate alcohol consumption—*only one or two drinks per week*—will not hurt a fetus. On the other hand, excessive alcohol consumption while pregnant causes fetal alcohol syndrome, which is serious and results in developmental problems and birth defects.[3] Our personal and professional opinion about this issue is to take the conservative approach and not to drink alcohol at all while you're pregnant. (See Chapter 1, page 75.)

Will taking antidepressants harm my baby?

Most antidepressants can be taken safely in pregnancy. Previous data linked antidepressants to a rare birth defect, but that finding has been refuted. If a woman cannot function without antidepressants, we believe that the risk to the mom of not taking antidepressants is greater than any risk to the baby. Deciding whether to take antidepressants is something that should be worked out between you, your obstetrician, and your psychiatrist or general physician. (See Chapter 1, page 27.)

What medications are okay if I get a headache or a cold?

We recommend over-the-counter acetaminophen (Tylenol), pseudo-ephedrine (Sudafed), dextromethorphan (Robitussin), or antihista-mines (Benadryl) during your pregnancy for headaches or a cold. Avoid medications containing ibuprofen (such as Motrin, Advil, Aleve). See Figure 1-1 on page 28 for a list of medications that are safe and unsafe.

Activities

Will petting a cat hurt my fetus?

Nothing is wrong with touching or playing with cats. However, *you must avoid changing the cat litter box.* Cats come into contact with the parasite Toxoplasma, usually from eating an infected rat or mouse, and that parasite is excreted through cat feces. If the pregnant mom touches or inhales cat excrement, she can be exposed to the parasite and pass it to the baby, causing miscarriage, stillbirth, blindness, or mental retardation. According to the Center for Disease Control, of the four million babies born annually, about two thousand are af-fected with congenital toxoplasmosis.[4] (See Chapter 2, page 85.)

When is it safe to travel during my pregnancy?

Travel by car or plane is safe throughout pregnancy. Flying does not cause miscarriage or birth defects. Because plane cabins are pressur-ized, the altitude is not dangerous to your baby. Whether you're trav-eling in a plane, bus, train, or car, however, sitting for long periods of time can cause blood clots to form in the legs. Pregnant women are more susceptible to blood clots because of their added pregnancy weight and elevated hormone levels. We recommend wearing support stockings and walking around to stretch your legs every two hours.

We don't recommend that women—especially high-risk moms—travel too far from their obstetrician, midwife, or hospital as they ap-proach their due date. The possibility of premature birth, although remote, means that after the twenty-fourth week, you'll want to be near a place with a NICU and the proper care. (See Chapter 5, page 190.)

Can I exercise during my pregnancy?

If you're fit and have been working out on a regular basis before pregnancy, you can continue to exercise. If you do cardiovascular exercises, get a heart rate monitor and make sure that your heartrate is less than 140 beats per minute to ensure that blood isn't shunted to your working muscles and away from your uterus and baby. Be cautious with certain types of exercise, such as jumping or any other physical activity where you could fall or injure yourself and the baby. If you were sedentary before pregnancy, stick to light exercise such as long walks or prenatal yoga. You should aim to exercise thirty minutes per day, five times per week. (See Chapter 2, page 76.)

How can I strengthen my back?

For back strengthening, we recommend prenatal yoga. (See Chapter 2, page 78.)

Can I use a steam room or hot tub?

Studies have linked extreme heat exposure during pregnancy with birth defects such as spina bifida. The American College of Obstetricians and Gynecologists recommends that pregnant women avoid hot tubs, saunas, or steam rooms where the temperatures are above 102.2 degrees. (See Chapter 2, page 83.)

Can I have sex while I am pregnant?

The answer is an enthusiastic yes—right up until the end, in fact—unless your doctor advises against it or you have a high-risk condition such as placenta previa, premature rupture of membranes, or preterm labor, where sexual intercourse could be dangerous. (See Chapter 2, page 87.)

Can I perm, color, or highlight my hair? Get manicures and pedicures?

No evidence exists that exposure to any of these products causes birth defects. Many women have had hair and nail treatments when they didn't know they were pregnant, with no consequence for the baby. (See Chapter 2, page 84.)

Do I need to worry about dry cleaning chemicals?

It is fine to dry clean your clothes. Dry cleaning chemicals have not been studied in extensive scientific trials, but at this point, you are in no obvious danger from casual exposure to these chemicals.

What can happen to a baby if the mom has a car accident or falls?

Falling down is common during pregnancy. Women may find they lose their balance easily or can't see their feet and miss a step. Usually, falling on your bottom or side won't hurt the baby because it is well protected behind the thick muscular wall of the uterus. Likewise, a minor fender-bender usually won't hurt the baby. However, if you fall directly on your abdomen or are in a more serious car accident in which your abdomen hits the steering wheel, the air bag deploys, or the abdomen is squeezed by the lap belt, you must be evaluated in the hospital. Direct abdominal trauma can cause the placenta to detach from the uterus (placental abruption). This condition is usually accompanied by pain and bleeding. Similarly, a fall from a high distance, such as from a horse, or a kick or punch to the stomach can be dangerous to your baby, and you should be evaluated by your doctor.

Whether the accident is slight or severe, it's always important to check in with your doctor—better safe than sorry. (See Chapter 2, page 89.)

Can I have an X-ray while pregnant?

You should have a CT scan or X-rays if medically necessary to diagnose an illness or injury. For example, a general surgeon may order a CT scan to determine whether a pregnant mom has appendicitis. Obstetric ultrasounds and MRIs do not use radiation, so they are safe at all times. (See Chapter 2, page 89.)

Is it safe to be around computers while pregnant?

There is no evidence that being in close proximity to a computer will harm your baby. If you need to use a laptop, we recommend placing it on a table or using a barrier between your skin and the computer so that the abdomen doesn't overheat.

Are microwaves bad for my baby?

No medical evidence exists that microwaves are harmful for you or your baby. Microwaves do not contain radiation. They use a high-frequency wave, much like a radio signal, to move the water molecules in your food, causing friction and heat. They do not change the molecular structure of your food and won't damage your baby either.

What about dental work while I'm pregnant?

Most dental work and procedures, including teeth cleaning, cavity filling, and root canals, are safe in pregnancy. You can even get an X-ray if necessary if you wear the lead shield over your abdomen. Using local anesthesia, such as novacaine, is safe as well. For postprocedure pain, you can take Tylenol. Antibiotics such as penicillin and cephalosporins are also safe. (See Chapter 2, page 84.)

Labor and Delivery

Will I be having my baby normally (vaginal, head-down delivery)?

The short answer is, we don't know yet. The birth route is based on a number of factors, including the size of the baby, its position in the uterus and birth canal, the effectiveness of the contractions in opening the cervix, and whether or not the mother has any complications that might render a vaginal birth dangerous. Usually we don't know how the baby will be born until the very end of the pregnancy. (See Chapter 5, page 200.)

My baby already dropped, so will I deliver early?

The exact time that labor begins is not related to the position of your baby inside your body. Babies may drop earlier if you have had babies before or if your abdominal muscles are more lax. (See Chapter 5, page 214.)

Can I figure out when my labor will start?

We still don't completely understand the cascade of events that lead up to the start of labor, so we cannot pinpoint the day that it will begin. The due date is merely an estimate, with 80 percent of mothers delivering in the five weeks surrounding the magical date. (See Chapter 3, page 101.)

How do I know if my baby has the umbilical cord wrapped around his or her neck?

You may not know if the baby has the cord around its neck until birth, leaving many women worried that something bad will happen to the baby or that they may need a cesarean delivery. The truth is that 25 percent of babies have the cord around the neck at the time of delivery. The cord is long and the uterus is small, so a wrapped cord happens easily.

Sometimes, an ultrasound can show whether the cord is wrapped around the neck or another body part, but the baby usually changes position and corrects the situation between ultrasound and delivery. Plus we cannot do anything about a twisted cord in utero. In most cases, moms go on to have natural births without any problem, but some babies do end up needing to be delivered by cesarean. (See Chapter 5, page 201.)

Is it better to have an episiotomy than to tear when you're giving birth?

For most women, natural stretching and tearing is preferred. In the past, the standard was for everybody to get an episiotomy, but recent studies prove that spontaneous lacerations heal just as well, if not better, than episiotomies. The blood supply to that area is ample, so healing is surprisingly rapid. (See Chapter 6, page 247.)

Why did my legs become swollen after delivery?

Pregnancy causes an increase of blood and fluid volume in the body. A large percentage of this blood is coursing through the uterine blood vessels to feed your baby. After the baby and placenta are delivered, the excess fluid has nowhere else to go, so it leaks into your tissues. Walking around generally helps to squeeze the fluid out of the soft tissue and back into the bloodstream, but often, a woman's legs stay swollen for a few weeks. (See Chapter 7, page 295.)

Why is my hair falling out after the birth of my baby?

About three months after delivery, some moms will experience the postpartum effluvium, which is a fancy way of saying hair loss. Women describe their hair coming out in clumps or finding their brush full of hair. This phenomenon has nothing to do with whether or not you're getting enough vitamins, as many believe. The stress your body goes through during labor causes more hair to move from the growth phase into the resting phase, resulting in hair loss. The postpartum effluvium is temporary and does not require treatment.

Frequently Repeated Myths

When our patients come to us with questions, they sometimes come in the form of urban legends, old wives' tales, and myths. In this section, we list the ones we hear most often. Nothing would please us more than to put these myths to rest once and for all.

First babies always come late.
We hear lots of rumors about due dates. The due date is just an estimate. Only *5 percent of babies* are born on their due date. The due date is set at 280 days (40 weeks) from the first day of the last period, approximately 256 days from conception.

Like the peak on a bell curve, most deliveries are clustered around the due date, but there will always be outliers. Anytime from thirty-seven weeks to forty-two weeks is considered full-term. Whether you were born late or early or whether your sister delivered early doesn't matter. When the baby comes depends on that specific baby. The only pattern we sometimes see is that women who deliver late tend to be late with each baby, and if you are early, you may be early with each baby. (See Chapter 5, page 213.)

You can tell if you're having a boy or girl by your belly shape.
The myth goes like this: You will have a girl if you are carrying your baby wide, and a boy if you are carrying the baby low. There's no truth to either. Or rather, due to the law of averages, you could say it will be true about 50 percent of the time!

The way that you carry a baby has nothing to do with the sex of the baby. It just has to do with your anatomy and the way the baby positions itself when you're carrying.

If you are vomiting or having bad heartburn a lot, you will have a hairy baby.

In one small study of 64 pregnant women, heartburn was linked to hairy babies. But we haven't seen this correlation in our practice and our informal studies! (See Chapter 4, page 149.)

Certain foods will help induce labor.

An urban legend in Los Angeles is that a certain Tujunga Village restaurant serves a salad with a balsamic vinaigrette that magically helps to induce labor. If you go to this restaurant, you will most certainly see a number of pregnant women (some of them from our practice) eating salads. Although this rumor undoubtedly increased sales of "The Salad," no food has been proven to induce labor. (See Chapter 6, page 249.)

Don't wear high heels when you're pregnant

High heels are absolutely okay to wear. We have yet to see any studies to confirm the claim that high heels contribute to varicose veins, either. As obstetricians, we're more concerned about the fact that as you get more and more pregnant, your center of gravity changes and you become less steady on your heels. We tell patients that if they are going to wear high heels, just be careful not to fall.

Don't raise your arms over your head, especially in the later months, because you could strangle the baby with the umbilical cord.

Some of our patients have also been told that they shouldn't stretch or bend, for the same reason. If stretching or bending were actually dangerous, our hunter-gatherer ancestors would have been in big trouble. A mother's bodily movement does not affect what's going on inside her uterus. You wouldn't believe how many times we hear things like this! (See Chapter 5, page 201.)

Cocoa butter prevents stretch marks.

If only this myth were true. No cream can prevent stretch marks; their formation mostly has to do with a woman's collagen and how well the skin stretches, which is usually a genetic issue. Cocoa butter is a great moisturizer, but like all creams, it does not get absorbed into the dermis, which is where stretch marks occur. Some women get a red, itchy rash in the third trimester from rubbing too much cocoa butter on their bellies.

If your mother had an easy pregnancy and delivery, so will you.
Sorry, no. But the good news is, it goes the other way, too: If your mom had a hard time delivering you, you won't necessarily have a rocky pregnancy.

A special brand of over-the-counter test guarantees it will tell me the gender of my baby by ten weeks of pregnancy.
Even a broken watch is right twice a day, and any gender test will be right 50 percent of the time. As of this writing, no 100 percent reliable over-the-counter gender tests are on the market.

Due to changes in gravitational pull, more spontaneous births occur when the moon is full.
The phases of the moon do not relate to the onset of labor. An analysis of thousands of patients found that birthdays were evenly distributed among all days of the lunar cycle.

If you look at a woman from behind and cannot tell that she's pregnant, she's having a boy. If she's carrying "wide on the side," she's having a girl.
Hilarious ... and wrong.

notes

chapter 1

1. Centrum Vitamins. http://www.centrum.com/productdetail.aspx?brand productid=40 (accessed October 5, 2010).

2. S. G. Gabbe, J. R. Niebyl, and J. L. Simpson, *Obstetrics: Normal and Problem Pregnancies* (Philadelphia: Churchill Livingstone Elsevier, 2007): 1134.

3. B. Jeffreys, "Maternal deaths linked to obesity," *BBC News* (December 4, 2007). http://news.bbc.co.uk/2/hi/health/7121566.stm (accessed February 4, 2011).

4. F. G. Cunningham, K. J. Leveno, S. L. Bloom, et al., *Williams Obstetrics,* 23rd ed. (New York: McGraw Hill, 2010): 1167.

5. K. Dow, J. R. Harris, C. Roy, "Pregnancy after breast-conserving surgery and radiation therapy for breast cancer," *Journal of the National Cancer Institute Monographs* 16 (1994): 131–137.

6. "Pregnancy and the Drug Dilemma." *FDA Consumer* magazine, 35 (May–June 2001). http://www.perinatology.com/Archive/FDA%20CAT.htm (accessed October 1, 2010); *Physician's Desk Reference,* 57th ed. (Montvale, NJ: Thomson PDR; 2003); G. G. Briggs, R. K. Freeman and S. J. Yaffe, *Drugs in Pregnancy and Lactation,* 6th ed. (Baltimore, MD: Williams & Wilkins, 2002).

7. S. Ascheim and B. Zondek, "Hpophysenvorderlappen hormone und ovarial hormore im Harn von Schwangeren," *Klin Wochenschr* 6 (1927): 3–21.

8. "A Timeline of Pregnancy Testing," Office of History, National Institute of Health. https://history.nih.gov/ (accessed November 1, 2010).

9. E. R. Love, S. Bhattacharya, N.C. Smith, and S. Bhattacharya, "Effect of interpregnancy interval on outcomes of pregnancy after miscarriage: retrospective analysis of hospital episode statistics in Scotland," 341 *British Medical Journal* (2010).

chapter 2

1. "Protein in your pregnancy diet," BabyCenter Medical Advisory Board (December 2009). http://www.babycenter.com/0_protein-in-your-pregnancy -diet_1690.bc (accessed January 19, 2011).

2. All nutritional information from the USDA Products and Services' "Reports on Single Nutrients" and specific web sites. USDA Products and Services, http://www.ars.usda.gov/Services/docs.htm?docid=20958 (accessed: December 2, 2010)

3. "Metabolic and Bariatric Surgery Fact Sheet," American Society of Metabolic and Bariatric Surgery. http://www.asmbs.org/Newsite07/media/ASMBS _Metabolic_Bariatric_Surgery_Overview_FINAL_09.pdf (accessed February 4, 2011); "New study finds social and economic actors play major role in determining who gets bariatric surgery," American Society of Metabolic and Bariatric Surgery Press Release (June 25, 2009). http://www.asmbs.org/ Newsite07/media/asmbs_fs_obesity.pdf (accessed February 4, 2011).

4. D. Forman, "Are nitrates a significant risk factor in human cancer?" *Cancer Surveys* 8, Issue 2 (1989): 443–458; D. Forman, S. Al-Dabbagh, and R. Doll, "Nitrates, nitrites, and gastric cancer in Great Britain," *Nature* 313 (February 21, 1985): 620–625.

5. Center for Food Safety, "An Evaluation of Sushi and Sashimi Microbiological Surveillance, 1997–1999," Hong Kong (December 30, 2006). http://www. cfs.gov.hk/english/programme/programme_rafs/programme_rafs_fm_01_09_ sshk.html (accessed November 1, 2010).

6. J. Kline, P. Shrout, Z. Stein, et al., "Drinking during pregnancy and spontaneous abortion," *Lancet* 2 (1980): 176.

chapter 3

1. S. G. Gabbe, J. R. Niebyl, and J. L. Simpson, *Obstetrics: Normal and Problem Pregnancies* (Philadelphia: Churchill Livingstone Elsevier, 2007): 18.

2. I. Donald et al., "Investigation of Abdominal Masses by Pulsed Ultrasound," *Lancet* 1(1958): 1188–1195.

3. L. Dodds, D. Fell, K. S. Joseph, V. Allen, and B. Butler, "Outcomes of pregnancies complicated by hyperemesis gavidaru," *Obstetrics and Gynecology* 107 (February 2006): 285–292.

4. T. Vutyavanich, T. Kraisarin, and R. Ruangsri, "Ginger for nausea and vomiting in pregnancy: randomized, double-masked, placebo-controlled trial," *Obstetrics and Gynecology* 97 (2001): 577–582; T. Vutyavanich, S. Wongtra-ngan, and R. Ruangsri, "Pyridoxine for nausea and vomiting of pregnancy: a randomized, double-blind, placebo-controlled trial," *American Journal of Obstetrics Gynecology* 173 (1995): 991–994.

5. California Department of Public Health, "Midtrimester Risk for Chromosome Abnormalities," *The California Prenatal Screening Program: Provider Handbook* (March 2009): Appendix G.

chapter 4

1. F. G. Cunningham, K. J. Leveno, S. L. Bloom, et al., *Williams Obstetrics,* 23rd ed. (New York: McGraw Hill, 2010): 83.

2. T. Kurki, A. Sivonen, et al., "Bacterial Vaginosis in Early Pregnancy and Pregnancy Outcome," *Obstetrics and Gynecology* 80 (August 1992): 173–177.

3. K. A. Costigan, H. L. Sipsma, and J. A. DiPietro, "Pregnancy Folklore Revisited: The Case of Heartburn and Hair," *Birth: Issues in Perinatal Care* 33 (December 2006): 311–314.

4. H. C. Butcher and J. G. Schmidt, "Does routine ultrasound scanning improve outcome in pregnancy? Meta-analysis of various outcome measures," *British Medical Journal* 307 (July 1993): 13–17.

chapter 5

1. Center for Disease Control, "Group B Strep Prevention Report." http://www.cdc.gov/groupbstrep/about/prevention.html (accessed January 19, 2011).

2. M. K. Yancy and P. Duff, "An analysis of the cost-effectiveness of selected protocols for the prevention of neonatal group B streptococcal infection," *Obstetrics and Gynecology* 83 (1994): 367.

3. R. Usher, F. McLean, "Intrauterine growth of live-born Caucasian infants at sea level: Standards obtained from measurements in 7 dimensions of infants born between 25 and 44 weeks," *Journal of Pediatrics* 74 (June 1969): 901–910.

4. R. Reid, J. Ivery, et al., "Fetal complications of obstetric cholestasis," *British Medical Journal* 1 (April 1976): 870–872.

5. F. Cardini and H. Weixin, "Moxibustion for Correction of a Breech Presentation: A Randomized Controlled Study," *The Journal of the American Medical Association* 282 (1999): 1329–1330.

6. California Disability Law. http://www.dpa.ca.gov/benefits/health/workcomp/pubs/disability/page8.shtm (accessed October 14, 2010).

7. T. O'Connor, J. Heron, et al., "Maternal antenatal anxiety and behavioural/emotional problems in children: a test of a programming hypothesis," *The Journal of Child Psychology and Psychiatry* 44 (October 2003): 1025–1036.

8. S. Morkved, K. Bo, et al., "Pelvic floor muscle training during pregnancy to prevent urinary incontinence: A single-blind randomized controlled trial," *Obstetrics and Gynecology* 101 (February 2003): 313–319.

9. You might want to check out *Baby Bargains* by Denise and Alan Fields for great deals on baby products.

10. http://www.youtube.com/watch?v=taDqKWWPDAY&feature=&p=461B360881B0A83B&index=0&playnext=1 (accessed January 19, 2011).

chapter 6

1. F. Menacker et al., "Trends in Cesarean Rates for First Births and Repeat Cesarean Rates for Low-Risk Women: United States, 1990–2003," CDC's National Vital Statistics Report. http://www.cdc.gov/nchs/data/nvsr/nvsr54/nvsr54_04.pdf (accessed October 12, 2010); P. J. Mancuso et al., "Timing of Birth After Spontaneous Onset of Labor." http://www.ncbi.nlm.nih.gov/pubmed/15051554 (accessed October 12, 2010); O. Goldstick et al., "The Circadian Rhythm of 'Urgent' Operative Deliveries." http://www.ncbi.nlm.nih.gov/pubmed/12929294 (accessed October 12, 2010).

2. H. A. Allott and C. R. Palmer, "Sweeping of Membranes: A valid procedure in stimulating the onset of labor?" *British Journal of Obstetrics and Gynecology* 100 (October 1993): 889–890.

3. L. Summers, "Methods of Cervical Ripening and Labor Induction," *Journal of Nurse-Midwifery* 42 (March–April, 1997): 71–85.

4. J. Zhang et al., "Does Epidural Analgesia Prolong Labor and Increase Risk of Cesarean Delivery? A Natural Experiment," *American Journal of Obstetrics & Gynecology* 185 (July 2011): 128–134.

5. K. Papagani et al., "Doula Support and Attitudes of Intrapartum Nurses: A Qualitative Study from the Patient's Perspective," *The Journal of Perinatal Education* 15 (Winter 2006): 11–18.

6. From Unicef's maternal mortality statistics. http://www.unicef.org/index.php (accessed February 10, 2011).

chapter 7

1. J. Mannella, "Short-Term Effects of Maternal Alcohol Consumption on Lactational Performance," *Alcoholism: Clinical and Experimental Research* 22 (October 2008): 1389–1392.

2. C. W. Schauberger, B. L. Rooney, and L. M. Brimer, "Factors that influence weight loss in the puerperium," *Obstetrics and Gynecology* 79 (March 1992): 424–429.

3. U.S. Census Bureau, "Women More Likely to Work During Pregnancy." http://www.census.gov/newsroom/releases/archives/employment_occupations/cb08–33.html (accessed on January 9, 2011).

chapter 8

1. D. Vandermolen, V. Ratts, et al., "Metformin increases the ovulatory rate and pregnancy rate from clomiphene citrate in patients with polycystic ovary syndrome who are resistant to clomiphene citrate alone," *Fertility and Sterility* 75 (February 2001): 310–315.

2. L. Seperoff and M. Fritz, *Clinical Gynecologic Endocrinology and Infertilty.* 8th ed., (Philadelphia: Lippincott Williams & Wilkins, 2010).

3. "Assisted Reproductive technology (ART)," Centers for Disease Control and Prevention. http://www.cdc.gov/art/ (accessed February 11, 2011).

4. J. Boldt et al., "Success rates following intracytoplasmic sperm injection are improved by using ZIFT vs. IVF for embryo transfer," *Journal of Assisted Reproduction and Genetics* 13, no. 10 (November 1996): 782–785.

5. B. Eiben, I. Bartels, S. Bahr-Prosch, et al., "Cytogenetic analysis of 750 spontaneous abortions with the direct-preparation method of chronic villi and its implications for studying genetic causes of pregnancy wastage," *The American Journal of Human Genetics* 47 (October 1990): 656–663.

6. L. A. Bartlett, C. J. Berg, et al.,"Risk Factors for Legal Induced Abortion-Related Mortality in the United States," *Obstetrics and Gynecology* 103 (April 2004): 729–737.

chapter 9

1. M. Heron, D. L. Hoyert, S. L. Murphy, J. Xu, K. D. Kochanek, and B. Tejada-Vera, "Deaths: Final Data for 2006," *National Vital Statistic Reports* 57 (April 17, 2009). http://www.cdc.gov/nchs/data/nvsr/nvsr57/nvsr57_14.pdf (accessed February 14, 2011); "Maternal mortality" Fact sheet, World Health Organization (November 2010). http://www.who.int/mediacentre/factsheets/fs348/en/ (accessed February 14, 2011).

2. UNICEF's maternal mortality statistics. http://www.unicef.org/index.php (accessed February 10, 2011).

3. S. G. Gabbe, J. R. Niebyl, and J. L. Simpson, *Normal and Problem Pregnancies* (Philadelphia: Churchill Livingstone Elsevier, 2007): 650.

4. A. Jacobs, "Overview of Postpartum Hemorrhage" (September 2010). http://www.uptodate.com/contents/overview-of-postpartum-hemorrhage (accessed February 14, 2011).

5. A. B. Caughey, J. R. Butler. "Posterm Pregnancy." emedicine.com (September, 2010). http://emedicine.medscape.com/article/261369-overview (accessed February 25, 2011).

chapter 11

1. D. M. Stamilio, E. DeFranco, E. Pare, et al., "Short Interpregnancy Interval: Risk of Uterine Rupture and Complications of Vaginal Birth after Cesarean Delivery," *Obstetrics and Gynecology* 110 (November 2007): 1075–1082.

2. S. Cnattingius, L.B. Signorello, G. Anneren, et al., "Caffeine Intake and

the Risk of First-Trimester Spontaneous Abortion," *The New England Journal of Medicine* 343 (December 2000): 1839–1845.

3. Y. J. Kelly, A. Sacker, R. Gray, J. Kelly, D. Wolke, J. Headl, and M. A. Quigley, "Light Drinking During Pregnancy: Still No Increased Risk for Socioemotional Difficulties or Cognitive Defects at 5 Years of Age?" *Journal of Epidemiology and Community Health* (October 5, 2010). http://jech.bmj.com/content/early/2010/09/13/jech.2009.103002.abstract (accessed October 18, 2011).

4. "Whether the rates of congenital infection in these studies are representative of the entire population is unknown. However, if these rates were extrapolated to the approximately four million live births in the United States each year, an estimated four hundred to four thousand infants would be born each year with congenital toxoplasmosis." A. Lopez, V. J. Diets, M. Wilson, T. R. Navin, and J. L. Jones, "Preventing Congenital Toxoplasmosis." http://www.cdc.gov/mmwr/preview/mmwrhtml/rr4902a5.htm (accessed January 5, 2011).

glossary

The 5-1-1 rule: Our suggested guideline of when to call your doctor or go to the hospital when labor ensues. If you are having contractions every five minutes, with each contraction lasting about one minute and those regular minute-long contractions have repeated consistently for one hour, you should call your doctor.

Acrochordon: A small benign skin tumor, also known as a skin tag, that appears as a flesh-colored bump. These tags occur anywhere on the body but especially on the neck and under the arms.

Amniocentesis: A procedure in which a small amount of amniotic fluid is withdrawn by a needle through the abdomen. If performed in the second trimester (between fifteen to twenty weeks), the amniotic fluid can be examined to determine fetal genetic abnormalities, such as Down syndrome. If performed in the late third trimester, the amniotic fluid can be examined to determine fetal lung maturity.

Amniotic fluid index (AFI): An ultrasound measurement of the amount of amniotic fluid surrounding the fetus.

Amniotomy: The artificial rupture of the amniotic sac (bag of water). This procedure is performed with a device called an amniohook (a long handle with a small plastic hook at the end). Amniotomy can be used for labor induction.

Anembryonic gestation: A pregnancy in which the fetus does not develop. On ultrasound, an amniotic sac can be seen without signs of a fetus. Also known as blighted ovum.

Anemia: A medical condition in which the body lacks healthy red blood cells. Because red blood cells carry oxygen, this condition is associated with dizziness, fatigue, shortness of breath, headache, and increased heart rate.

Anovulation: When you don't release an egg from the ovary. If you don't ovulate, you can't become pregnant because there is no egg to be fertilized. Anovulation is the cause of infertility in 15 percent of infertile couples.

Antepartum testing: Exams to check the well-being of the fetus. The most common method of antepartum testing is the modified biophysical profile, consisting of a nonstress test and the amniotic fluid index.

Apgar score: An evaluation of five characteristics of your newborn—appearance (color), pulse (heart rate), grimace, activity, and respiration—after one minute, five minutes, and ten minutes of life.

Appendicitis: A bacterial infection in the appendix. Symptoms of appendicitis include right-sided abdominal pain, decreased appetite, fever, diarrhea, nausea, and vomiting.

Asthma: A chronic disease of the lungs due to muscle spasm and inflammation of the airways.

Autosomal dominant disorders: A genetic disease caused by the inheritance of a defective gene from one parent.

Autosomal recessive disorders: A genetic disease caused by the inheritance of a defective gene from both parents.

Bacterial vaginosis (BV): A bacterial vaginal infection caused by an imbalance of the normal bacterial flora in the vagina. BV is not sexually transmitted and is characterized by discharge with a fishy odor.

Basal body temperature (BBT): The body's lowest temperature attained during rest. Because ovulation causes an increase of 0.4 to 1.0 degrees in the basal body temperature, monitoring the BBT throughout the menstrual cycle can predict the time of egg release.

Bishop's score: A scoring system used to predict if labor induction would be successful. The Bishop's score evaluates five characteristics: cervical dilation, cervical effacement, station of the fetal head, cervical consistency, and cervical position.

Bloody show: Bleeding that accompanies the release of the mucous plug at the beginning of the labor process.

Braxton Hicks contractions: Uterine contractions that do not cause cervical change. Also known as false labor.

Breech presentation: The fetal presention in which the feet or buttocks enter the birth canal first.

Candidiasis: A vaginal infection caused by yeast, most commonly *Candida albicans*. Symptoms include vaginal itching and burning along with a thick, white discharge.

Caput succedaneum: The swelling of a newborn's scalp directly over the cervical opening during labor.

Carrier: A person who has one copy of an autosomal recessive gene defect and is not affected by the disease. A carrier can pass the abnormal gene to his or her offspring.

Cerclage: A stitch placed around the cervix to hold it closed as a treatment for cervical insufficiency.

Cerebral palsy: A permanent disorder affecting movement, causing physical disabilities. Cerebral palsy is caused by injuries or abnormalities to the motor system of the brain, which can happen during pregnancy, labor, or early childhood.

Cervical dilation: Describes how far the cervix has opened. Complete cervical dilation is when the cervix is open ten centimeters.

Cervical insufficiency: A second trimester pregnancy complication in which the cervix weakens and dilates, usually resulting in a miscarriage.

Cervical length test: An ultrasound measurement of the length of the cervix used to diagnose and assess cervical insufficiency and preterm labor.

Cervical position: A component of the Bishop's score that describes the orientation of the cervix in the vagina. Before labor, the cervix is posterior, pointing toward the back of the vagina. As labor ensues, the cervix is anterior, angling toward the front.

Cervix: The lowest part of the uterus that opens into the vagina.

Cesarean delivery: A surgical procedure in which an incision is made in the mother's abdomen and uterus to allow delivery of a baby.

Chemical pregnancy: A pregnancy that ends shortly after conception, resulting in miscarriage. In a chemical pregnancy, the pregnancy test is positive but there is no evidence of the pregnancy on an ultrasound.

Cholestasis of pregnancy: A medical condition in which the pregnancy hormones cause the flow of bile to slow within the liver. Cholestasis typically occurs in the third trimester and is characterized by total body itching and elevated bile acids in the blood.

Chorionic villus sampling (CVS): A medical procedure in which a small amount of placental tissue is removed either vaginally or abdominally between ten and thirteen weeks of pregnancy. The tissue can be analyzed to determine whether the fetus has a genetic or chromosomal disorder.

Chronic hypertension: A form of high blood pressure (blood pressure higher than 140/90) that is present before pregnancy.

Colostrum: A form of breast milk produced in late pregnancy and during the first five days after delivery. Also known as premilk, colostrum contains protein and antibodies but less fat than regular milk.

Complete blood cell (CBC) count: A blood test that measures the number of white blood cells (for fighting infection), red blood cells (for carrying oxygen), and platelets (for blood clotting).

Consistency: A component of the Bishop's score that describes whether the cervix is soft or firm.

Costochondritis: A painful inflammation between the ribs, especially in the rib joints.

Cystic fibrosis: An autosomal recessive disease that affects a baby's lungs and digestive system. A defective gene causes the body to produce unusually thick, sticky mucous that clogs the lungs, causing life-threatening infections and difficulty breathing.

Deep vein thrombosis (DVT): A blood clot in the deep veins of the leg, usually the calf.

Diabetes: A metabolic disease characterized by high blood sugar caused by decreased insulin production from the pancreas or by insulin resistance.

Dilation and curettage (D&C): A surgical procedure in which the cervix is dilated (opened) and pregnancy tissue is removed.

Docosahexaenoic acid (DHA): An omega-3 fatty acid important for brain and eye development in the fetus.

Doppler: An electronic instrument that uses sound waves to measure the baby's heartbeat after twelve weeks of gestation.

Doula: A woman who is trained and experienced in childbirth and provides continuous physical, emotional, and informational support to a woman during labor, birth, and the immediate postpartum period.

Down syndrome (Trisomy 21): A genetic disorder in which there is an extra chromosome 21 and characterized by certain facial features, mental retardation, and a higher risk of heart and intestinal birth defects.

Eclampsia: A life-threatening complication of pregnancy characterized by preeclampsia (high blood pressure) and seizures.

Ectopic pregnancy: A pregnancy that develops outside the uterus, most commonly in the fallopian tube.

Effacement: The shortening, or thinning, of the cervix associated with labor.

Epidural: A form of regional pain relief that delivers medications through a small catheter or tubing in the epidural space (in front of the nerves of the spine) to lessen the pain of labor.

Episiotomy: An incision near the vaginal opening to allow for delivery of the baby's head. The incision is usually made from the bottom of the vaginal opening toward the anus.

External cephalic version (ECV): A procedure to attempt to turn a breech or transverse baby manually to the head-down position.

Fetal alcohol syndrome (FAS): A disorder caused by consumption of excessive amounts of alcohol during pregnancy and characterized by distinct facial features, short stature, and learning disabilities.

Fetal demise: A baby that has died in the uterus at any stage of the pregnancy.

Fetal fibronectin (FFN): A protein produced by fetal cells near the placenta that acts as a glue to attach the amniotic sac to the uterus. FFN is present in the cervical and vaginal secretions of women who are at higher risk for preterm delivery.

Fetal scalp electrode (FSE): A device placed directly on the fetal scalp during labor to monitor the fetal heart rate.

Folic acid: A B-complex vitamin essential for all cell function. Low levels of folic acid are linked to the development of birth defects such as neural tube defects and cleft lip and palate.

Follicles: Tiny cysts inside the ovaries where your eggs are found.

Forceps: A metal instrument that resembles large salad servers and is used to facilitate a vaginal delivery by applying traction to the fetal head.

Fundal height: A measurement, in centimeters, from the mom's pubic bone to the fundus, or top of her uterus. This measurement is used to track the baby's growth after twenty weeks of gestation.

Gemete intrafallopian transfer (GIFT): An assisted reproductive technology (infertility treatment) in which a woman's eggs and her partner's sperm are placed in the fallopian tube.

Group B streptococcus (GBS): A bacteria that lives in the genitourinary or gastrointestinal tracts of some women. GBS can cause serious infections in the newborn, so all women are screened for the bacteria before labor. Also known as Streptococcus agalactiae.

Hemorrhoids: Enlarged rectal veins that cause swelling, pain, and itching around the anus.

Human chorionic gonadotropin (hCG): A hormone made by fetal tissue that is present in maternal blood and urine. The beta-subunit of hCG can be detected by pregnancy tests.

Hypertension: *See* chronic hypertension.

Hyperthyroidism: A disease caused by overproduction of thyroid hormone, most commonly an autoimmune disorder known as Grave's Disease. Symptoms include a rapid heart rate, bulging eyes (exopthalmus), increased body temperature, and weight loss.

Hypothyroidism: A disease caused by insufficient amounts of thyroid hormone. Symptoms include dry skin, slow heart rate, weight gain, fatigue, and menstrual cycle irregularities.

In vitro fertilization (IVF): An infertility treatment in which hormone injections cause multiple eggs to be produced in the ovaries. The eggs are then removed in a surgical procedure and fertilized with the partner's sperm in a laboratory. The resulting embryos are placed into the woman's uterus.

Inferior vena cava: A large vein that returns blood from the abdomen and legs to the heart. The vein is located on the right side of your spine.

Intrauterine growth restriction (IUGR): A pregnancy complication in which the fetus does not grow normally and the fetal weight is less than the tenth percentile.

Intrauterine insemination (IUI): An infertility treatment for male factor infertility. A semen specimen is washed and placed directly into the woman's uterus with a small catheter.

Intrauterine pressure catheter (IUPC): A thin, sterile tube placed inside the uterus during labor to measure the strength and frequency of uterine contractions.

Jaundice: A yellow discoloration of the skin and whites of the eyes that occurs when bilirubin (a by-product of the breakdown of red blood cells) builds up in a baby's body. Jaundice happens when there is excessive breakdown of red blood cells or when the immature liver cannot metabolize the by-product.

Kegels: Exercises that strengthen the pelvic floor muscles to control urinary incontinence.

L&D floor: The labor and delivery unit, where you deliver your baby in the hospital.

Leopold's maneuvers: The palpation of the pregnant uterus to determine an estimate of the baby's size and position.

Leukorrhea: A heavy, clear, white, or watery vaginal discharge common in pregnancy due to elevated estrogen levels.

Lie: The relationship between the spine of the fetus and the spine of the mother. If they are parallel, the fetus is in longitudinal lie.

Linea nigra: The dark line (hyperpigmentation) that appears down the middle of a pregnant woman's abdomen. Linea nigra is caused by elevated pregnancy hormones.

Listeria: A bacterium found in unpasteurized dairy and uncooked meats that can cause flu-like symptoms, muscle pain, vomiting, and seizures. In pregnancy, Listeria can cause miscarriage, preterm labor, or stillbirth.

Lochia alba: A yellow or white vaginal discharge that occurs four to six weeks after delivery.

Lochia serosa: A red-brown discharge that may have a foul odor and lasts for the first three to four weeks after delivery.

Lordosis: An inward curvature to the lower spine.

Macrosomia: A newborn with an excessive birth weight of more than forty-five hundred grams (ten pounds).

Mastitis: A bacterial infection of the breast associated with fever, red and tender skin over the breast, and body aches.

Meconium: The first bowel movement of a newborn.

Meconium aspiration syndrome: A condition in which a newborn breathes meconium into its lungs during delivery, resulting in pneumonia or respiratory distress.

Membrane stripping: A procedure in which the obstetrician or midwife separates the amniotic membranes from the cervix vaginally to release natural hormones that can potentially stimulate labor.

Metoclopramide (Reglan): A prescription medication that can increase milk production by increasing prolactin levels.

Midwife: A health care professional who provides care to women in pregnancy and childbirth.

Molding: The temporary form of the baby's skull that results from pressure in the birth canal.

Moxibustion: A traditional Chinese treatment that involves burning an herb near the small toe to stimulate a breech baby to change to vertex presentation.

Mucous plug: A protective mucous in the cervix that blocks bacteria from entering the amniotic sac. It is usually released before the onset of labor.

Multiparous: A woman who has given birth to a child (or children) before.

Neonatal intensive care unit (NICU): A place in the hospital where premature infants or sick neonates are cared for.

Nesting: A primal instinct among all mammals and birds that directs them to prepare a sheltered, safe place in which to give birth.

Neural tube defects (NTD): A birth defect of the brain or spinal cord in which the fetal spinal column doesn't close completely or the brain doesn't develop normally.

Neuropathies: Damage or inflammation to a nerve that results in altered sensation or function.

Nonstress test (NST): A component of antepartum testing in which the fetal heart rate and uterine activity are recorded with an external fetal monitor to determine fetal well-being.

Nuchal cord: An umbilical cord that is looped around the baby's neck.

Nulliparous: A woman who has never delivered a baby.

Occiput anterior (OA): The position of the fetal head in the birth canal in which the face is toward the mother's spine.

Occiput posterior (OP): The position of the fetal head in the birth canal in which the face is toward the mother's pubic bone.

Ovulation: The release of an egg from the ovary.

Ovulation induction: A fertility treatment that utilizes medication to cause the ovaries to release eggs.

Oxytocin: A hormone made in the pituitary gland that causes uterine contractions and milk letdown.

Perinatologist: An obstetrician who specializes in high-risk pregnancies.

Pica: A condition in which a person craves starch, clay, ice, and dirt.

Pitocin: The synthetic equivalent of oxytocin used to stimulate uterine contractions.

Placenta accreta: A placenta that is abnormally attached to the uterine lining.

Placenta increta: A placenta that is abnormally attached to the uterine muscle.

Placenta percreta: A placenta that is abnormally attached to the uterus and has grown through the lining, muscle, and surface of the uterus.

Placenta previa: A placenta that is near or covering the cervical canal. Because the cervix is the opening out of the uterus during a vaginal delivery, patients with placenta previa require a cesarean delivery.

Placental abruption: The separation of the placenta from the wall of the uterus before the delivery of the fetus. Because oxygen and nutrition are passed from the mother to the fetus through the placenta, abruption can lead to oxygen deprivation, fetal distress, and even fetal death.

Polycystic ovarian syndrome (PCOS): A condition, now known as hyperandrogenic chronic anovulation, in which a hormonal imbalance causes irregular menstrual cycles, infertility, increased hair growth (hirsuitism), and high glucose levels.

Polyhydramnios: An excessive amount of amniotic fluid.

Position: The orientation of the baby's head in the birth canal. *See also* occiput posterior and occiput anterior.

Postpartum blues: A transient phase of depressive mood that can include tearfulness, anxiety, irritation, difficulty concentrating, and restlessness. Postpartum blues can start two to three days after delivery and last up to four weeks. It differs from postpartum depression in its intensity, severity, and duration. Also called baby blues.

Postpartum depression (PPD): Intense feelings of sadness, anxiety, or despair in the postpartum period. These feelings are so intense that they interfere with the mother's ability to function.

Preeclampsia: A form of high blood pressure caused by pregnancy and diagnosed by the findings of persistently elevated blood pressure (higher than 140/90) and protein in the urine.

Pregnancy rhinitis: Nasal congestion caused by pregnancy hormones.

Premature rupture of membranes (PROM): A condition of pregnancy when the bag of water breaks before contractions have begun. PROM occurs in about 10 percent of pregnancies at term, and 3 percent of preterm pregnancies.

Presentation: The part of the baby that is coming out first. A vertex fetus is head-first, and a breech fetus is buttocks or feet first.

Preterm birth: Any birth that occurs before thirty-seven weeks. One in every eight babies in the United States is born prematurely.

Prolactin: A hormone made in the pituitary gland of the brain that stimulates the breast to produce milk.

Prostaglandins: Chemicals that regulate the contraction and relaxation of smooth muscles cells. In pregnancy, prostaglandins prepare the cervix for labor, causing effacement, softening, and dilation. Synthetic prostaglandins are used for labor induction.

Prurigo: Tiny, itchy red bumps that can occur during pregnancy.

Pruritic urticarial papules and plaques of pregnancy (PUPPP): An extremely itchy red rash that is unique to pregnancy, starts on the abdomen, and can spread all over the body.

Ptyalism: A condition that can occur during pregnancy in which there is an overproduction of saliva.

Pubic symphysis: The joint that unites the two pubic bones.

Quad test: A blood test offered to pregnant women between fifteen weeks and twenty weeks of pregnancy that screens for Down syndrome (Trisomy 21), Trisomy 18, neural tube defects, abdominal wall defects, and a rare cholesterol defect in the baby called Smith-Lemli-Opitz Syndrome (SLOS).

Quickening: The first time that a baby's movements are felt by its mother.

Round ligament pain: A dull, achy pain that runs through the groin and is caused by stretching of the round ligaments as a result of a rapidly growing uterus.

Seizure disorder: A neurological disorder that results in convulsions (or epilepsy) due to abnormal electrical activity in the brain with or without loss of consciousness.

Shoulder dystocia: An obstetric emergency where the baby's head has delivered but the shoulders are stuck behind the mom's pubic bone, potentially causing injury to both the mother and the baby.

Sickle-cell anemia: An inherited red blood cell disorder that results in crescent, sickle-shaped red blood cells due to abnormal hemoglobin, the protein that carries oxygen in the red blood cells. These sickle cells can cause anemia and episodes of pain. Sickle-cell anemia affects primarily African Americans.

Spina bifida: A neural tube defect in which there is incomplete closure of the baby's spine. Spina bifida may cause paralysis and deformities of the legs.

Spinal anesthesia: A form of anesthesia in which pain medication is placed directly into the compartment containing spinal fluid. A spinal takes effect more quickly than an epidural, and is the type of anesthesia commonly used during a scheduled cesarean delivery.

Station: How high or low the baby's head is in the birth canal.

Stillbirth: Fetal death that occurs after twenty weeks of pregnancy.

Striae gravidarum: A skin condition that occurs when the second layer of skin (dermis) tears due to extreme stretching. Striae are commonly seen in the late second trimester and third trimester of pregnancy. Also know as stretch marks.

Tay-Sachs disease: An autosomal recessive disorder caused by a genetic mutation that results in an enzyme deficiency of hexosaminidase A. Infants affected with Tay-Sachs disease have severe developmental delays, seizures, and blindness.

Teratogens: Any agent that can cause a birth defect in a fetus.

Thalassemia: An inherited blood disorder that results in an abnormal form of hemoglobin, the protein that carries oxygen in red blood cells. Thalassemia is characterized by excessive destruction of red blood cells and anemia.

Thyroid disease: A family of diseases caused by dysfunction of the thyroid gland. *See* hypothyroidism and hyperthyroidism.

Toxoplasma gondii: A parasite that can be present in cats' feces and raw or undercooked meat and unwashed vegetables. If a woman is infected for the first time while pregnant, toxoplasma can cause fetal birth defects and mental retardation.

Trichomonas: A microscopic sexually transmitted parasite that causes a foamy vaginal discharge with odor, itching, and irritation.

Trisomy 18: A genetic disorder in which there is an extra chromosome 18, resulting in severe mental retardation and multiple physical problems, such as heart defects and small brains, both of which can be life threatening.

Umbilical artery velocimetry: Ultrasound measurement of blood flow through the umbilical artery. This antepartum test evaluates fetal well-being.

Umbilical cord: Connection between the baby and the placenta. The umbilical cord contains two arteries and one vein. The vein transports oxygen and nutrients from mother to the baby while the two arteries in the umbilical cord carry waste materials and carbon dioxide back to the placenta to filter them through the mother.

Umbilical cord prolapse: An obstetric emergency in which the umbilical cord slips out through the cervix before the delivery of the baby, usually necessitating emergency cesarean delivery.

Umbilical hernia: A protrusion of part of the intestines around the belly button caused by weakening of the tissues in this area.

Uterine atony: The failure of the uterus to contract normally after the delivery of the baby and placenta, resulting in a soft uterus that continues to bleed excessively.

Vacuum extractor: A handheld plastic soft-cup placed on the baby's head to assist the delivery of the baby while the mom is pushing.

Vaginal birth after cesarean (VBAC): Delivering a baby vaginally after a previous baby had been delivered by cesarean.

Varicose veins: Swollen veins most commonly found in the legs, vulva, or anus due to slow blood flow.

Vernix: A white cheese-like protective substance that covers the fetal skin.

Vertex presentation: A baby in the head-down position. Also known as cephalic presentation.

Zygote intrafallopian transfer (ZIFT): Assisted reproductive technique in which one or more embryo are surgically placed directly into the fallopian tubes.

acknowledgments

WE COULD NOT HAVE WRITTEN THIS BOOK without the countless women who have allowed us into their lives in such an intimate and personal way. From our very first patients at Los Angeles County Hospital to the women we still see every day in our private practice, we thank you for the honor of attending your births, for trusting us with your care, and teaching us more than we ever expected. You will never know just how much you have enriched our lives.

First, let us express our thanks to the patients who directly contributed to our book by sharing their personal stories: Leticia Espinoza, Christina Bebes, Jennifer Polenzani, Pete Cummin, Joanna Stevens, Alex Kang, Stacey Lynn, Krishna Rao, Cynthia Rivera, Moon Kim, Michelle Rodriguez, Jasmine Vergara, Teresa Carlson, Janelle Walker, Leigh Ruth, Rachel McDermott, Ghina Rodriguez, Jennifer Astacio, Christia Karp, Cruzita Hernandez, Ralinda Watts, Sunhee Lee, Christine Joseph, and Robyn Hansen. Thank you, too, to the women who allowed us to photograph their beautiful babies along the way: Amy Talkington, Sue Jean Chang, Chante Hardy, Corey Carter, Erin Kolpek, Georgina Moncho, Jessamyn Piehl, Miho Travi, Tonya Tooley, and Maria Julia Castro.

It has also been encouraging to have received so much support from colleagues within our profession. We would like to thank those who added their personal thoughts: Dr. Cliff Bochner, Dr. John Jain, Carmen Bornn, Aleksandra Evanguelidi, and Jinnie Noh, RN. We would also like to acknowledge our amazing professors at the University of Southern California, especially our chairman Dr. Daniel Mishell and Dr. Paul Brenner. They taught us how to think critically and evaluate the evidence as well as to become compassionate and caring physicians.

The opportunity to write this book was born out of our experience on our TV show *Deliver Me*. By working on this show, we found a new platform, and a new confidence in ourselves, for educating women about their bodies and their pregnancies. We were touched by the strength and perseverance of our patients who chose to share their lives with the world. We are grateful to the team which made *Deliver Me* possible: Eric Schiff, Shannon O'Rourke, Robyn Salzman-Pinkerton, Inga Kleinrichert, Carol Marren, the crew at Banyan Productions, our writers and editors, and to Alon Ornstein of Discovery Health and the Oprah Winfrey Network.

We were honored to write this book with our co-author Melissa Jo Peltier. Her enthusiasm for the project and ability to bring our ideas to life made this a wonderful collaboration. Also from MPH Entertainment, we'd like to thank Mark Hufnail and Jim Milio—who now know more about pregnancy than they ever wanted—Ben Stagg, Jackie Younce, and our illustrator Victoria Parr. We would not be here today without our agents Neil Stearns and Damon Frank from Venture IAB. They believed in us from the beginning, and for that, we will always be thankful.

We are fortunate to deliver babies at Good Samaritan Hospital in Los Angeles. We work with the most dedicated and caring nursing staff and are supported by the finest physicians. We thank them, and Andy Leeka, the hospital's president, for making this a safe and comfortable environment for our patients to bring their babies into the world.

Our extended family is our office staff. They take care of our patients, and us, with compassion, concern, and love. We are especially grateful for Silvia Cifuentes, Daisy Lira, Barbie Montera, Patty Ponce, Dora Casillas, Karina Carranza, and Lizette Flores.

And finally, the three of us have truly been blessed in our lives. We are surrounded by supportive partners, healthy children, and inspiring patients and colleagues. Through our Mommy Docs foundation, we hope to express our gratitude by giving back to women's health.

From Allison: Finally, I would like to thank my parents Pat and Bob Hill and my children Luke and Kate who have taught me how to be a mother. And to my best friend and love Eric Pulier who has believed in me, inspired me, and enriched my life in so many ways, I am forever grateful.

From Yvonne: I would like to thank my husband Bob who has been my partner through all the years of medical training, cheering me on and holding down the fort during all the nights on call, always standing by when I had to put him second. My children Kylie and Ryan have had to be unselfish by giving up their Mommy in the middle of the night or in the middle of a basketball game, always waiting eagerly for my return from a delivery. Because of their love and caring, I have been able to undertake this incredible journey of providing women's health care, delivering babies and now educating women through our book.

From Alane: I would like to thank my two boys, Matthew and Max, who motivate me everyday to be a better human being and to live a meaningful life. They have taught me to love and give unconditionally. And to my partner and husband, John, thank you for standing by me and supporting me the past 27 years. I would not be here without you.

In addition, Melissa Jo Peltier wishes to thank: our terrific literary agent, Scott Miller at Trident Media Group; our supporters at Perseus, editor Katie McHugh and prodution editor, Christine E. Marra, my staff and partners at MPH Entertainment, and my husband John Gray who brings me daily joy. Thanks especially to Allison, Yvonne, and Alane—what a pleasure to work with three such brilliant, passionate, professional and yet always fun women! I'm proud and grateful to have been a part of your achievement.

index

a

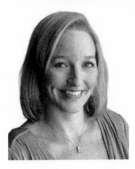

YVONNE BOHN, MD, attended UCLA where she majored in Psychobiology and received her MD from USC Medical School. She completed her residency in OB/GYN at USC Women and Children's Hospital. Dr. Bohn worked as an Assistant Clinical Professor at USC for three years before joining Drs. Hill and Park to start their practice. Board-certified and a Fellow of the American College of OB/GYN, Dr. Bohn has been in private practice for ten years. She lives in Los Angeles with her children, Ryan and Kylie, and her husband, Bob.

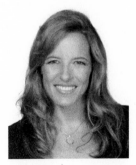

ALLISON HILL, MD, received a BS in Biology from the University of Notre Dame and her MD from Loyola University in Chicago. She completed her residency in OB/GYN at Los Angeles County–USC School of Medicine, where she met Drs. Park and Bohn. Dr. Hill is board-certified and a Fellow of the American College of OB/GYN. She has been in private practice in Los Angeles for ten years. She is the mother of two children, Luke and Kate.

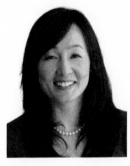

ALANE PARK, MD, was born in Seoul, Korea, and moved to the United States when she was eight years old. She completed her undergraduate studies in biochemistry at University of California–Berkeley, participated in medical research at UCLA, and received her MD from USC Medical School. Dr. Park completed her residency in OB/GYN at USC, where she met

Drs. Hill and Bohn. Dr. Park is board-certified and a Fellow of the American College of OB/GYN. Dr. Park lives with her husband and two sons, Matt and Max, in Los Angeles.

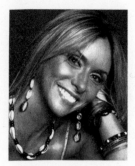

MELISSA JO PELTIER, co-author of five *New York Times* bestsellers with "Dog Whisperer" Cesar Millan, has been honored for her film and television writing, producing, and directing with an Emmy, a Humanitas, a Peabody, several Writer's Guild of America nominations, and more than fifty other awards, nominations, and honors. She lives in New York with her husband, writer-director John Gray, and stepdaughter, Caitlin.